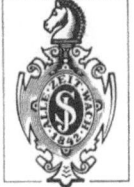

Stuart L. Stanton (Ed.)

Principles of Gynaecological Surgery

With 152 Figures

Springer-Verlag
London Berlin Heidelberg New York
Paris Tokyo

Stuart L. Stanton, FRCS, FRCOG,
Senior Lecturer, Department of Obstetrics and Gynaecology,
St. George's Hospital Medical School, London, and Consultant
Gynaecologist, St. George's and St. James's Hospitals, London

British Library Cataloguing in Publication Data
Stanton, Stuart L.
Principles of gynaecological surgery.
1. Gynecology, Operative
I. Title
618.1'059   RG104

Library of Congress Cataloging-in-Publication Data
Principles of gynaecological surgery
Includes bibliographies and index.
1. Gynecology, Operative. I. Stanton, Stuart L. [DNLM: 1. Genitalia, Female—surgery. WP 660 P957]
RG104.P75 1987 618.1'059 87-9524

ISBN-13: 978-1-4471-1448-2   e-ISBN-13: 978-1-4471-1446-8
DOI: 10.1007/978-1-4471-1446-8

© Springer-Verlag Berlin Heidelberg 1987
Softcover reprint of the hardcover 1st edition 1987

2128/3916–543210

John Dickinson, FRCS, FRCOG (1909–   )

Obstetric physician, St. Thomas' Hospital, London
Gynaecological Surgeon, Hospital for Women, Soho Square, London
Visiting Gynaecologist, Potters Bar Hospital

Gynaecologist, Surgeon and Teacher: who first taught me
the intricacies of gynaecological surgery and whose sympathetic
approach, humour and patience have guided me thereafter

Preface

For a long time I have felt that the present gynaecological training for registrars lacked familiarisation and understanding of the basic principles of surgery. This is due to several factors. Firstly, the historical separation of gynaecology from general surgery which led to our development as an independent speciality (and which Victor Bonney foretold to our detriment when he opposed the formation of the College of Obstetricians and Gynaecologists as a separate body from the College of Surgeons). Secondly, a vast improvement in medical management of many gynaecological conditions has made surgical practice dull and an unquestioning daily routine with little or no surgical instruction for many junior staff. Thirdly, the arrival of subspecialisation has exacerbated this, as complicated surgery may be referred out by the general gynaecologist. Finally, the trend in further education towards writing an MD rather than taking an FRCS degree. The arguments for and against were set out in an editorial in the *British Journal of Obstetrics and Gynaecology* (1983), later taken to task in the ensuing correspondence. That editorial, together with the difficulty in finding up-to-date articles on surgical principles in one volume, were the catalysts for this book. With the help of colleagues from other disciplines, I have attempted to present recent advances side-by-side with modern-day gynaecological practice.

In dividing this book into the three sections of preoperative, operative and postoperative, I have chosen growing points and aspects of gynaecological surgery which we need to be aware of as practising gynaecologists. Discussion with the patient is an important part of preoperative preparation and vital in the prevention of litigation. I have long been concerned with the elderly and disabled, who have very special needs relating to surgery which are often neglected. Many recent advances have occurred with imaging techniques and an up-to-date synopsis of these advances and their indications are presented in the chapter on imaging. The frequent encounter with a trainee who either failed to carry out an abdominal laparotomy at the time of pelvic surgery or was unaware of a systematic approach to laparotomy, motivated inclusion of a chapter on this topic. Surgical instruments can be very personal items and in preparing this chapter I was conscious of much innovation in surgical design which has not yet made its impact on our surgical practice. The remaining chapters deal with diverse topics such as laser, microsurgery, complications of surgery and psychiatric sequelae of surgery—all of which are reasonably within the ambit of gynaecological training.

I am also conscious of the debt to those surgeons who taught me and to those books which left their mark on me. I refer particularly to John Dickinson, to whom this book is dedicated and who taught me and many others the rudiments of surgery and the patience to assist. The opening words of Victor Bonney's *Principles of Gynaecological Surgery* are surely a model for all time: "The keystones of the surgeon's bearing should be self-control and, while it is his duty to keep a general eye upon all that takes place in the operating theatre and without hesitation to correct mistakes, he should guard against becoming irritable or losing his temper. The man who, when confronted with a difficulty, loses self-control, has mistaken his vocation, however dextrous he may be, or however learned in the technical details of his art. The habit of abusing assistants, the instruments. or the anaesthetists, so easy to acquire and so hard to lose, is not to be commended."

I would thank my colleagues at St. George's and St. James's Hospitals, those colleagues who have referred patients to my care, and research fellows and registrars whose constructive criticisms I welcome. I would also like to acknowledge the wisdom and surgical experience of Harold Ellis who helped me in planning this volume.

I thank and acknowledge Robert Lane, whose high standard of illustration has made my task much easier, Pat Philpott of the Department of Photography at St. James's Hospital and Jon Larsson of the Audiovisual Department of St. George's Hospital, for professional photographic skills, John Studd for the stimulating discussion on the FRCS and the MD, Michael Jackson, who as London Editor of Springer-Verlag has always been helpful, enthusiastic and resourceful, and Nora Galvin, who has patiently typed and corrected manuscripts and helped edit and collate the final text.

Finally, I thank those who taught me what to do and those who taught me what not to do.

June, 1987   Stuart L. Stanton

Contents

Contributors

Elizabeth Bellamy, MB, BS, DMRD, FRCR, MRCP
Consultant Radiologist, Ashford Hospital, London Road, Ashford, Middlesex TW15 3AA

Timothy E. Bucknall, MS, FRCS
Consultant General Surgeon, The General Hospital, Burton on Trent, Staffordshire DE14 3QH

David Cosgrove, MRCP
Consultant in Nuclear Medicine and Ultrasound, Royal Marsden Hospital, Downs Road, Sutton, Surrey SM2 5PT

John Dormandy, FRCS
Consultant Surgeon, Department of Vascular Surgery, St. James's Hospital, Sarsfeld Road, London SW12 8HW, and St. George's Hospital, London

Dennis Gath, DM, FRCP, FRCPsych
Clinical Reader in Psychiatry, University Department of Psychiatry, Warneford Hospital, Oxford OX3 7JX

Paul Hilton, MD, BS, MRCOG
Senior Lecturer and Honorary Consultant, Department of Obstetrics and Gynaecology, Princess Mary Maternity Hospital, Newcastle upon Tyne NE2 3BD

Susan Iles, MA, DPhil, BM, BCh, MRCPsych
Wellcome Research Fellow in Mental Health, Honorary Senior Registrar, University Department of Psychiatry, Warneford Hospital, Oxford OX3 7JX

Joseph Jordan, MD, FRCOG
Consultant Gynaecologist, The Birmingham and Midland Hospital for Women, Showell Green Lane, Sparkhill, Birmingham B11 4HL

Andrew F. Kent, BSc(Hons), MB, BCh
General Practitioner trainee, Corbett House Surgery, Avondale Road, Bristol BS5 9QX (formerly SHO in Gynaecology, St. James's Hospital, London)

Philippa Keyes-Evans, MB, BS, DA, FFARCS
Consultant Anaesthetist, Isle of Thanet District Hospital, St. Peter's Road, Margate, Kent

Michael Knight, MS, FRCS
Consultant Surgeon, St. George's Hospital, Blackshaw Road, London SW17 0QT, and St.
James's Hospital, London

Julian M. Leigh, MD, FFARCS
Consultant Anaesthetist, Director—Intensive Care Unit, Royal Surrey County Hospital,
Egerton Road, Park Barn, Guildford, Surrey GU2 5XX

John M. Monaghan, MB, ChB, FRCS (Ed), FRCOG
Consultant Surgeon, Regional Department of Gynaecological Oncology, Queen Elizabeth
Hospital, Sheriff Hill, Gateshead, Tyne and Wear NE9 6SX

Anthony R. Mundy, MS, FRCS, MRCP
Consultant Urological Surgeon, Guy's Hospital, St. Thomas Street, London SE1 9RT,
and Senior Lecturer, Institute of Urology, London

Malcolm Pearce, FRCS, MRCOG
Senior Lecturer, Department of Obstetrics and Gynaecology, St. George's Hospital Medical
School, Cranmer Terrace, London SW17 0RE

Anthony P. Rubin, MB, BChir, FFARCS
Consultant Anaesthetist, Charing Cross Hospital, Fulham Palace Road, London W6 8RF

Philip James Sanderson, PhD, FRCPath, MB, DipBact
Consultant Microbiologist, Department of Microbiology, Edgware General Hospital,
Edgware, Middlesex HA8 0AD

Stuart L. Stanton, FRCS, FRCOG
Senior Lecturer and Consultant Gynaecologist, St. George's Hospital Medical School,
Cranmer Terrace, London SW17 0RE, and St. James's Hospital, London

Jean-Pierre Van Besouw, BSc(Hons), MB, BS, FFARCS(Eng)
Senior Registrar, Department of Anaesthetics, St. Bartholomew's Hospital, West Smithfield,
London EC1

Robert M. L. Winston, MD, FRCOG
Reader in Fertility Studies, Institute of Obstetrics and Gynaecology, Hammersmith Hospital,
Du Cane Road, London W12 0HS

Section A:

PREOPERATIVE

1 · Preoperative Preparation of the Patient

Jean-Pierre Van Besouw, Andrew F. Kent and Stuart L. Stanton

The true position is that an error of judgement may or may not be negligent; it depends on the nature of the error. If it is one that would not have been made by a reasonably competent professional man professing to have the standards and type of skill that the defendant holds himself out as having and acting with ordinary care then it is negligent. If on the other hand it is an error that such a man acting with ordinary care might have made then it is not negligent.

Lord Fraser
House of Lords

Counselling and Information for Patients and Relatives

There are several reasons for counselling a patient about her treatment. Firstly, it is her right to make a reasoned choice and she will need information to do this. Secondly, counselling will allay her anxiety about the procedure. Thirdly, the patient should sign a consent form, which gives express rather than implied consent. To do this, she will need to know the nature of her medical condition, the choice of treatment, the need for surgery, the prognosis or success rate and equally important—the chance, nature and extent of complications.

There can be little dispute about the first reason: communication between patient and doctor in the past has been inadequate. Today, we are aware that counselling the patient is an important part of preoperative preparation and begins with the first visit, when the patient is told that treatment is required. Counselling is undertaken again as part of preoperative "clerking". It is very much the responsibility and training of the doctor.

Alleviation of anxiety by preoperative explanation is well documented (Wilson-Barnett 1984) and methods are constantly being refined to decrease anxiety levels and to cope with the influence of personality variables on recovery from surgery (Mathews and Ridgeway 1981). In addition to providing information about pre- and postoperative routine and the operation itself, techniques such as cognitive coping should be employed (Ridgeway and Mathews 1982), where patients are encouraged to dwell on the more positive aspects of their hospital stay and to talk through common worries.

The routine and extent of counselling will depend on many factors, including the patient's physical and mental state, intellectual capacity, grasp of the situation and reason for the procedure of operation, and the questions asked by the patient. It will also depend on the prevailing state of medical litigation: in the United States, this is alarmingly high, often leading to "defensive medicine" being practised, in which many unnecessary investigations are performed and surgery is often premature and more major than might otherwise be undertaken in a less litigiously orientated society. Preoperative counselling there can take over an hour, with every conceivable complication being discussed.

Under English law, there is fortunately no requirement to discuss *every* possible complication and side effect, although judges are tending to require more detailed explanations to be given to patients than were required a few years ago. In the Sidaway case, decided by the House of Lords in 1985 (Sidaway 1985), it was affirmed that a decision about degree of disclosure of risks, best calculated to assist the patient in making a rational choice about treatment, must primarily be a matter of clinical judgement. The doctor retains the discretion to limit information which would not deter the patient from undergoing treatment to the ultimate detriment of her health.

It may be relevant to involve the patient's relatives in counselling: firstly, because the patient may not take in all the details at once and a relative or friend is useful to help recall information and sometimes to aid in decision making. Secondly, with the elderly and mentally frail, consent of the relatives may be required and they should be aware of the procedure and stages in recovery and prognosis, particularly if malignancy is present. Thirdly, if the relatives have been party to decision making, they are less likely to resort to litigation, should that subject arise later.

Information may be imparted by discussion with the medical and paramedical team, via local or nationally produced information pamphlets, from the hospital, Royal Colleges or public institutions (e.g. Health Education Council). It should be lucid, in suitable language and not patronising. If producing a pamphlet oneself for patient education, it may be wise to add a disclaimer, similar to that used by the American College of Obstetricians and Gynaecologists—"The information in this pamphlet does not dictate an exclusive course of treatment or procedure to be followed and should not be construed as excluding other acceptable methods of practice." Because of increased consumer and patient interest, it may be prudent to liaise with rather than to ignore patient organisations.

In the Royal College of Obstetricians and Gynaecologists' study group on litigation and obstetrics and gynaecology (1985), the following recommendations were made:

1. Communication between patients and doctors must be adequate.
2. Preoperative discussion with the patient should be full and noted in the hospital records.
3. The patient should be informed of likely operative complications. Not every conceivable com-

plication should be discussed, but the patient's questions should be answered truthfully.
4. A postoperative appointment should be offered to discuss any problems which may have arisen.
5. Opinions of senior staff and operative notes, including details of any complications, must be fully documented.

Informed Consent

It is technically an assault to operate on a patient without her consent. Why, apart from legal considerations, should a doctor bother to obtain consent? Justice Kirby (1983) defines consent as a "right of self-determination: the principle or value choice of autonomy of the person". To consent, the individual requires sufficient information to be given to her. In England, anyone of sound mind and over 16 years of age can give legally valid consent for surgical or medical treatment. Under the age of 16 years, a parent, guardian, local authority (if the child is in care) or High Court (if the child is a ward of the Court) can give consent. In the case of contraception and termination of pregnancy, the medical practitioner is advised by the General Medical Council that he or she ought to obtain parental consent, but if the patient wishes confidentiality, this should be respected and the doctor should use his or her judgement: before agreeing to contraception or termination, consultation with another colleague would be wise.

If the doctor is not satisfied and decides to disclose the information learned from the consultation, he or she should inform the patient accordingly.

Consent may be given orally or in writing. Both should be documented. The former may lead to difficulties some years later, if witnesses to oral consent are dead or untraceable. Consent forms should be simple (Fig. 1.1), stating the procedure, that explanation has been given and that the patient has consented. It is signed by the patient and the doctor who has explained the procedure. Sterilisation procedures require a disclaimer, stating that there is a possibility of failure (Fig. 1.2). However, both forms are no more than pieces of written evidence, duly witnessed. The most important part of the consent is the explanation and preamble to the signature.

Consent for the mentally handicapped is more complex. These patients are protected by the provisions of the Mental Health Act 1983, which does not give power to consent to medical treatment, i.e. the patient's consent is ultimately required, except

---

GENERAL CONSENT FORM

I,.. of..
(name and address of person giving consent)

     *hereby consent to undergo

OR

     *hereby consent to .... undergoing
                                            (name of patient)

the operation/treatment of ....

the nature and purpose of which have been explained to me

by Dr./Mr. ....

I also consent to such further or alternative operative measures or treatment as may be found
necessary during the course of the operation or treatment and to the administration of general
or other anaesthetics for any of these purposes.

No assurance has been given to me that the operation/treatment will be performed or
administered by any particular practitioner.

Date ....   Signature of ....
                                       Patient/parent/guardian*

I confirm that I have explained the nature and purpose of this operation/treatment to the
person(s) who signed the above form of consent.

Date ....   Signature ....
                                          Medical Practitioner

*Delete whichever is inapplicable

Fig. 1.1. Sample consent form for gynaecological surgery.

for urgent and life-saving treatment. Most patients with an intelligence quotient of between 50 and 75 are able to give consent. This should be taken without coercion and with full discussion, involving parents, psychiatrist and general practitioner; in this way consent is usually achieved by a consensus. If the patient is severely handicapped (IQ of less than 50), and she cannot give informed consent, a guardianship order can be granted: however, this does *not* give consent to medical treatment. Here, unfortunately, the law is particularly vague. If the patient is less than 16 years of age, then a guardianship order can be invoked, although the guardian is unable to insist on or give consent for treatment. For both categories, the courts would judge that the reasons for treatment are "good

faith" and "duty of care". Alternatively, the next-of-kin can be asked for agreement, although legally a relative cannot give valid consent for another adult. If such agreement is withheld, the consultant in charge of the patient should seek a second opinion from another medical colleague and then act in what he or she considers to be the best interest of the patient (Editorial, Royal College of Psychiatrists 1986).

When sterilisation or termination of pregnancy is involved, if consent to treatment cannot be given by the patient, then a consensus opinion (as described above) may have to be resorted to. In the case of minors, there is some authority that a non-therapeutic procedure, if irreversible and of no benefit to the subject, may be unlawful.

STERILISATION

CONSENT BY PATIENT

I,.. of..
(name and address of patient)

....

hereby consent to undergo the operation of...

....

the nature and purpose of which have been explained to me

by Dr./Mr. ....

I have been told that the intention of the operation is to render me sterile and incapable of
further parenthood. I understand that there is a possibility that I may not become or remain
sterile.

I also consent to the administration of a general, local or other anaesthetic.

No assurance has been given to me that the operation will be performed by any particular
surgeon.

Date ....   Signature ....
                                                                                    Patient

I confirm that I have explained to the patient the nature and purpose of this operation.

Date ....   Signature ....
                                                                              Medical Practitioner

---

Fig. 1.2. Sample consent form for sterilisation.

Principles of Preoperative Assessment

Preoperative preparation for surgery begins once the surgeon has placed the patient's name on the waiting list. In this section the principles underlying patient suitability for anaesthesia will be discussed and the steps outlined that can improve the outcome for patients with coexisting medical conditions likely to increase the morbidity of surgery and anaesthesia.

In an ideal world, patients would be referred to anaesthetic outpatient clinics for assessment and relevant investigations. Those patients with intercurrent disease could have their treatment regimens altered where appropriate, and the suitability of

patients for day case surgery assessed, a decision often left to the gynaecologist (Burn 1976).

However, the more common practice in the National Health Service is for patients to be admitted the day before operation with blanket investigation and insufficient time to change therapy prior to surgery. It is therefore important that the gynaecologist is aware of the precepts of preoperative assessment and the relevant action to take.

Objectives

1. Evaluation of physical status
2. Relevant investigations
3. Evaluation of current medication and introduction of therapy as necessary

4. Discussion of perioperative events and alleviation of patient's anxiety

Evaluation of Physical Status

The assignment of a physical status category to patients based upon history and examination acts as a useful "language" when conferring information to the anaesthetist on their preoperative visit. The most widely used system is that recommended by the American Society of Anaesthesiologists (Table 1.1), in which patients are placed into one of five categories; however, although this system gives an indication of the physical status of the patient prior to surgery, it is not a good prognosticator of postoperative morbidity as the intended surgery is not taken into consideration (Keats 1978).

Table 1.1. Classification of physical status. (American Society of Anaesthesiologists 1963)

Status

ASA 1. Normal healthy patient—no known organic, biochemical or psychiatric disease
ASA 2. Patient with mild to moderate systemic disease
ASA 3. Patient with severe systemic disease that limits normal activity
ASA 4. Patient with severe systemic disease that is a consistent threat to life
ASA 5. Patient who is moribund and unlikely to survive 24 h

The addition of the letter E, e.g. 2(E), indicates those patients in whom emergency surgery is undertaken

History

It is important in the preoperative preparation to take a detailed history with particular emphasis on those points relevant to the course of surgery and anaesthesia. This should include details of the presenting complaint, current medication and past medical history. The anaesthetist will be interested in any cardiorespiratory problems, as well as any adverse reactions to anaesthesia the patient may have suffered during previous surgery. Some of the more important questions are outlined in Table 1.2 and their relevance to surgery and anaesthesia detailed in subsequent sections.

Examination

The physical examination from a gynaecological and anaesthetic viewpoint is primarily directed at

Table 1.2. Important questions in an anaesthetic preoperative assessment

Cardiovascular	Angina pectoris
	Myocardial infarction
	Rheumatic fever
	Systemic vascular disease
Respiratory	Acute coryza
	Exercise tolerance
	Dyspnoea and orthopnoea
	Asthma and allergic lung diseases
	Bronchitis; cough and sputum production
	Pulmonary infection
	Pulmonary surgery
	Smoking
Nervous system	Epilepsy
	Neuromuscular disease
	Neuropathy
	Psychiatric disease including treatment
Liver	Alcohol consumption
	Hepatitis
Endocrine	Diabetes mellitus
	Thyroid disease
	Adrenal disease
Genitourinary	Renal disease
	Sexually transmitted diseases
	Menstrual history
Previous anaesthesia	Nausea and vomiting
	Adverse reactions
	Postspinal headache
	Familial problems with anaesthesia

the genital tract and the cardiovascular and respiratory systems; however, the importance of a full examination documented in the notes by the house surgeon cannot be overemphasised. The anaesthetist will be interested in the signs of respiratory disease including the nature and pattern of respiration, the presence of abnormal breath sounds plus additional evidence of respiratory disease, e.g. tracheal deviation and cyanosis. Simple bedside tests of respiratory function, e.g. peak expiratory flow measurement, can be useful indicators of respiratory reserve.

Cardiovascular examination should include assessment of heart rate and rhythm, and auscultation for cardiac murmurs, in particular diastolic murmurs and the presence of third or fourth heart sounds. Measurement of arterial blood pressure is essential and should be repeated at least twice, at intervals, if found to be elevated.

More detailed examination of other systems is dictated by the presence of any intercurrent disease, e.g. neurological assessment of the patient with multiple sclerosis and assessment of joint mobility in patients with arthritis, particularly if leg stirrups are to be employed.

Intercurrent Medical Disease, Surgery and Anaesthesia

It is not possible, nor intended, to give a comprehensive account of the effects of medical conditions on the course of surgery and anaesthesia, but to give an overview of those problems commonly encountered in patients presenting for surgery and the steps one can take to ensure that they are in the best possible condition prior to operation.

Cardiovascular Disease (Foex 1981)

The presence of cardiovascular disease is associated with an increase in morbidity and mortality during surgery and anaesthesia. The assessment of the severity of the condition and the instigation of measures to reduce the incidence of complications is therefore an essential part of preoperative assessment.

Ischaemic Heart Disease

The incidence of ischaemic heart disease is high in this country and patients may present with a spectrum of conditions from angina pectoris to myocardial infarction. The presence of coronary artery disease is associated with a significant increase in perioperative mortality and morbidity including a marked increase in postoperative infarction in these individuals presenting for surgery within 3 months of myocardial infarction. The development of angina pectoris occurs when the oxygen demands of the myocardium exceed the oxygen delivery. In the preoperative assessment of those patients the frequency and duration of attacks, along with the efficacy of current medication, should be noted and where control of symptoms is inadequate, referral to a cardiologist for evaluation and treatment is advisable.

Hypertension

Hypertension is difficult to define as it represents the upper end of a spectrum of blood pressure within a population; however, the World Health Organisation definition of a persistently elevated systolic pressure greater than 160 mm Hg and/or a diastolic pressure greater than 95 mm Hg serve as good guidelines. By these criteria one would expect approximately 15% of the population to suffer from hypertensive disease.

Preoperative evaluation of the hypertensive patient should aim to determine the adequacy of blood pressure control, to review current therapy, to evaluate the effects of surgery on that therapy and to assess any major organ dysfunction associated with the condition, e.g. coronary artery disease, renal disease or cerebrovascular disease.

If persistent hypertension is present, then instigation of appropriate antihypertensive therapy is indicated, as normalisation of blood pressure in the hypertensive patient is associated with a significant reduction in morbidity and mortality.

Valvular Heart Disease

Valvular heart disease may be congenital or acquired. The commonest lesions affect the left side of the heart and produce haemodynamic disturbances of left ventricular function which may be pressure related, i.e. mitral and aortic stenosis, or volume related, i.e. mitral and aortic regurgitation.

The degree of cardiac reserve can be ascertained by evaluation of the patient's exercise tolerance, and it is important to appreciate the effects of compensatory mechanisms, e.g. cardiac hypertrophy, in maintaining normal cardiac output.

All these patients should have prophylactic antibiotic therapy prior to surgery in order to prevent the development of bacterial endocarditis. In gynaecological surgery the recommended regimen as laid down by the American Heart Association (1977) is gentamycin 1·5 mg/kg i.v. and ampicillin 1 g i.v. both 30 min prior to operation and repeated twice at 8-h intervals after surgery. In penicillin-sensitive individuals erythromycin lactobionate 500 mg i.v. can be substituted for ampicillin. In the United Kingdom pivampicillin is now preferred to ampicillin.

Arrhythmias

The presence of ischaemic heart disease is frequently associated with the development of arrhythmias and conduction defects, e.g. atrial fibrillation and bundle branch block. Events in the perioperative period, e.g. hypoxia, hypercarbia, the use of volatile anaesthetic agents and alterations of pH, may exacerbate these arrhythmias and produce marked haemodynamic disturbance. Where concerned, appropriate treatment with antidys-rhythmic drugs or referral for prophylactic cardiac pacing should be undertaken.

Respiratory Disease

The function of the lungs is to provide an interface for exchange of oxygen and carbon dioxide between blood and air, necessary to meet the metabolic requirements of the body. Pulmonary disease results in a decrease in the efficiency of this exchange, which in combination with the effects of surgery and anaesthesia on pulmonary function may lead to an increase in postoperative morbidity and mortality (Fowkes et al. 1982).

Upper Respiratory Tract Infections

There is seldom necessity for patients with upper respiratory tract infections to undergo elective surgery. The infection combined with the immuno-suppressive effects of anaesthesia, postoperative inhibition of coughing and the sedative effects of anaesthetic agents increase the risk of developing a postoperative pneumonia. It is therefore advisable to withhold surgery until recovery is complete.

Obstructive Lung Disease

These are a heterogeneous group of conditions from bronchitis to asthma which may be acute or chronic, reversible or irreversible and which together constitute the largest group of respiratory disease.

Preoperative preparation should aim to assess the severity of the condition, using clinical judgement, simple spirometry—measurement of vital capacity and forced expiratory volume in 1 s (FEV 1)—and blood gas analysis (Rigg and Jones 1978). On the results of these tests appropriate therapy may be instigated. This should include advice on stopping smoking, preoperative physiotherapy and breathing exercises and the use of bronchodilator therapy—in these cases where reversibility is demonstrated—together with antibiotics for the treatment of any acute exacerbations. It is advisable to repeat these tests after treatment, and to delay surgery until the patient is in the optimum condition. In those patients with severe pulmonary disease, i.e. FEV 1, $<25\%-50\%$ predicted and $PaO_2 < 9.3$ kPa, the possibility of surgery under regional or local anaesthesia should be discussed.

Diseases of the Nervous System

Epilepsy

Epilepsy is an expression of a disorder of neuronal function resulting from the excessive synchronous discharge from a focal area of neuronal hyper-excitability. This may present as an expression of a local event, e.g. temporal lobe epilepsy, or spread to the entire cerebral cortex resulting in a generalised seizure. It is advisable for patients to continue with anticonvulsant therapy in the perioperative period and for the anaesthetist to be informed, as a number of anaesthetic agents predispose to seizure activity.

Multiple Sclerosis

This is a progressive disease of young adults (15–40 years) characterised by random and multiple sites of demyelination of neurones within the brain and spinal cord. It is manifest by visual disturbance, cerebellar problems with resulting disturbance of gait, and spinal cord demyelination with limb par-aesthesia and urinary incontinence—for which the patient may be referred to the gynaecologist for assessment and possible surgery. It is important to document the degree of neurological impairment prior to surgery and to explain to the patient that the stress associated with surgery has been shown to exacerbate the condition in the postoperative period.

Endocrine Disease and Obesity

There are many endocrine conditions which a patient may have who presents for surgery; their management is dealt with in the subsequent sections on the influence of pre-existing medication. One important condition to consider, however, is the effect of obesity on the course of surgery and anaesthesia. Obesity can be defined as body fat content in excess of 30% in the female or where the ratio of weight (kg) over height (m^2) is greater than 30. Patients in this category present a considerable risk to surgery, associated with abnormalities of respiratory and cardiovascular physiology as well as technical problems with access for surgery and problems with postoperative mobilisation (Vaughn 1983).

Appropriate dietary advice in the outpatient clinic with regular follow-up by a dietician prior to surgery is advocated in order to reduce some of these problems.

Haematological Disorders

Anaemia

Anaemia is an acute or chronic reduction in the number of circulating erythrocytes manifest as a decrease in the concentration of haemoglobin and a concomitant reduction in the oxygen-carrying capacity of the blood. In the majority of patients the cause of this may be known, e.g. menorrhagia; however, where this is unclear relevant investigations prior to surgery to elucidate the cause are essential.

In patients with chronic anaemia, compensatory changes including a shift to the right of the oxyhaemoglobin dissociation curve increasing oxygen release at a tissue level and an increase in cardiac output take place in order to maintain oxygen availability (AvO_2).

The necessity for a minimum preoperative haemoglobin of 10 g/dl is based on a physiological necessity for a minimum AvO_2 of 250 ml oxygen/min.

Oxygen availability = cardiac output × haemoglobin × % haemoglobin saturation × haemoglobin-carrying capacity for oxygen.

If the Hb = 15 g/dl, AvO_2 = 5000 ml/min × 15/100 g/dl × 95/100 × 1·38 ml/O_2/g haemoglobin, which = 983 ml O_2/min.

For a haemoglobin of 10 g/dl the AvO_2 is decreased to 655 ml O_2/min; if during the course of surgery any of the other variables are reduced, e.g. cardiac output secondary to hypovolaemia or the myocardial depressant affects of anaesthetics, the AvO_2 will be further reduced and approach a level where tissue oxygen availability will be impaired.

Therefore in those individuals where the haemoglobin is less than 10 g/dl and the cause identified, preoperative transfusion 48 h prior to surgery is indicated in order to allow redistribution of the fluid and electrolyte load and reactivation of the 2–3 DPG in the stored blood.

Sickle Cell Disease

Described by J. B. Herrick in 1910, sickle cell disease is an inherited group of disorders ranging from benign sickle cell trait to a severe form of sickle cell anaemia, characterised by the substitution of normal haemoglobin A by abnormal haemoglobin S. The symptoms of the disease are related to the inability of the HbS to withstand hypoxia, which results in the reduced haemoglobin forming tactoids which cause disruption and eventual rupture of the red cell. This leads to microvascular occlusion with infarctions and organ damage.

Sickle cell trait, the heterozygous form of the condition, generally presents little problem as far as surgery and anaesthesia are concerned; conversely the sickle cell anaemia presents a grave threat to the patient in the perioperative period, and preoperative exchange transfusion is indicated in those individuals where the haemoglobin is less than 8 g/dl.

Thalassaemia

This is a collective term for a group of inherited disorders associated with a reduction or lack of production of structurally normal components of the haemoglobin molecule, i.e. β-thalassaemia and a diminution of beta globulin production and α-thalassaemia and reduction of alpha globulin synthesis. Similar preoperative considerations to those for sickle cell disease should be taken.

Relevant Investigations Prior to Surgery

Haematology

A full blood count is considered to be a minimum preoperative requirement prior to surgery, supplemented in patients of negroid or Mediterranean extraction by a sickle test and if necessary by haemoglobin electrophoresis.

Where perioperative transfusion is envisaged, blood may be sent for grouping—including the rhesus group—and cross-matched preferably 24 h prior to surgery.

In patients with abnormalities of clotting, e.g. on anticoagulant therapy, or those with liver disease, full clotting profiles should be sent and appropriate corrective therapy instituted prior to surgery.

Biochemistry

Biochemical analysis of patients' urine is generally performed by the nursing staff on admission or in the outpatient clinic, using one of the many multitest dipstick kits available. These detect glycosuria, proteinuria, etc. and, if abnormal, warrant further investigation.

Serum multiple analysis (SMA) for abnormalities of urea, electrolytes and liver function are indicated where:

1. Renal function may be impaired, i.e. by virtue of the primary gynaecological pathology, e.g. late-stage carcinoma of the cervix, or secondary to systemic disease
2. Current medication includes drugs likely to affect serum electrolytes, e.g. diuretic therapy, corticosteroids
3. Hepatic or bony secondaries are suspected
4. Postoperative nephrotoxic cytotoxic therapy is contemplated
5. Postoperative enteral or parenteral nutrition is envisaged

Microbiology

A midstream urine specimen should be sent for microscopic examination and culture to exclude urinary tract infection prior to any urogynaecological procedure.

In those patients where pelvic inflammatory disease (PID) is suspected or where tubal surgery is to be undertaken with a previous history of PID, swabs from the vagina, cervix and urethra should be sent for microscopy culture and sensitivity studies.

Virology

In those individuals where hepatitis B virus infection is suspected, e.g. drug abusers or those with a previous history of hepatitis, testing for hepatitis surface antigen (HBsAg) is necessary. Similarly, testing for HIV (AIDS virus) is nesessary in homosexuals, drug abusers and patients from areas with endemic AIDS.

Radiological Investigations

Many of these are dictated by the nature of the presenting complaint and the anticipated surgery, e.g. lymphangiography in pelvic carcinoma or ultrasound of the liver if hepatic secondaries are suspected, and are further dealt with in Chap. 5.

Preoperative chest X-ray is only indicated in those individuals where underlying pulmonary or cardiac disease is present or in those individuals, e.g. immigrants, where exposure to tuberculosis may be suspected.

Routine electrocardiographic examination (ECG) is only necessary if cardiovascular disease is present; an abnormal ECG is associated with an increased operative risk.

Influences of Pre-existing Medication

Corticosteroids

Patients treated with systemic corticosteroids develop suppression of the hypothalamic-pituitary-adrenal axis (HPA). High levels of corticosteroids suppress hypothalamic production of corticotrophin-releasing factor (CRF) and anterior pituitary release of adrenocorticotrophic hormone (ACTH), and eventually low levels of ACTH lead to adrenocortical atrophy. (Patients treated with ACTH and similar analogues develop HPA suppression.) The degree of suppression depends on dosage and duration of treatment, but some adrenal suppression can occur within 1 week of starting corticosteroids. On stopping corticosteroids, recovery may take several months. It is usually considered that patients who have been off treatment with corticosteroids for 18 months have a normal response to stress.

A surgical operation acts as a stress to the body and the normal response involves an increased output of corticosteroids. It has been estimated that a major surgical operation results in the output of an extra 200–400 mg cortisol. Therefore in patients undergoing surgery who potentially have a suppressed HPA axis additional corticosteroids must be given to avoid the risk of adrenocortical insufficiency.

Patients undergoing minor procedures may be managed by an increase in the daily dose of corticosteroid or ACTH, or by the monitoring of vital signs and treating with hydrocortisone if features suggestive of adrenocortical insufficiency arise. For major surgery it is usual to give cover in the form of hydrocortisone, usually 100–200 mg with the premed and then 50–100 mg four times daily reducing to a daily maintenance dose over several days if there are no complications. Recently it has been questioned whether additional corticosteroids are always necessary to cover surgery (Lloyd 1981).

Patients treated with topical steroids, e.g. to the skin or rectum, occasionally absorb sufficient quantities to cause adrenal suppression.

Other patients who also require corticosteroid cover for surgical procedures include those who have been hypophysectomised, those without functional adrenocortical tissue and patients receiving adrenolytic therapy—aminoglutethimide, metyrapone and trilostane.

Contraceptive Steroids

Women taking the combined oral contraceptive have a higher incidence of deep venous thrombosis (DVT) when compared with non-pill users. This risk is increased by anaesthesia, surgery and the accompanying immobilisation. It has been estimated that among pill takers undergoing major surgery, the relative risk of DVT was twice that of non-users (Stabel 1981). However, the reduction in the dosage of the oestrogen component of these preparations since this work suggests that the real risk may now be less.

Oestrogens have been shown to increase the plasma concentration of several clotting factors as well as decreasing antifibrinolytic activity and the level of antithrombin III, factors which all increase the tendency to thrombosis. These changes in the coagulation and fibrinolytic systems have reverted entirely to normal 6 weeks after discontinuation of the oestrogen pill (Von Kaulla 1971) but epidemiological evidence suggests that the excess risk of DVT reverts to normal in less than 1 month (Vessey 1970).

Current opinion therefore is that the combined oral contraceptive should be discontinued 1 month prior to major surgery, restarting at the first menses, at least 2 weeks postoperatively (Guillebaud 1985). It is important that the patient is counselled in alternative contraceptive measures or unwanted pregnancy may result (Carter 1985). This risk of DVT following minor surgery—including laparoscopy—is extremely small and any extra risk from the oral contraceptive is more than outweighed by the risk of pregnancy—it is therefore recommended that the pill should be continued.

Where patients continue to take the pill up to the time of surgery, e.g. emergency surgery, prophylactic low-dose heparin should be considered, particularly if there are other risk factors such as obesity and smoking.

Oestrogens given for hormone replacement therapy in postmenopausal patients should similarly be discontinued.

Progestogens do not cause changes which favour venous thrombosis and therefore the constraints of the combined pill do not apply.

Insulin and Oral Hypoglycaemic Drugs

As previously discussed, the effect of anaesthesia and surgery causes a stress reaction which results in outpouring of catabolic hormones—catecholamines, corticosteroids and glucagon. One of the metabolic effects of these is to stimulate glycogenolysis and gluconeogenesis resulting in glucose liberation. These hormones also cause an increase in lipolysis, which under normal circumstances is offset by the antilipolytic effect of the increased secretion of insulin which occurs as a result of the hyperglycaemia. The resultant effect is depletion of liver glycogen and protein catabolism. Untreated type 1 (insulin-dependent) diabetics subjected to such stress would become hyperglycaemic, ketoacidotic and catabolic. Type II (non-insulin-dependent) diabetics have some residual insulin secretion so these effects would be less profound and they do not usually become ketoacidotic.

The perioperative management of diabetes aims to avoid these problems:

Type I diabetics—for all surgery involving general anaesthesia, the patients should be admitted several days preoperatively and stabilised on short-acting insulins. Numerous different regimens of perioperative management are in use. However, the simplest consists of the omission of the insulin dose on the day of operation, in place of which an infusion of 10% glucose potassium and soluble insulin is established. Alternatively an infusion of glucose and potassium may be supplemented by soluble insulin administered separately intravenously by a pump or by a regular small subcutaneous injection. These are continued until the patient is eating again. All regimens require regular and careful monitoring of glucose and potassium. Suitable regimens are suggested by Alberti and Hockaday (1983).

Type II diabetics—for minor surgery it is often sufficient to omit the oral hypoglycaemic agent on the morning of the operation, checking the blood sugar before, during and after the operation. The hyperglycaemic effect of the operation usually counteracts the residual effect of the previous day's dose even when a long-acting agent such as chlorpropamide is used. If there are problems or the operation becomes prolonged the patient is managed as for type I diabetes (see above). For major surgery the oral agent is discontinued on the day of operation: the alternative is to change several days preoperatively from a long-acting agent and stabilise on a short-acting insulin. The patient is then managed as discussed for type I diabetes. The infusion is discontinued and the oral agent reintroduced once the patient is eating normally again.

Drugs Acting on the Cardiovascular System

Patients whose cardiovascular disease is controlled with drugs should in general continue on their medication over the operative period. Abrupt withdrawal of clonidine (for hypertension) can cause profound rebound sympathetic overactivity with anxiety, sweating, tremor and severe hypertension: this may occur after only one or two missed doses. It is therefore essential that it is continued over the operative period, parenterally if necessary. Patients receiving potassium-losing diuretics whether or not being given potassium supplements, should have their plasma potassium estimated, and hypokalaemia corrected preoperatively.

When patients who are anticoagulated require surgery, and the need for anticoagulation is short term, e.g. following a deep vein thrombosis, it is often easiest where possible to postpone the surgery until the need for full anticoagulation has passed. When the need for anticoagulation is long term, e.g. patients with prosthetic heart valves, it is important to liaise with the physician supervising such treatment. In general the patient is admitted several days prior to operation to allow adjustment of the degree of anticoagulation. A British corrected ratio (BCR) in the range 2–3 is considered suitable for surgery. Postoperatively, anticoagulation is maintained with intravenous heparin until the patient is once again able to take the oral agent. When an anticoagulated patient requires emergency surgery the BCR is adjusted to the suitable range by the administration of fresh frozen plasma.

Drugs Acting on the Nervous System

Monoamine Oxidase Inhibitors (MAOIs)

Drugs of this group are used in the treatment of depression resistant to other agents. Their therapeutic effects are believed to result from the inhibition of central nervous system monoamine oxidase, leading to an increase in central catecholamines and 5-hydroxytryptamine. Their peripheral effects, however, include MAO inhibition, inhibition of hepatic drug oxidation and a variable degree of sympathetic blockade, making anaesthesia and surgery fraught with difficulties. Sympathomimetics may cause a hypertensive crisis, opiates (particularly pethidine) may cause profound hypotension and barbituates are metabolised at a variable and unpredictable rate. These problems can be overcome by withdrawing the drug at least

2 weeks before surgery; this must always be done in liaison with the prescribing psychiatrist.

Tricyclic and Quadricyclic Antidepressants and Major Tranquillisers

It is safe for patients to continue on these drugs provided that the anaesthetist is aware that they are being given and thus the anaesthetic may be varied appropriately. Sudden cessation of administration of these agents may result in an acute exacerbation of the psychiatric illness. In the case of patients suffering from a psychotic illness stabilised on an oral major tranquilliser it may be worth considering giving it parenterally over the operative period.

Lithium

It is usual practice to withdraw lithium approximately 1 week prior to major surgery, because of the risk of toxicity should there be an electrolyte imbalance or deterioration in renal function. This risk must be balanced against the possible relapse of the affective disorder for which it is prescribed and hence liaison with the psychiatrist is essential. No change in well-controlled lithium therapy is necessary for minor surgery unless muscle paralysis is envisaged as part of the anaesthetic technique. In these cases it is important that the anaesthetist be aware that the patient is on lithium therapy.

Anticonvulsants

It is important that patients continue to receive their anticonvulsant medication over the operative period—it is usual to give the dose orally on the day of surgery, then parenterally until the patient can take it again by mouth.

Sodium valproate (Epilim) deserves particular mention because in addition to its anticonvulsant properties it interferes with haemostasis. This drug causes depression of platelet counts (including frank thrombocytopenia) in a dose-related fashion, and it has been reported on occasions to cause impairment of platelet aggregation and minor defects of coagulation, including hypofibrinogenaemia. It is therefore recommended that patients taking sodium valproate who require surgery should have a platelet count and coagulation screen—prothrombin time, activated partial thromboplastin time and a fibrinogen titre.

Smoking (Jones 1985)

Although not strictly medication, the effects of smoking on perioperative events and the necessity to encourage patients to stop smoking prior to surgery are important in the preoperative preparation of the patient.

Cigarettes have a number of deleterious effects on the patients:

1. Cardiovascular system—reduction in oxygen availability secondary to carbon monoxide binding to haemoglobin
2. Respiratory system—impairment of mucociliary clearance and hyperreactivity of small airways, increasing the predisposition to postoperative chest infection
3. Immune system—reductions in neutrophil chemotaxis and immunoglobulin concentrations
4. Increase in platelet aggregatability

Patients should be encouraged to stop smoking at least 6 weeks prior to surgery, in order to improve pulmonary function and definitely to stop for the 48 h prior to surgery in order to eliminate carbon monoxide and improve oxygen availability.

Alcohol (Edwards 1985)

It is important to appreciate the effects of alcohol on surgical morbidity and to ascertain any alcohol-related problems in the preoperative preparations of the patient.

Surgery is associated with an increased risk to the heavy drinker due to diminution of the stress response, impaired immunity, abnormalities of electrolyte control, etc. Development of the alcoholic withdrawal syndrome may occur within 8 h of abstention and treatment with infusion of alcohol may be necessary.

In the alcoholic with systemic manifestations of the condition, e.g. a bleeding diathesis, pretreatment with parenteral vitamins and correction of clotting abnormalities are necessary. The preoperative administration of steroids in those alcoholics with severe impairment of the stress response should be considered.

Day Case Surgery

When considering patients for day case surgery one must consider two aspects. Firstly is the procedure suitable to be undertaken? Ideally it should be of short duration, less than 1 h and be associated with a low incidence of perioperative and postoperative complications, in particular a low incidence of postoperative pain. Suitable gynaecological procedures include dilatation and curettage, suction termination of pregnancy and diagnostic laparoscopy (Thurlow 1983).

Patient suitability for day case surgery is generally limited to those within ASA categories 1 and 2; however, consideration of patients in ASA class 3, especially where the patient is well known to surgeon and anaesthetist, e.g. check cystoscopy should be given.

Skilled surgery and anaesthesia are essential and these cases should not be delegated to an inexperienced surgeon or anaesthetist. Preoperative assessment is generally undertaken in the gynaecological clinic and a knowledge of the constraints of day case surgery is essential in order to prevent undue cancellation due to patient unsuitability; where the surgeon is unclear prior consultation with an anaesthetist is advised.

The principles of preoperative assessment are as outlined above for inpatients.

Adequate information about preparation for anaesthesia including the withholding of food and drink for at least 6 h and detailed instructions about discharge from hospital should be given. This should include the importance of an escort to accompany and to look after the patient at home. The importance of not driving vehicles, operating machinery or taking unprescribed drugs or alcohol for 24 h should be stressed.

Special Cases

Jehovah's Witnesses

Jehovah's Witnesses are a fundamentalist sect formed in the United States in the 1870s. In recent years the numbers have increased substantially and it is now estimated that there are some 83 000 in the United Kingdom (Clarke 1982).

Their beliefs are based entirely on their own unique interpretation of the Bible and contradict those of the major churches. A minor part of their doctrine is taken to imply that blood transfusion should be forbidden as violating God's law. Jehovah's Witnesses accept medical treatment in all other respects, and make no attempt to argue against the medical indications for blood transfusion. They are willing to take responsibility for their lives and accept that the constraints they place on their medical attendants may lead to their death. To this end, Health Authorities (with the guidance of the defence societies) have produced forms consenting to treatment but stating that blood transfusion is unacceptable and that the doctor will be absolved of any consequences of its omission. The legal value of these documents has been questioned (Casale 1979; Palmer 1980).

The individual doctor must decide if he is willing to treat such a patient, given the constraints placed on his or her management. The techniques of haemodilution and autotransfusion, which are acceptable to Jehovah's Witnesses, have been developed and these facilitate surgery. It must be remembered that to administer blood against the wishes of the patient would constitute assault. The situation with regard to children is different by virtue of the Childrens and Young Persons Act, 1933.

The Medical Defence Union and the Medical Protection Society stress that they are always happy to offer advice in such circumstances, but whatever decision is taken they will give full support to the individual doctor if that decision is subsequently challenged.

Acknowledgements. We should like to acknowledge and thank Professor Joan Bicknell, Department of Psychiatry of Mental Handicap, St. George's Hospital Medical School, for her helpful advice on consent for the mentally handicapped.

References

Alberti KGMM, Hockaday TDR (1983) Diabetes mellitus. In: Weatherall DJ, Ledingham JG, Warrell DA (eds) Oxford textbook of medicine, vol 1. Oxford University Press, Chap 9, pp 5–49

American Society of Anaesthesiologists (1963) New Classification of Physical Status. Anaesthesiology 24:111

Burn JMB (1976) Preoperative assessment clinics. Proceedings Royal Society of Medicine 69:734–736

Carter RJ, Pryce J (1985) Risk of pregnancy while waiting for an operation. Br Med J 291:516

Casale F (1979) Blood transfusion and Jehovah's Witnesses. Br Med J 1:1796

Clarke JMF (1982) Surgery in Jehovah's Witnesses. Br J Hosp Med 27:497–500

Editorial, Royal College of Psychiatrists (1986) Interim guidelines on the consent to medical and surgical treatment, contraception, sterilisation and abortion in the mentally handicapped, vol 10, pp 184–185

Edwards R (1985) Anaesthesia and alcohol. Br Med J 291:423–424

Foex P (1981) Pre-operative assessment of the patient with cardiovascular disease. Br J Anaesth 53:731–744

Fowkes JR, Lunn J, Farrow SC (1982) Epidemiology in anaesthesia: mortality risk in patients with co-existing physical disease. Br J Anaesth 54:819–825

Guillebaud J (1985) Surgery and the pill. Br Med J 291:498–499

Jones RM (1985) Smoking before surgery: the case for stopping. Br Med J 290:1763–1764

Keats AS (1978) The ASA classification of physical status: a recapitulation. Anaesthesiology 49:233–236

Kirby MD (1983) Informed consent: what does it mean? J Med Ethics 9:69–75

Lloyd EL (1981) A rational regimen for perioperative steroid supplements and a clinical assessment of the requirements. Ann R Coll Surg Engl 63:54–57

Mathews A, Ridgeway V (1981) Personality and surgical recovery. Br J Clin Psychol 20:243–260

Palmer RN (1980) Consent, confidentiality, disclosure of medical records. The Medical Protection Society, 50 Hallam St, London, W1N 6DE

Ridgeway V, Mathews A (1982) Psychological preparation for surgery: a comparison of methods. Br J Clin Psychol 21:271–280

Rigg JR, Jones NL (1978) Clinical assessment of respiratory function. Br J Anaesth 50:3–13

RCOG 14th Study Group (1985) "Litigation and obstetrics and gynaecology". In: Chamberlain G, Orr C, Sharp F (eds). Royal College of Obstetricians and Gynaecologists, London, p 311

Sidaway (1985) Sidaway v. Board of Governors of Bethlem Royal Hospital and Maudsley Hospital. Weekly Law Reports 2:480

Stabel BV (1981) Oral contraceptives and cardiovascular disease (1). N Engl J Med 305:612–618

Stabel BV (1981) Oral contraceptives and cardiovascular disease (2). N Engl J Med 305:672–677

Thurlow A (1983) Outpatient anaesthesia: current concepts. In: Mazze RI (ed) Clinics in anaesthesiology, vol 1, part 2. Saunders, Philadelphia, pp 397–413

Vaughn RW (1983) Anaesthesia for the morbidly obese. In: Mazze RI (ed) Clinics in anaesthesiology, vol 1, part 2. Saunders, pp 337–355

Vessey MP, Doll R, Fairburn AS, Glober G (1970) Post-operative thromboembolism and the use of oral contraceptives. Br Med J iii:123–126

Von Kaulla E, Droegmueller W, Aoki N, Von Kaulla KN (1971) Antithrombin III depression and thrombin generation acceleration in women taking oral contraceptives. Am J Obs Gynec 109:868–873

Wilson-Barnett J (1984) Interventions to alleviate patients' stress: a review. J Psychosom Res 28:63–72

Further Reading

Steven J (ed) (1986) Pre-operative assessment. Holt-Saunders, London (Clinics in anaesthesiology, vol 4, part 3)

2 · Management of the Elderly or Disabled Patient

Stuart L. Stanton

Senescence begins
and middle age ends
the day your descendants
outnumber your friends.
Ogden Nash

Introduction

Care of the elderly is germane to gynaecology today: 10% of the female population are over 65 years of age and this incidence is increasing. Life expectancy at 80 years is 6·5 years, at 85 years it is 5 years and at 90 years it is 3·5 years. For some departments, the current incidence of major surgery is highest in the 60- to 65-year-old age group (Mattingly and Thompson 1985) and about 30% of major gynaecological surgery is found between 70 and 90 years of age (Lewis 1968). The average female life span is now 78 years. Anaesthesia and postoperative care are much improved and many more patients expect to live out the winter of their lives with dignity and independence. Nonetheless, in the elderly there is still a mortality rate of 3·4% for general major elective surgery (Filzwieser and List 1983) and 2% for major gynaecological surgery (Lewis 1968). Morbidity in the elderly is due to urinary tract infection, ileus, deep venous thrombosis, pulmonary emboli and respiratory infection and can be as high as 65·7% (Seymour and Pringle 1983).

Although the elderly are defined as being over 65 years of age, most surgical studies in the literature refer to the elderly as being over 70 years old.

Over the past decade, greater emphasis has been given to the special needs of the disabled person and recognition that more attention is required for their pre- and postoperative care.

Pathophysiology in Relation to Surgery

The changes seen in old age represent cellular age changes in some tissues, rather than a specific disease of old age. The central nervous system is fundamental to ageing, largely because the cells are thought to be irreplaceable and also due to the coordinating role of this system. Closely linked with this system is the endocrine system, which controls the arrival of puberty and the menopause. The decline in ovarian function is matched by a change in function of the adrenal gland. There is also a change in immune function with age: an increasing number of autoantibodies are found in supposedly healthy older individuals and it has been suggested that ageing is due to a long-term minor-grade histoincompatibility reached in the cell population.

Most of the pathophysiology disorders which affect surgery are cardiovascular in origin. Heart disease is responsible for over one-third of all deaths over the age of 65 years, largely due to ischaemia. Surgery is especially influenced by hypertension and cardiac disease. Over 65 years, about 80% of women will have an upper limit of systolic blood pressure of 190 mm Hg and a diastolic blood pressure of 100 mm Hg. Untreated hypertension may suddenly fall when the patient undergoes anaesthesia during surgery, and transient rises in blood pressure in response to intubation are more likely to occur with hypertensive than normotensive patients. Cardiac disease may be precipitated by the stress of anaesthesia in surgery, leading to congestive cardiac failure. Conduction defects may be intensified during surgery, so that any preoperative evidence of heart block should be taken seriously. Loss of elasticity in the cardiovascular system, due to degenerative change, means that sudden changes in posture or intrathoracic pressure may be poorly tolerated and inadequately compensated. The effects of haemorrhage and hypovolaemia are less well tolerated in the elderly and resuscitation after blood loss must be prompt and adequate.

Surgery and anaesthesia following a recent myocardial infarct causes an increased risk of a further episode of a myocardial ischaemia or pulmonary embolus and ought to be avoided within 3 months of a myocardial infarct, unless urgent.

Pulmonary function declines with age, as progressive weakness and loss of elasticity and elastic recoil affects primary and secondary muscles of respiration, leading to reduction of total and vital capacity. The total number of functional alveoli is also reduced and there is loss of compliance due to decrease in bronchiolar elastic tissue and to alveolar membrane thickening. This leads to hypoxaemia which will be precipitated by stress and will lead to impaired uptake of volatile anaesthetic agents, with delay in their excretion from the lungs (Sewell 1979).

Ageing in the central nervous system may begin as early as the twenties, with progressive deterioration more rapid after the 6th and 7th decades. Histological examination shows thickening of meninges and walls of perforating arterioles and intracellular deposits of lipofuscin granules. There is degeneration of the myelin sheath, leading to increased response to local anaesthetics: nerve cell degeneration results in impaired memory and mental confusion and susceptibility to hypotension and hypoxia.

Renal function is progressively impaired with advancing age, but the reserve of renal capacity is so large that considerable impairment can occur before renal deterioration becomes apparent. Deterioration is usually due to atherosclerosis, leading to a decreased renal blood supply, a decrease in the number of functioning nephrons and hyalinisation of the glomeruli. Thickening of the basement membrane of Bowman's capsule leads to diminished membrane permeability. The end result is a decrease in glomerular and tubular function, leading to reduced rate of drug elimination, with the plasma half-lives rising by as much as 50%, failure to concentrate urine and deal with a fluid load and a rise in blood urea and serum creatinine. Liver function deteriorates too with age: there is a steady loss of liver mass from 50 years onwards. Efficiency of metabolic pathways and production of hepatic enzymes decline with age. This leads to impaired extraction of substances from the portal venous blood flow and impaired detoxification. In addition, there is a reduction in plasma albumin concentration and reduced plasma binding, which increases the concentration of unbound bioavailable drug, i.e. standard doses of drugs will give rise to a higher blood and tissue concentration and these may remain in the body for longer periods than normal. For the anaesthetist, this can lead to overdosage and difficulty in reversing relaxing agents.

Wound healing is likely to be impaired: a decrease in skin collagen is a common finding after the menopause (Brincat et al. 1983) and results in atrophic skin changes with loss of subcutaneous tissue, loss of ligamentous strength and elasticity and an increase in the incidence of hernias.

Evaluation of Risks in the Elderly

Many surveys indicate the increase in morbidity due to major surgery in the elderly. Goldman et al. (1977), using multivariate discriminate analysis, have identified nine independent significant correlates of life-threatening and fatal cardiac complications: they include preoperative third heart sound or jugular venous distension, myocardial infarction in the preceding 6 months, more than five premature ventricular contractions per minute, rhythm other than sinus rhythm, age over 70 years, important valvular aortic stenosis, emergency operation and poor general condition. Emergency surgery has a higher mortality than elective surgery and upper abdominal has a higher mortality than lower abdominal surgery.

Non-cardiac risks have yet to be evaluated, but other factors, such as hypertension, diabetes, mitral valve disease and congestive heart failure, affect postoperative outcome (Schneider 1983).

Towards reducing higher mortality and morbidity associated with surgery in the elderly, Del Guercio and Cohn (1980) developed a preoperative staging based on invasive monitoring and showed that after standard anaesthetic assessment, a further 23% of patients would have been rejected on results derived from serial intracardiac and pulmonary artery pressures and blood pH and gas measurements.

Perhaps the first major screening should involve categorisation of the patient into the ASA physical status classification (Table 1.1, p. 7).

As dementia and decreased mobility are common amongst the elderly and may sometimes affect outcome, an attempt should be made objectively to grade these preoperatively (Tables 2.1, 2.2).

Table 2.1. Dementia score

1. Age
2. Time (to nearest hour)
3. Address for recall at end of test—this should be repeated by patient to ensure it has been heard correctly: 42 West Street
4. Year
5. Name of hospital
6. Recognition of two persons (doctor, nurse, etc.)
7. Date of birth (day and months sufficient)
8. Year of First World War
9. Name of present monarch
10. Count backwards 20–1
3b. Recall of address

Dementia score: /10

Table 2.2. Mobility score

1. Mobile
2. Walks with stick/frame
3. Confined to chair, but can stand
4. Cannot stand, but in chair
5. Bed bound

Mobility score: /10

Seymour and Pringle (1983) have evaluated postoperative morbidity in the elderly and found this was due to respiratory complications (40%), acute cardiac failure (10%), wound infection (16%) and thrombo-embolic disease (3·2%). Factors affecting morbidity included emergency rather than elective surgery, upper rather than lower gastrointestinal procedures and abdominal rather than non-abdominal operations in general. Preoperative fitness and activity led to less respiratory, cardiac and wound complications. They found an overall incidence of 10% of confusional states.

Additional adverse factors include weight loss, malignancy, steroid or cytotoxic therapy, diabetes mellitus, alcoholism and perioperative contamination (Schneider 1983).

The benefit of the preoperative anaesthetic clinic for the management of aged patients for elective surgery was demonstrated by Filzwieser and List (1983), who found that in a series of 500 consecutive surgical patients aged over 76 years, 6% of patients were in the ASA group III-IV: two-thirds had preoperative cardiovascular problems and one-third had respiratory disease. Forty-five per cent of patients were inadequately treated and required postponement of surgery for 2–5 days' medical treatment. The most frequent complications during operation were cardiovascular. The most frequent cause of death was postoperative renal failure and heart failure.

Preoperative Preparation and Management

The Elderly

There is no upper age limit for surgical eligibility. Rather, it is a question of does the patient wish surgery: the following should be answered:

1. Will the operation improve the quality of life?
2. Is the patient medically fit for surgery?
3. Which is the simplest and most effective procedure for the patient? (Sewell 1979).

A careful history and examination (including dementia and mobility scores, Tables 2.1, 2.2) should be completed and the patient's background, home circumstances and nature of support (such as relatives and friends and how much she will cope after she returns home after surgery) are assessed. It must be determined that the patient fully understands the implications of surgery.

Operative assessment ought to be a combined effort by the surgeon, geriatrician and anaesthetist and should include ECG, chest X-ray, full blood count, blood chemistry, liver function tests and blood gases. When indicated, lung function tests should be performed.

Drug prescribing in the elderly needs careful consideration. Elderly people are the largest consumers of medicines and frequently receive numerous (sometimes unnecessary) drugs for multiple disease (BNF 1986). The ageing nervous system shows increased susceptibility to opium alkaloids, sedatives and tranquillisers and these should always be used sparingly. The commonest drugs given to the elderly are hypotensives and diuretics and these may be responsible for many adverse reactions in the elderly, which can present in a very non-specific manner. This may be aggravated by poor compliance found in the elderly, who may have memory impairment, poor eyesight and difficulty in coping with complex drug regimes.

The common medical conditions which need recognition and management are cardiac failure, respiratory failure, neurological deterioration, diabetes mellitus and anaemia. Elderly patients requiring emergency surgery may be dehydrated, so an initial full blood count may not detect anaemia. Because postoperatively the elderly patient can slide insidiously into cardiovascular, respiratory, renal or neurological failure, and these are more likely to be promptly diagnosed and managed in a medical rather than surgical ward, it may be better to nurse elderly patients in the familiar surroundings of the geriatric ward, rather than in the acute gynaecological ward. In the former, they will at least be at less risk of developing confusional states, which may be associated with preoperative transfer to another ward. The likely acute surgical complications, namely, haemorrhage, urinary retention and wound dehiscence can be adequately detected by the joint care of the medical and surgical teams on the geriatric ward.

Preoperative counselling should be full and careful explanation of the procedure, the rate of recovery, its benefits and its risks is required, so that the patient and relatives fully understand. It is also important that the nursing staff are aware of the expected time scale of postoperative recovery.

Sedative premedication drugs are required only occasionally. Both opiates and atropine are to be avoided: the former because they cause respiratory depression and therefore have adverse effects on inhalation anaesthesia, and the latter because of retention of viscid secretions in the bronchial tree.

The Disabled

Preoperative counselling is similar to that for the elderly. With deaf patients, it is necessary to speak slowly and distinctly and have a light shining on your face, which is at the same level as theirs. It is important to ensure that the attendants know how to handle any hearing aid. For a patient currently having therapy for impaired vision, the current drug regime should be discussed with an ophthalmologist and advice taken about drugs which may be given by the anaesthetist, especially if the patient is likely to be off drug therapy for more than 8 h. A patient who has had eye surgery within 1 month should not have a mask placed on her face, either during surgery or to give postoperative oxygen.

The patient with ankylosing spondylitis or rheumatoid arthritis of the cervical spine needs careful preoperative assessment by the anaesthetist, because of the difficulties of intubation and the dangers of subluxation of the cervical spine.

Prevention of deep venous thrombosis is important: with 35% of all elderly patients at risk postoperatively, subcutaneous calcium heparin should be given as a 5000-IU dose with the premed and then three times daily until the patient is fully mobilised.

Operative Care

Attention should be paid when placing the elderly or disabled on the operating table to avoid pressure on prominent bony surfaces, which might lead to pressure sores and to ensure that no undue strain is placed on the cervical spine, hip or knee joints. Arthritis and joint deformities may make positioning difficult and limit surgical access. The surgeon may have to modify his technique to overcome this.

Full monitoring during anaesthesia is required and an accurate record of blood loss and intravenous food replacement is essential. All surgery should be expediently and carefully performed. The tissues in the elderly are particularly fragile and sharp and blunt dissection must be gentle. Full venous circulation should be maintained, using some Trendelenberg tilt and TED stockings.

Postoperative Care

The Elderly

The ward environment is important: seats and beds should be of adjustable height and the patient should be encouraged to be as mobile as possible. Small and regular doses of analgesia are important. It is necessary to avoid postoperative "stress", including pain, ischaemia, urinary retention and anxiety. It is wise to use an indwelling catheter (suprapubic preferably) for bladder neck surgery and posterior repairs, as the older patient usually takes longer to establish spontaneous micturition than her younger counterpart. Careful fluid replacement is necessary, with accurate input and output charting. Measurement of central venous pressure and hourly urine output are required in the more seriously ill patient. Hypertension or hypotension may result from uncontrolled pain. Hypertension may occur when anaesthetic agents are stopped: continuous sedation and analgesia will control this, but care should be exercised, so that the patient does not develop heart failure or have a cerebrovascular accident. Hypotension, leading to oliguria and anuria, is more serious and blood loss should be accurately replaced.

Respiratory conditions, particularly post-operative atelectasis, can account for 25%–40% of postoperative surgical deaths and these must be treated energetically with bronchoscopic aspiration at the bedside, physiotherapy and oxygen therapy.

Postoperative physiotherapy is necessary to ensure prompt mobilisation to avoid deep vein thrombosis and muscle weakness due to disuse.

Prophylactic subcutaneous heparin administration should be continued until the patient is fully mobile, usually on the 5th day.

Early discharge home or to convalescence is equally important for the elderly as for the younger patient and early discussion with relatives, general practitioner and district nurse is important, so that the patient is not alone at home, nor expected to cope on her own too early.

Provided the patient is fit and recovering satisfactorily, discharge a few days after surgery to a nursing home or a GP community hospital, with easy access to visitors and attended by a general practitioner, can be beneficial and should be encouraged (McGarry 1986).

The Disabled

Careful postoperative assessment, similar to the elderly, may be indicated. It is prudent to provide a special nurse for the blind or partially sighted in the immediate 8 h or so after anaesthesia. The mentally frail and elderly require careful and patient explanation by medical and nursing staff of the surgical procedure and its consequences: it is wrong to assume that the patient is either disinterested or unable to understand.

Care of the elderly and disabled is rewarding and of increasing importance in our "ageing" society, as more patients become aware of and eligible for the spectrum of surgical treatment.

Acknowledgements. I should like to thank Professor Peter Millard, Eleanor Peel Professor of Geriatrics at St. George's Hospital Medical School, for his helpful advice and criticism.

References

Brincat M, Moniz C, Studd JW, Darby A, Magos A, Cooper D (1983) Sex hormones and skin collagen content in postmenopausal women. Br Med J 287: 1337–1338

Del Guercio L, Cohn J (1980) Monitoring operative risk in the elderly. JAM Assoc 243: 1350–1355

Filzwieser G, List W (1983) Morbidity and mortality in elective geriatric surgery. In: Vickers M, Lunn J (eds) Mortality in anaesthesia. Proceedings of European Academy of Anaesthesiology, 1982. Springer, Berlin Heidelberg New York, pp 75–82

Goldman L, Caldera D, Nussbaum S et al. (1977) Multifactorial index of cardiac risk in non-cardiac surgical procedures. N Engl J Med 297: 845–850

Lewis A (1968) Major gynaecological surgery in the elderly: a review of 305 patients. J Int Fed Gynaec Obstet 6: 244–258

Mattingly RF, Thompson J (1985) Pre-operative care. In: Mattingly RF, Thompson J (eds) TeLinde's operative gynecology, 6th ed. J B Lippincott, Philadelphia, pp. 63–81

McGarry J (1986) Early pre-convalescent care after major gynaecological surgery. Health Trends 18: 7–8

Prasad A (ed) (1986) British National Formulary. Prescribing for the elderly, vol II. British Medical Association and Pharmaceutical Society of Great Britain, London, pp. 7–8

Schneider A (1983) Assessment of risk factors and surgical outcome. Surg Clin North Am 63: 1113–1126

Sewell I (1979) Surgery for the elderly, parts I and II. Hospital update. Sept, pp 791–812; Oct, pp 889–921

Seymour D, Pringle R (1983) Post-operative complications in the elderly surgical patient. Gerontology 29: 262–270

3 · Prevention and Treatment of Thromboembolism

John Dormandy

Aetiology and Pathology

All the essential pathology of venous thrombosis and pulmonary embolism was described by Virchow in the decade from 1846 to 1856. Thrombi form in the peripheral veins as a result of stasis, changes in the blood or damage to the venous endothelium. Virchow's famous triad has remained unchallenged and work in the past 130 years has merely elaborated and dissected its details. Virchow also described for the first time the true sequence of events leading to pulmonary embolism: the dis-

lodgement of peripheral venous thrombi. The relative importance of the three components of Virchow's triad in gynaecological surgery is illustrated in Figure 3.1.

Stasis

Stasis is the most important factor in the development of deep venous thrombosis (DVT) at the time of surgery. Investigations, such as radioactive-labelled fibrinogen scanning, have shown that venous thrombosis is initiated within a few hours of the

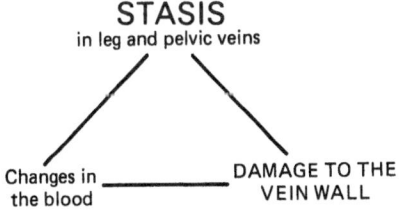

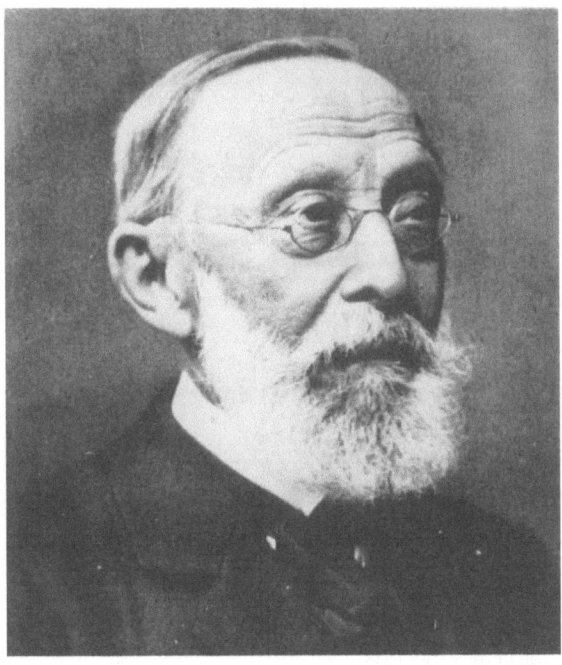

Fig. 3.1. Professor Rudolph Virchow (1821–1902) and his triad of basic causes of venous thrombosis: their relative importance in gynaecology.

operation, even though its clinical manifestations are usually delayed till the third to sixth postoperative day. Measurements of blood flow have shown that during anaesthesia, in at least some of the leg veins, blood is virtually static. Therefore the very high incidence of leg DVT associated with surgery and anaesthesia is due to the abnormal stasis of blood in the leg veins. For this reason, the most rational, if not necessarily the most effective, prophylactic measures are aimed at maintaining venous flow during and after surgery.

The birthplace of the thrombus is in the venous valve cusps; this is where the original nidus forms which given appropriate conditions grows into a macroscopic pathological thrombus. Figure 3.2 shows the flow patterns in a normal valve cusp, where there is typically a slowly rotating vortex with a static centre, even when there is movement of blood in the vein as a whole.

In varicose veins stasis will be even more pronounced. Blood can be stationary in these grossly dilated veins when the patient is fully conscious, explaining the higher incidence of DVT in patients with varicose veins.

Changes in the Blood

Maintaining the fluidity of the blood while at the same time protecting the integrity of the vascular space is one of the most important homeostatic mechanisms in the body. In health, there is a balance between haemostasis, which automatically plugs vessels when damaged and without which the surgeons would be quite incapable of carrying out the operation, and fibrinolysis which prevents the whole vascular system becoming solid. Pathological thrombosis results when this equilibrium is upset towards an exaggeration of the normal haemostatic processes. This can be precipitated by the stress of anaesthesia and surgery, a stress this homeostatic mechanism was not designed to withstand.

The details of activation of clotting factors leading to the formation of fibrin, platelet reactions and the lysis of fibrin are getting more complex every year. Figure 3.3 illustrates diagrammatically the basic features of these processes, their interaction, as well as the initial triggering role of vessel wall damage.

During anaesthesia and surgery the forces acting on both sides of the haemostasis-fibrinolysis balance are altered. The coagulation system is activated, primarily by tissue trauma. (The increased incidence of DVT in patients with cancer or receiving oestrogens may be explained by the greater activation of the clotting cascade in these circumstances.) The role of an increased activation of platelets in the pathogenesis of peroperative venous thrombosis is still speculative. On the other side of the balance, a decreasing level of plasminogen activator has been shown in the first 24 h following surgery. The continuing balance between thrombosis and fibrinolysis is illustrated by the fact that using the most sensitive test for DVT, it has been estimated that approximately 35% of small DVT completely disappear within 72 h. Clearly it could be argued that such transient phenomena are in no way pathological and should not correctly be called DVT.

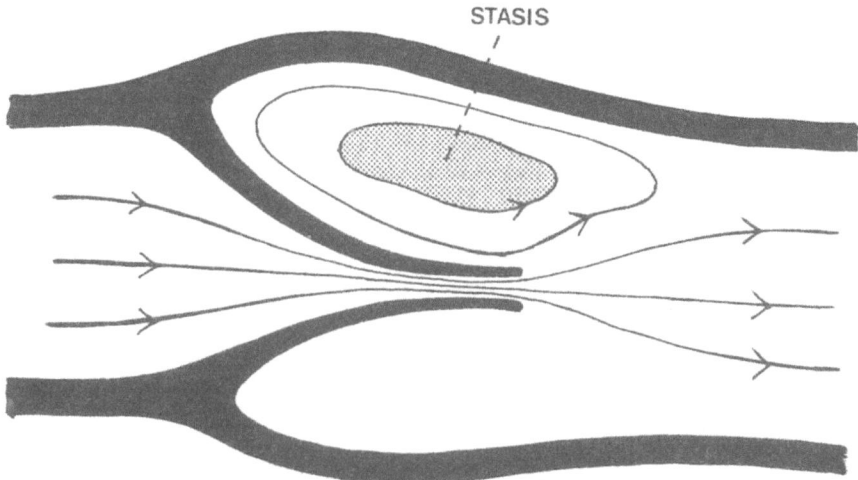

Fig. 3.2 Blood flow patterns around a vein valve, showing area of stasis in the valve cusp.

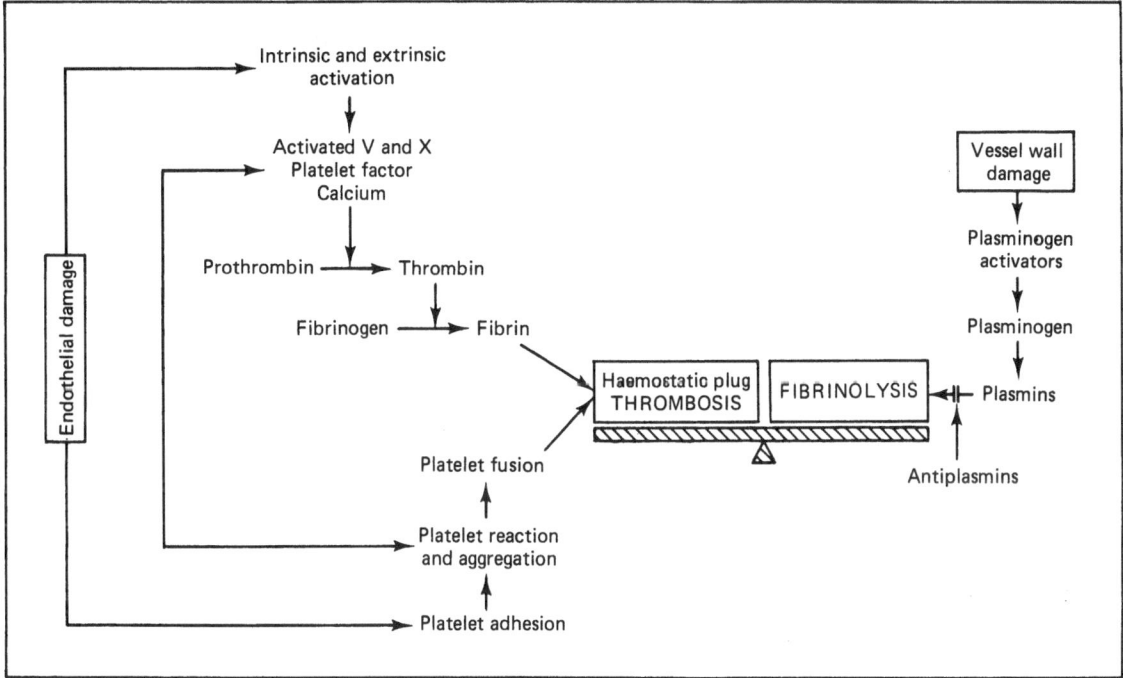

Fig. 3.3. Homeostatic mechanism maintaining balance between haemostasis and fibrinolysis.

Damage to the Vein Wall

It is difficult to assess the relative importance of this in the aetiology of venous thrombosis, but the mechanism must be through an activation of the clotting and platelet systems as illustrated in Fig. 3.3. Almost all our knowledge of postoperative venous thrombosis is based on studies of leg DVT, and damage to the vein walls simply as a result of lying on the operating table must nowadays be rare. However, in the case of gynaecological operations there may be significant direct damage to the pelvic veins, for instance by retractors. As there is no technique available for diagnosing pelvic DVT, except in the external and common iliac veins, the true incidence of pelvic DVT is not known, but it may be quite significant following gynaecological and general surgery. Almost all the clinical data comparing DVT in gynaecological and general surgery examine only the incidence in the leg and ignore a possible difference in the incidence of pelvic DVT. The same fundamental criticism applies to the interpretation of prophylactic trials.

Risk Factors

Whilst surgery itself is the major risk for the development of DVT, it is valuable to look at other factors within the surgical group so that the risk for an individual patient can be estimated and the advantage of preoperative prophylaxis evaluated. A number of studies have looked at this and suggest that significant risk factors in decreasing order of importance are (Clayton et al. 1976; Crandon et al. 1980):

Increasing age
Malignant disease
Previous thromboembolic disease
Use of oestrogen oral contraception
Prolonged bed rest
Obesity
Varicose veins

In most cases the additional risk clearly operates by enhancement of one of the primary mechanisms mentioned above, although the highly significant influence of age remains unexplained. Malignant tumours, particularly mucous adenocarcinoma, are thought to release free circulating thrombin. The resulting monomer complexes can be detected by the ethanol gel or the protamine sulphate test. If these tests remain positive for five consecutive days in the presence of venous thrombosis the risk of cancer is 60% (Edgington 1980). In the case of oral contraceptives, the risk is related to the oestrogen rather than progesterone content (Vessey 1982).

Bed rest and varicose veins clearly increase the risk of DVT by promoting stasis. In about 10% of cases of superficial thrombophlebitis the thrombus will extend into the deep venous system. Haematological diseases predisposing to DVT are not mentioned in the above list because they are exceedingly rare. They can, however, be an important risk and some, like polycythaemia and hyperfibrinogenaemia (giving a high ESR), can be suggested by the routine preoperative blood tests. In both these conditions the incidence of DVT is increased severalfold, presumably as a result of increased blood viscosity encouraging stasis. By contrast DVT is rare in anaemic subjects.

Incidence and Natural History

Incidence of Thromboembolic Disease Without Prophylaxis

The wealth of information about the incidence of postoperative leg DVT is matched by a complete ignorance about the incidence and natural history of pelvic DVT. The variations in the quoted incidence of DVT can be partly explained by differences in the populations studied and the sensitivity of the techniques used to detect it. Possibly some of the DVT detected by the very sensitive labelled fibrinogen techniques are within the normal physiological range. Only a few studies have looked specifically at gynaecological operations (Walsh et al. 1974; Clayton et al. 1976; Crandon et al. 1980).

Figure 3.4 attempts to summarise the evidence and shows the probable incidence of pathological DVT and the likelihood of their extension and embolisation. The figures represent the estimated incidence associated with all gynaecological operations in patients aged over 40. Younger patients have a very much lower risk unless they have malignant disease. Figure 3.4 illustrates therefore the natural history of perioperative thromboembolic disease in older gynaecological patients without prophylaxis.

Approximately 30% of patients over 40 years of age will develop a thrombus in the calf veins, although less than a third of these will spread into the femoropopliteal region. It is generally believed that only these latter thrombi are associated with a significant risk of embolisation. The incidence will vary according to the presence of associated risk factors and the type of operation. For instance, an abdominal hysterectomy will carry a higher risk than a vaginal hysterectomy (Walsh et al. 1974;

Verstraete and Vermylen 1984), possibly because of the improved drainage of the blood from the legs in the lithotomy position and increased trauma and stasis associated with an abdominal operation. The overall incidence of non-fatal PE, using the best available diagnostic techniques, is between 3% and 5% and about one out of ten of these will prove to be fatal. In the study by Walsh et al. (1974), the overall incidence of DVT was lower (14%) than those quoted in Figure 3.4 because many of their patients were aged under 40 years. They showed that 3% of all DVT appeared to start in the iliac veins, presumably because of local factors. There must have been other pelvic thrombi which could not be detected by the methods used. Almost half their patients with carcinoma of the ovary or uterus of all ages developed a DVT in the leg.

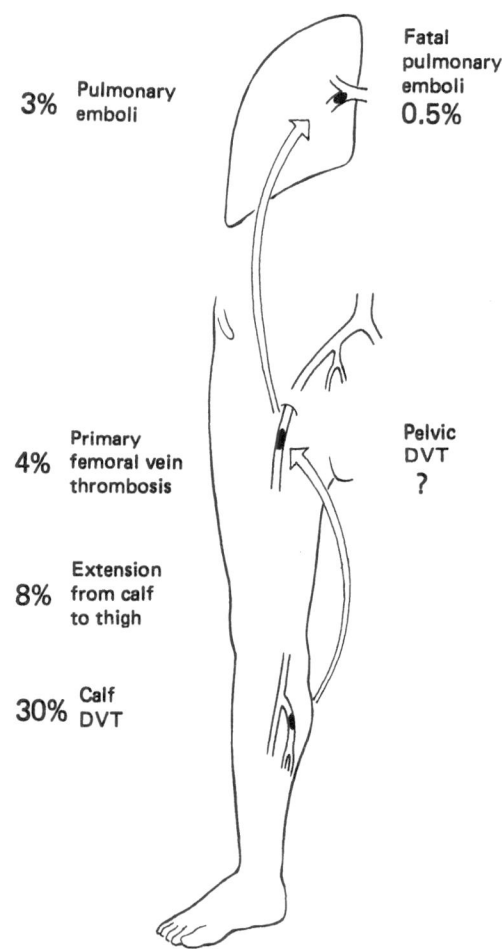

Fig. 3.4. Probable incidence of DVT and its complications following gynaecological operations in patients over 40 not receiving prophylactic treatment. In the presence of prophylaxis the figures are decreased to a third or quarter of the above.

Post-thrombotic Syndrome

The importance of the long-term local sequelae of leg DVT is often ignored, partly because these complications usually appear several years later and do not present to the surgeon performing the original operation. Family practitioners, dermatologists and vascular surgeons, however, are all too familiar with these long-term problems. Whether the original thrombus recanalises or not, the end result is likely to be abnormal venous hypertension, either due to obstruction of the deep veins or to destruction of the venous valves during the process of recanalisation. The effects of chronic venous hypertension will be maximal at the extremity of the leg and will result in impaired microcirculation and tissue hypoxia. The post-thrombotic syndrome is characterised by permanent irreversible trophic skin changes near the ankle, often leading to intractable ulceration. This is an important source of serious morbidity in the population and should not be allowed to be overshadowed in importance by the more acute and dramatic, but much less frequent, embolic complications of DVT. Oedema, which is the earliest change along the inexorable progression of the post-thrombotic leg, develops in about 30% of patients 3 years after DVT. The full post-thrombotic syndrome develops sooner or later in 10% of patients with DVT in the lower leg and 50% of patients with DVT above the popliteal (Verstraete and Vermylen 1984).

Diagnosis

The biggest advance in our knowledge of venous thromboembolic disease, since it was first described by Virchow, has been the improved techniques now available for its diagnosis. These have all been developed in the past 20 years and have led to the recognition of the true magnitude of the problem and have been an essential foundation for the development of proper prophylaxis and treatment.

Diagnosis of DVT

The classical symptoms and signs of pain, swelling, redness, warmth, tenderness, oedema and prominent superficial veins are unfortunately almost useless in making a correct clinical diagnosis. Even a clinical suspicion based on these criteria will miss at least half the true DVTs of the leg and will diagnose a DVT where none is present in also half the cases (Simpson et al. 1980; Gallus 1981). This sad reflection on classical clinical teaching is illustrated in Fig. 3.5. Moreover, it seems that DVT giving rise to the classical symptoms and signs are not necessarily the most dangerous; in the majority of patients with fatal pulmonary emboli, there were no clinical signs of a DVT (Nielsen et al. 1982). It is uncertain what gives rise to the false-positive signs, but at least some of the patients have a popliteal cyst, lymphoedema or calf haematoma, although these conditions cannot possibly explain all the cases of false-positive symptoms and signs.

The "gold standard" for the diagnosis of DVT is the ascending venogram. This must be carried out using one of the newer isotonic contrast media as the older substances frequently precipitated a thrombosis where none had previously existed. Although this procedure is now safe, it is still very time consuming and requires considerable experience in interpretation. (A venogram is much more difficult to interpret than an arteriogram and, in the future, venography may prove to be a false "gold standard".) The left side panel of Fig. 3.6 shows a DVT which few could miss; however, the venogram on the right also shows a DVT, which a day later could be equally dangerous.

The radioactive-labelled fibrinogen technique has been mentioned earlier and has been widely used in studies of the prophylaxis of DVT. Although it is also time consuming, it is easier to interpret than a venogram. Its principal disadvantage is that the fibrinogen (usually labelled with iodine-125) has to be injected before the bulk of the thrombus has formed and therefore cannot be used to detect DVT several days after surgery, unless the patient had been labelled and monitored since before the oper-

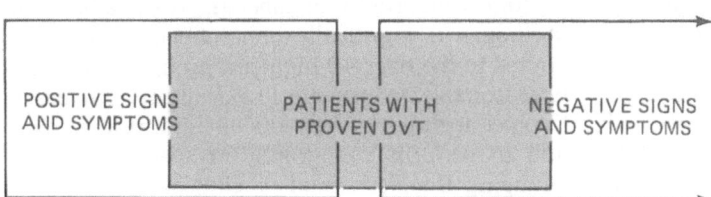

Fig. 3.5. Diagram illustrating the inaccuracy of clinical diagnosis of deep vein thrombosis. The *shaded area* represents the patients who had proven DVT on investigation.

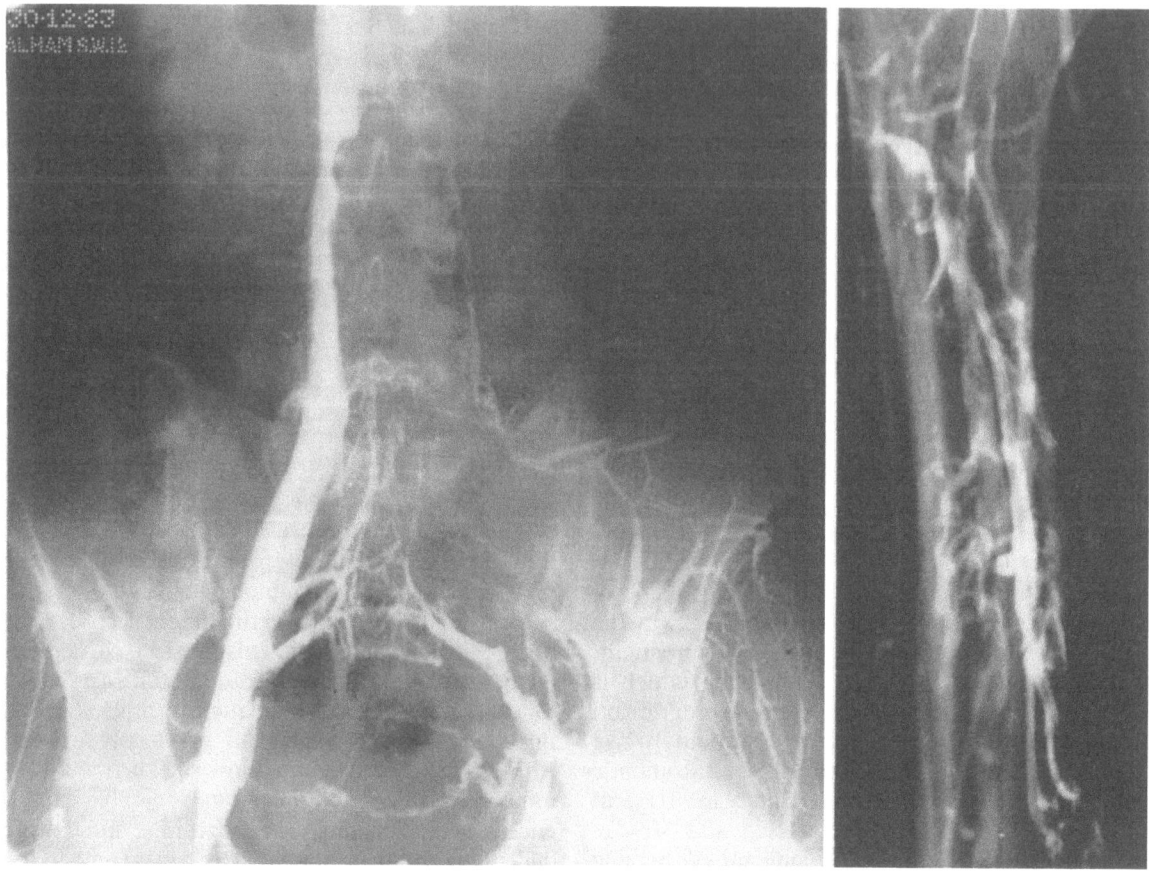

a   b

Fig. 3.6a,b. Two venograms showing **a** a massive DVT in the iliofemoral systems extending into the inferior vena cava on the left and **b** a small DVT in the calf region on the right.

ation. New techniques for diagnosis are being tested and introduced continuously. For instance, impedance plethysymography is proving to be surprisingly accurate, but unfortunately needs expensive special equipment and an experienced operator.

The only simple and cheap investigation which significantly improves on the accuracy of clinical diagnosis is the use of the Doppler ultrasonic flowmeter. In its simplest form it costs approximately 300 pounds sterling (in 1987) and its application can be learnt quickly and easily. Flow is detected in the femoral vein at the groin, thereby excluding thrombosis at that level. The characteristic changes in femoral flow during a Valsalva manœuvre will be lost if there is iliac vein thrombosis, whilst occlusion of the femoral or popliteal veins will abolish the typical rush of blood when the thigh or calf is suddenly compressed. The principal disadvantage of the technique is that inevitably it cannot diagnose thrombi that are non-occlusive; however, it could be argued that it is the large occlusive thrombus which is the most dangerous in terms of both PE and post-thrombotic syndrome.

Practical Recommendations for Diagnosing a DVT

Routine venography or labelling with radioactive fibrinogen is logistically impractical, even if it is limited to the over 40 high-risk group. Therefore it is reasonable to use the less-accurate, but easier Doppler technique daily on all high-risk patients and to perform venography on patients with a changing Doppler signal or clinical symptoms or signs. It cannot be emphasised too much that a positive diagnosis of leg DVT cannot and must not be made on purely clinical grounds.

Diagnosis of Pulmonary Emboli

In the case of major pulmonary emboli the classical symptoms and signs of sudden chest pain, severe dyspnoea, tachypnoea, cyanosis and raised jugular venous pressure, are much more reliable than the clinical diagnosis of DVT, provided false positives are excluded by a chest X-ray, ECG and measurement of arterial blood gases, which will exclude conditions like pneumothorax or myocardial infarction. Nevertheless, the problem of the clinical diagnosis of moderate, mild or recurrent small PE remains. Figure 3.7 shows a positive pulmonary angiogram, which is the "gold standard" for diagnosing PE. In studies where this was performed routinely on all cases suspected of having a PE, only 25%–30% were confirmed (Gallus 1981). Figure 3.8 shows a typical positive perfusion and ventilation lung (VQ) scan, which has become a practical non-invasive and reasonably accurate alternative to pulmonary angiography. A clear mismatch between perfusion and ventilation of an area of the lung is diagnostic of PE.

Practical Recommendation for Diagnosing a PE

All patients with a clinical suspicion of PE and where common alternative diagnosis has been excluded should have a perfusion-ventilation lung scan. Only if this is positive should a diagnosis of PE be accepted. Pulmonary angiograms can then be reserved for cases with equivocal scans.

Prophylaxis of Thromboembolic Disease

Prophylaxis is the most controversial aspect of thromboembolic disease and the subject of scores of clinical trials. These are often inconclusive and frequently generate the strong emotional feeling evoked in clinicians when there is a lack of scientific proof. The problems revolve around two questions:

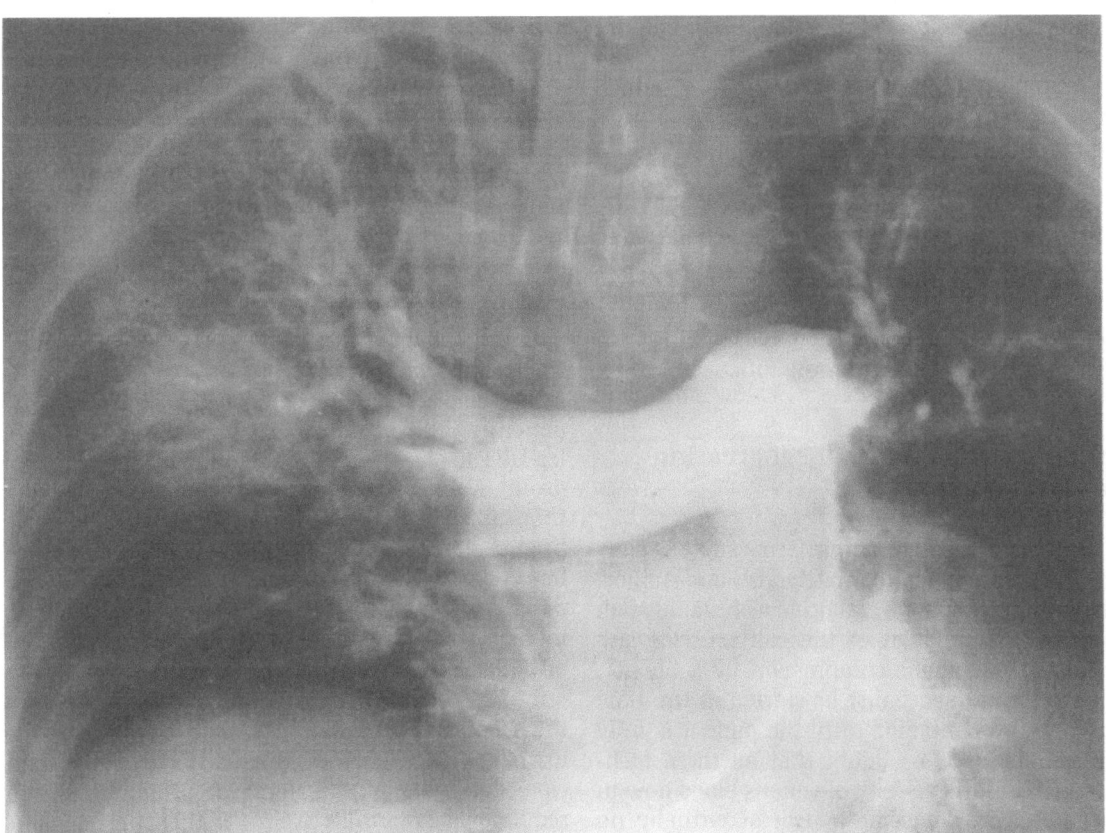

Fig. 3.7. Pulmonary angiogram showing a large pulmonary embolus in the right pulmonary artery and some additional small filling defects. Pulmonary angiography is the "gold standard" for the diagnosis of pulmonary emboli.

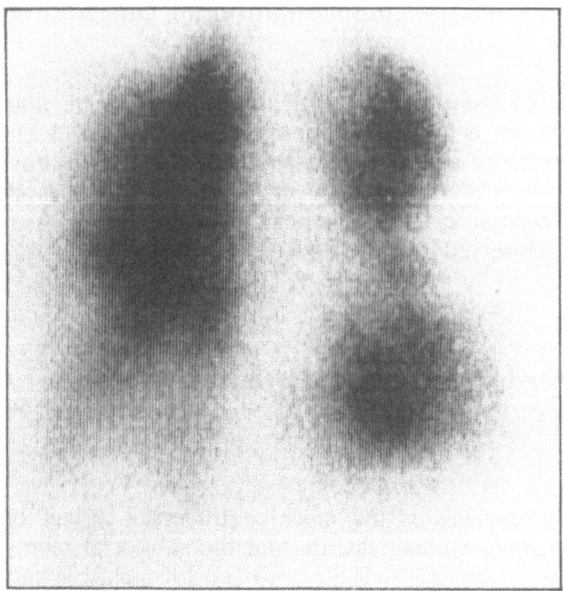
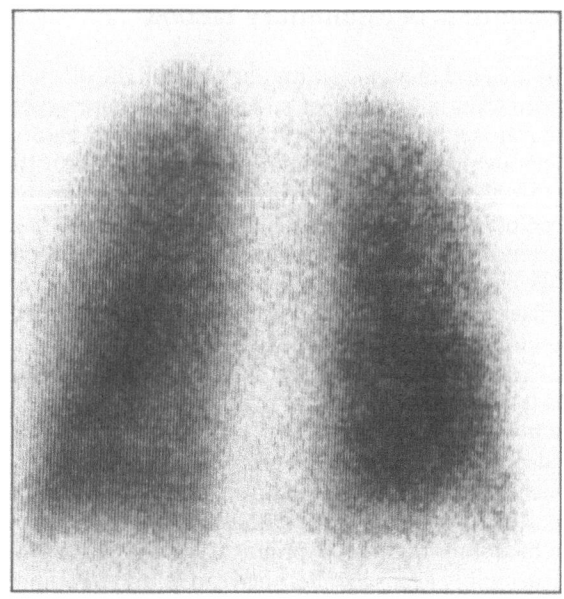

Fig. 3.8a,b. Lung perfusion a and ventilation scan b, showing an area of mismatch.

Is prophylaxis worthwhile in any preoperative patient, and if so which patient? Secondly, which prophylactic regime strikes the best balance between efficacy and risk?

The established prophylactic techniques which need to be considered fall into four major groups. In order of increasing effectiveness and, sadly, also increasing risk, available methods are:

1. Mechanical measures accelerating venous blood flow
2. Low-dose heparin
3. Dextrans
4. Full anticoagulation with oral anticoagulants

Mechanical Techniques for Increasing Venous Blood Flow

This may take relatively simple forms such as elevation of the legs (to approximately 20°) and support stockings, or rather more elaborate techniques such as electrical stimulation of the calf muscles and intermittent pneumatic compression by a "boot". In all cases treatment must be started at the time of surgery and continued until the patient is fully ambulant. There is no doubt that all these techniques increase the velocity of venous blood flow in the legs and provide some benefit at virtually no risk. Pneumatic compression may also provide some benefit by stimulating the release of plasminogen activator, which may explain why it

decreases the incidence of leg DVT even when it is applied to the arms. Clinical trials have shown that any of these techniques will reduce the incidence of DVT to approximately one-third to one-half of a control untreated group. There is, however, considerable doubt whether they decrease the incidence of DVT in the high-risk groups and whether they have any effect on the incidence of PE, one of the main objectives of treatment.

Low-Dose Heparin

There is no doubt that 5000 units of heparin 2 h before surgery and repeated 8–12 hourly till the patient is fully ambulant reduces the incidence of leg DVT to about a quarter compared with a control group (Kakkar 1981). In controlled trials involving thousands of patients, low-dose heparin has also been shown probably to decrease the number of PE, but it has still not convincingly demonstrated a decrease in mortality. There is a small but definite increase in bleeding during and after operation, although this may not be the case if heparin is given only 12 hourly. Professor Mitchell has summarised the sceptical and purist argument against routine use of low-dose heparin (Mitchell 1979). If the principal rationale of this form of prophylaxis is a reduction in mortality from PE, then this remains to be proven. Whilst this may be true, the weight of evidence is very much in favour of supposing that it does. Moreover, there is a considerable morbidity attached to multiple non-fatal PE causing permanent lung damage and leg DVT causing post-thrombotic syndrome, and both PE and DVT have been shown to be reduced by low-dose heparin.

The search is continuing for modifications of the standard regime, for instance by lowering the dose of heparin, and adding other drugs like dihydro-ergotamine, which may have an even greater prophylactic effect and possibly less effect on bleeding.

Dextrans

Infusion of either dextran 40 or dextran 70 is effective in reducing the incidence of leg DVT and PE, although the evidence that they decrease the incidence of fatal PE is also inconclusive. The benefits may be as great as with low-dose heparin but certainly no greater. On the other hand, the incidence of complications including bleeding, allergic reactions and pulmonary oedema make it less safe than low-dose heparin. For these reasons it is less accepted for routine use.

Full Anticoagulation with Oral Anticoagulants

This is the most effective regime for the prevention of DVT and PE, some studies showing up to a tenfold

decrease in the latter. But this only applies if anti-coagulation is adequate, which requires careful monitoring. However, it is rarely used for routine prophylaxis because of the very real increase in operative haemorrhage.

Practical Recommendations

Figure 3.9 illustrates a possible practical scheme for the prophylaxis of DVT in gynaecological operations. Not all the recommendations are of definite proven value and often there is no evidence specifically related to gynaecological operations. On the basis of present evidence the suggestions probably strike a reasonable balance between decreasing the incidence of complications from DVT and minimising side effects from the prophylactic technique itself.

The first step is to remove those risk factors which can be eliminated, for instance stopping oral contraceptives containing oestrogen and screening patients for polycythaemia and thrombocythaemia. If the patient is under 40 years of age and has no major risk factors such as malignancy or previous thromboembolic disease then it is probably unnecessary to apply any form of prophylaxis.

In the remaining cases prophylaxis with low-dose heparin should be routinely instituted, with the exception of two groups of patients: Patients undergoing operations where haemorrhage is a particular

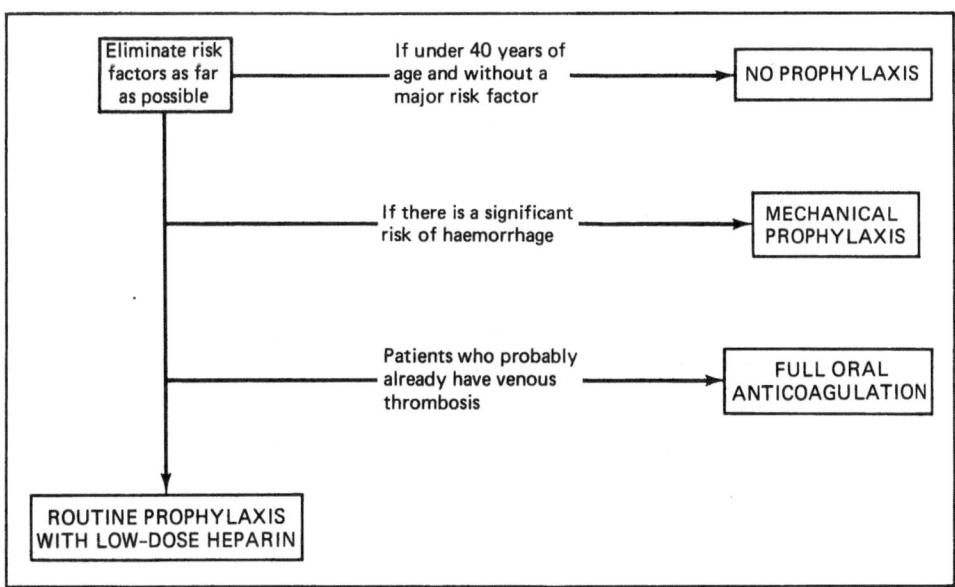

Fig. 3.9. A practical scheme for the prophylaxis of thromboembolic disease.

problem should have some form of simple mechanical prophylaxis. This is especially the case if large
raw areas of oozing are anticipated. The second
special group are those patients who already have
venous thrombosis prior to surgery. This is probably
commoner than generally realised, particularly in
patients with malignant disease who have already
been in bed for several days before surgery. Such
patients should be screened preoperatively, using a
Doppler flowmeter in the first instance, and if
venous thrombosis is confirmed the risk of extension
and embolism following surgery is so high that full
anticoagulation with oral agents may be justified.

Treatment of Thromboembolism

Only patients with *proven* DVT or PE should be
treated for these conditions. Unfortunately, in the
past many patients who do not have these complications have received treatment, even full anti-

coagulation, because no attempt was made to prove
the diagnosis.

It is difficult in this area to get definite guidance
from good clinical studies because it is now thought
to be unethical to leave patients with proven DVT
untreated and studies using historical controls are
irretrievably biased to favour the treatment group
(Moser and Lemoine 1981). Some experts in fact
conclude that there is no good scientific evidence
that the standard treatment of DVT with full anticoagulation is useful (Lowe and Prentice 1985).
Nevertheless, the balance of available evidence is
that full anticoagulation, which undoubtedly works
in prophylaxis, is probably also useful in the treatment of venous thrombosis presumably by preventing extension of the thrombosis and allowing
the normal fibrinolytic process to proceed unchallenged by further thrombosis.

Routine Treatment of DVT

It is important to emphasise again that treatment
should not be initiated without definite evidence

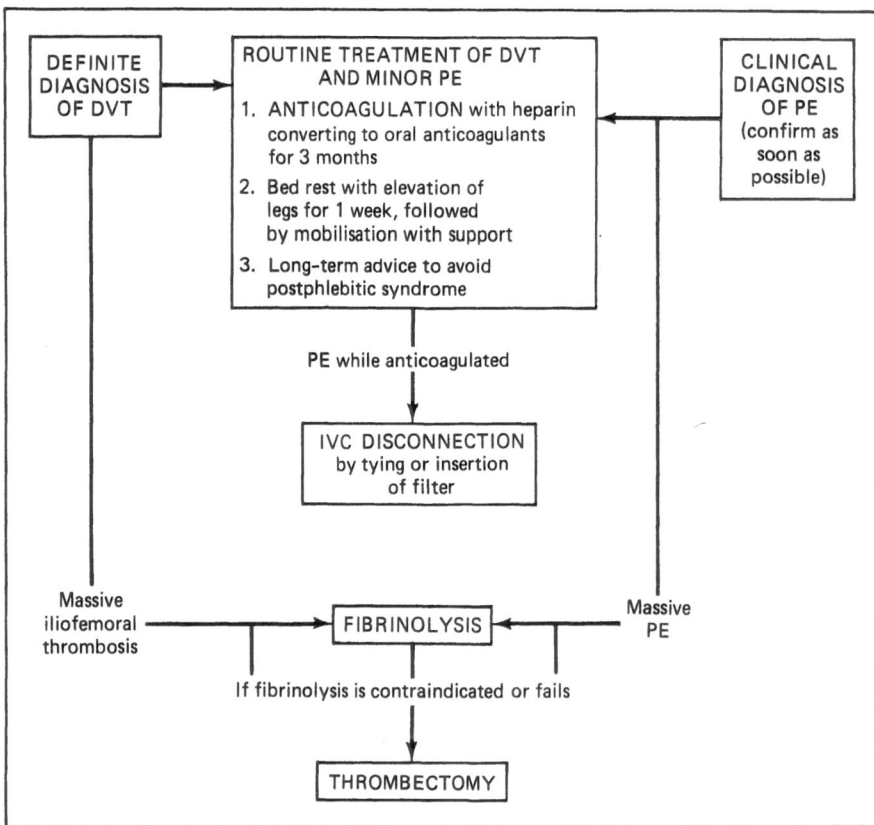

Fig. 3.10 Outline of a practical scheme for the management of proven thromboembolic disease.

that the patient indeed has a DVT. Figure 3.10 outlines a practical routine scheme for the management of peripheral DVT and some of its complications. The treatment of some special cases will also be outlined.

The first aim of treatment is to try and prevent the dislodgement of all or part of the thrombus with consequent pulmonary embolisation. It is generally believed that decreasing mobility of the patient by more or less complete bed rest may significantly help in the first few days before the thrombus has become firmly anchored and in practice this is usually continued for a week. As bed rest and decreased venous flow in the leg is known to predispose to thrombosis, bed rest should be combined with elevation of the legs to about 15° as well as the application of well-fitting support stockings. After a week, mobilisation is advised as the risks of embolisation are then decreased and the aim is to encourage lysis and the development of collaterals.

The best way to achieve the second aim of treatment, to prevent extension of the thrombus, is full anticoagulation. Oral anticoagulants take several days to have full effect and treatment in the first few days has to rely on intravenous heparin. Immediate heparinisation in patients with proven DVT reduces the incidence of both non-fatal and fatal emboli by a factor of 5–10 (Verstraete and Verymylen 1984). Anticoagulation is naturally contraindicated in patients with proven peptic ulcer, hypertension or other diseases associated with bleeding complications. Intravenous heparin should be started with a bolus of 5000 IU (65 IU/kg)/h. A more consistent and therefore safer level of anticoagulation can be achieved by constant infusion, but if this is not possible 10 000 IU every 6 h is an alternative starting dose. (Heparin must not be mixed in the infusion fluid with antibiotics or morphine derivatives.) There is considerable individual variation in the effect of heparin and it is essential to check and adjust the dosage on the basis of at least daily tests. The most appropriate tests are the partial thromboplastin time or thrombin time. If bleeding complications develop, anticoagulation will spontaneously cease over a few hours as the biological half-life of heparin is only 6 h. Immediate reversal of anticoagulation can be achieved using the antagonist protamine chloride. Heparin should be continued until full oral anticoagulation has been achieved, usually in 2–4 days.

Recently some reports have drawn attention to the dangers of occult bleeding during anticoagulant therapy. Particularly relevant to gynaecological surgery is the risk of retroperitoneal haemorrhage. The appreciation of these potential hazards makes the current practice of occasionally treating DVT

without a definite diagnosis particularly regrettable.

There is no risk attached to the temporary simultaneous use of heparin and an oral anticoagulant; the latter can therefore also be commenced as soon as the diagnosis of a DVT is confirmed. A practical and commonly used regime is 10 mg warfarin (or the equivalent dose of another coumarin derivative) on the 1st day and 5 mg on the 2nd day. Subsequent dosage should be adjusted according to the prothrombin time or thrombotest. The results of these tests are often expressed differently; the optimal therapeutic range is a prolongation of the prothrombin time by a factor between 4·8 and 2·8, which corresponds to a thrombotest value between 5% and 10%. There is a very long list of drugs, including aspirin, danol and metronidazole, which often potentiate anticoagulants. Vitamin K will reverse the anticoagulant effect of coumarins and can be given orally or intravenously according to urgency. The biological half-life of warfarin is 1–3 days.

The long-term aim of the treatment of DVT is to prevent the post-thrombotic syndrome. Although there are no precise studies on this, the optimal treatment is currently thought to be oral anticoagulation for 3 months and encouragement of regular exercise with proper support hosiery until all symptoms and signs have disappeared.

Treatment of Complicated DVT— Fibrinolysis and Surgery

The only indication for direct surgery on the veins to remove the thrombus mechanically is in massive iliofemoral thrombosis where the venous outflow from the legs is so obstructed that the viability of the leg is jeopardised. This rare condition (sometimes called phlegmasia caerulea dolens) is characterised by gross swelling, discoloration, coldness and severe pain up to the groin. An alternative treatment is systemic fibrinolysis, although this is absolutely contraindicated for 10 days following any form of surgery.

There is a small group of patients with DVT who will continue to form thrombi and continue to embolise despite adequate anticoagulation. In these patients some form of mechanical disconnection of the venous system is indicated. The earlier practice of tying the femoral vein has largely been abandoned because it did nothing for iliac vein thrombosis and those patients who also have contralateral leg thrombosis. The optimal treatment is the percutaneous insertion of an inferior vena cava filter, but if the necessary facilities are not available simply tying the inferior vena cava can be life saving.

Treatment of Pulmonary Emboli

The aim of treatment is similar to that of venous thrombosis, that is rapid and complete anticoagulation to prevent extension of the thrombosis. It is particularly important to achieve complete and sustained anticoagulation with intravenous heparin. Because of the acute danger to life it may be necessary to begin treatment on the basis of a clinical diagnosis, although if in doubt confirmation by angiography or scan should be attempted as soon as practicable.

Some of the manifestations of pulmonary emboli are due to venous and humoral reflexes causing vasoconstrictions and bronchospasm. If present, these effects can be partly treated by an infusion of isoprenaline (2 mg/kg per minute) or dopamine (2–10 μg/kg per minute). Pain should be relieved by morphine.

The treatment of complicated DVT or PE is best carried out in special units equipped with specialised haematological and surgical facilities necessary for fibrinolytic therapy or surgery should it become necessary. This may be indicated if the patient's haemodynamic status deteriorates rapidly and threatens to be fatal.

References

Clayton JK, Anderson JA, McNicol GP (1976) Preoperative prediction of postoperative deep vein thrombosis. Br Med J 2:910–912

Crandon AJ, Peel KR, Anderson JA, Thompson V, McNicol GP (1980) Prophylaxis of postoperative deep vein thrombosis: selective use of low-dose heparin in high risk patients. Br Med J 2:345–347

Edgington TS (1980) Activation of the coagulation system in association with neoplasia. J Lab Clin Med 96:1

Gallus AS (1981) Established venous thrombosis and pulmonary embolism. Clin Haematol 10:583–611

Kakkar VV (1981) Prevention of venous thromboembolism. In: Bloom AL, Thomas DP (eds) Haemostasis and thrombosis. Churchill Livingstone, Edinburgh

Lowe GDO, Prentice CRM (1985) Hemostasis and thrombosis. In: Walter Bowie EH, Sharp AA (eds) Butterworths, London, pp 284–318

Mitchell JRA (1979) Can we really prevent post-operative pulmonary emboli? Br Med J 2:1523–1524

Moser, KM, Lemoine JR (1981) Is embolic risk conditioned by location of deep venous thrombosis? Ann Intern Med 94:439–444

Nielsen HK, Geday E, Bechgaard, Husted SE (1982) Anticoagulant therapy and pulmonary embolism. Lancet 1:278

Simpson FG, Robinson PJ, Bark M, Losowsky MS (1980) Prospective study of thrombophlebitis and pseudothrombophlebitis. Lancet 1:331–333

Verstraete M, Vermylen J (1984) Thrombosis. Pergamon, Oxford

Vessey MP (1982) Oral contraception and cardiovascular disease: some questions and answers. Br Med J 284:615–616

Walsh JJ, Bonnar J, Wright FW (1974) A study of pulmonary embolism and deep leg vein thrombosis after major gynaecological surgery using labelled fibrinogen, phlebography and lung scanning. J Obstet Gynaecol Br Commonwealth 81:311–314

4 · Prevention and Treatment of Surgical Sepsis

Philip James Sanderson

Aetiology and Prevention of Surgical Sepsis

Sources of Organisms

Sepsis originates when organisms are able to grow and produce toxins with subsequent tissue destruction. Reaction to the presence of microbial products by humoral and cellular defences may lead to further damage. Microbes, in general, are destroyed by the combined action of polymorphs and antibodies. Steroids and cytotoxic agents may affect the function of polymorphs in killing bacteria, and in immunodeficient patients humoral defences may be reduced. Elderly patients and those with malignancy, diabetes and intercurrent infection seem less able to resist the hazards of infection associated with surgery.

Bacteria normally colonise the mouth, gastrointestinal tract, vagina and skin, forming the normal flora of these regions. Colonisation by bacteria of these sites involves different groups of bacteria and is a complex interrelationship between the bacteria themselves and the host. The competition for nutrients, for growth space and the production of antibacterial substances by the normal flora contribute to resisting invasion by pathogens, with subsequent infection or sepsis. On the other hand, the deposition of bacteria in a previously sterile tissue or cavity, in a haematoma or around a foreign material, encourages their growth as warmth, nutrients and space are provided unimpeded.

Sepsis arising at the site of an operation or in the operation wound usually results from organisms deposited in the tissues at the time of operation. The incision of the vagina or gut, which normally contain a bacterial flora, may seed the field of operation with microbes. In addition organisms inhabiting the skin or hair follicles and sweat glands of the patient may also enter the wound. These are *endogenous* sources of bacteria from the patient's own normal flora.

An equally important source of contamination of the operation field is *exogenous*, predominantly organisms of the skin flora of the operating team and other members of staff in the operating theatre, as well as organisms from possible environmental sources. The human skin sheds large numbers of dead skin scales, and about one in ten carry viable bacteria of the skin flora, namely *Staphylococcus epidermidis*, diphtheroids and micrococci. Skin scales are released by friction with clothing mainly from the bathing trunk area and emanate from trouser openings at the ankles, from below skirts and through pores in the fabric of clothing. Theatre clothing is little different from outdoor clothing in this respect, and scales soon adhere to the fabric from which they can be released by shaking. Liberated scales are entrained in the theatre air currents and in conventionally ventilated theatres the turbulent air flows may lead to their deposition in the tissues exposed by operation.

Prevention of Endogenous Infection During Operation

Infection by endogenous organisms or the patient's skin and vaginal flora is reduced by local antisepsis.

Skin Disinfection

Removal of body hair is probably unnecessary for bacteriological reasons, but is surgically convenient. Shaving immediately before operation is associated with less postoperative wound infection than shaving some hours before (Cruse and Foord 1973), since bacteria do not then have time to multiply in the abrasions caused by the razor. Depilatory creams are bacteriologically safer than shaving (Seropian and Reynolds 1971) but may lead to skin reactions in some patients. Antiseptics should be applied to the skin at the site of the incision with a rubbing motion, working progressively outwards, over a period of 2 min. A second application with a fresh swab is more valuable than allowing the first to dry. Appropriated antiseptics are chlorhexidine gluconate 0·5% in 70% alcohol or iodine 1% in 70% alcohol.

Vaginal Disinfection

The vaginal flora consists mainly of lactobacilli, *Staphylococcus epidermidis*, micrococci, diphtheroids and anaerobes. The latter have increased in prominence as culture methods have improved and *Bacteroides fragilis* and anaerobic cocci predominate. Haemolytic streptococci of group B are often found, and *Escherichia coli*, other coliforms, *Staphylococcus aureus* and *Clostridium welchii* may appear.

Disinfection of the vaginal mucosa before operation is best achieved by using a preparation of iodine or chlorhexidine. Creams and gels will provide a longer action, but iodine is slowly absorbed from the vagina (Vorherr et al. 1980). Povidone iodine in a vaginal douche and aqueous chlorhexidine with cetrimide are used widely. A preliminary application an hour or two before operation, with an immediate preoperative application by swab, may have more effect than a single treatment just before surgery, since organisms can be recovered from the incised vaginal edge after a single preparation (George et al. 1975). Vaginal hysterectomy is followed by a higher incidence of postoperative pyrexia and pelvic inflammation than abdominal hysterectomy, and operations through the vagina should be regarded as taking place in a contaminated field.

There is no doubt that organisms of the skin and vaginal flora are able to cause postoperative sepsis. Their elimination by preoperative antisepsis is important, requiring effective agents carefully applied.

Other Sources of Infection in the Patient

Patients who are carriers of *Staphylococcus aureus* have an increased incidence of postoperative sepsis. The organism is carried in the nose of 5%–25% of the general population, with lesser rates in the axillae and perineum but rarely on the dry skin. Septic skin lesions are usually due to this organism and should be eliminated before operation, but preoperative swabbing of a healthy patient is not normally worthwhile. Urinary tract infection should be treated if symptoms are present, as should chest infection or infection elsewhere, and operation postponed until recovery.

The use of antibiotic prophylaxis to prevent infection will be described below.

Prevention of Exogenous Infection During Operation

Theatre Ventilation

The predominant source of organisms in the air of operating rooms is the skin flora of persons in the room. These organisms are of low pathogenicity except in immunosuppressed patients, implant and transplant surgery, but it is possible for some *Staphylococcus aureus* carriers to disperse these organisms into the air. Similarly, haemolytic streptococci of group A (*Streptococcus pyogenes*) can be dispersed in theatre air currents as may coliforms, clostridia and fungi if an accessible source is present.

Proper theatre ventilation provides some protection from the danger of airborne exogenous infection. In a conventionally ventilated theatre, air should be filtered and introduced from the ceiling at a rate of 20 air changes per hour. This provides plenum ventilation at positive pressure so that air flows outwards from the preparation and operating rooms towards the scrub and anaesthetic rooms and corridors. Air from these areas should flow to disposal and sluice rooms. Air flows are preserved only if doors are kept closed and staff movements are kept to a minimum. This system is designed primarily to prevent contaminated air from the hospital and other areas entering operating rooms. Bacteriological sampling should reveal not more than 35 colony forming units per cubic metre.

Conventional ventilation cannot prevent turbulent air currents within the theatre; opening doors, movements of staff and body warmth destroy the weak downward flow. Consequently bacteria-carrying particles can be swept upwards from lower levels to the wound. Unidirectional downward air flow with ultra clean air from a ceiling fitment provides uncontaminated air over the site of operation and has been shown to reduce sepsis in hip implant surgery (Lidwell et al. 1982). Whether these units are of benefit in gynaecological surgery has not been investigated, but their costs would be harder to justify than in implant surgery.

Theatre Design and Maintenance

The layout of rooms within the theatre suite and the air supply to them should ensure air flow from the cleanest to less clean and then to dirty areas. Access to the rest of the hospital should be protected by lobbies and double doors. Walls and floors require hard, resistant surfaces without cracks or gaps at junctions of different surfaces. Corners and floor to wall junctions should be rounded, and shelves and ledges avoided. Doors should fit closely and air exit grilles provided with weighted vents so that the extent of outward airflow can be seen at a glance.

Floors, the operating table, trolleys and stools require cleaning and a wipe over with disinfectant after each session. Walls should be cleaned if visibly dirty and regularly cleaned every 3 or 6 months. The ventilation ducting should be inspected and the filters changed according to a planned maintenance schedule. The autoclaves of a theatre sterile supply unit, or CSSD, require accurate monitoring and checks of each cycle by a named person. A surgeon is wise to enquire that these features of theatre maintenance, which often lie outside the aegis of the theatre staff, are being carried out.

Theatre Clothing

The ritual of changing from outdoor clothing into theatre garb has little or no effect of the shedding of bacteria from the body. Elastic closures at the wrist and ankles reduce bacterial dispersal and are worthwhile. More effect is achieved by wearing densely woven underpants or body exhaust suits, but these are uncomfortable or impractical. Improvements in theatre clothing design are being made and disposable items may become more acceptable. If the cotton fabric is wetted gowns become pervious to bacteria and "strike through" occurs; in an operation where contact with fluids or excess blood is likely a waterproof apron beneath a surgical gown should be worn.

Surgical *face masks* composed of paper or cotton do not prevent emission of bacteria from the throat or mouth and masks incorporating an impervious "cellophane" layer will only deflect bacteria. The value of wearing a mask during an operation is to prevent deposition of bacteria-carrying droplets from the mouth into the operation site. This is a rational, rather than a bacteriologically proven, reason for the continued use of masks in theatres. Their use during ward procedures when deeper tissues are not exposed is being abandoned. Friction of the mask with facial skin will release skin scales and masks should remain untouched throughout the operation. Masks should be changed between each operation and when they become damp.

Changing *footwear* for operations is more of a ritual than a rational procedure. Boots and clogs should be washed regularly and fit the wearer, so that excess air in the boots is not pumped upwards. Wearing linen or plastic shoe covers within the theatre suite is of doubtful value. Floor mats with sticky or disinfectant surfaces do not protect theatre floors from contamination.

Head hair and beards should be completely covered with impervious material although hair itself releases few bacteria. Friction of the edges of the covering material with skin should be avoided.

Personal jewellery should be removed before operation. Bacteria have been shown to accumulate beneath wedding rings, but this has not been associated with an increased risk of infection.

Handwashing

The consistent use of antiseptics for handwashing by surgeons and nurses produces a lasting antibacterial effect on the skin. This will reduce the "resident" skin bacteria in the hair follicles and sweat glands, which may reappear at the skin surface during operation. The "transient" flora is more easily eliminated by a social handwash, using only soap and water. Nails should be kept clean and short and the surrounding skin healthy. Only the first handwashing of the session requires scrubbing with a nailbrush; continued use of hard bristles will damage the skin and may allow bacterial multiplication. Appropriate lathering antiseptics are 4% chlorhexidine in detergent and povidone iodine in detergent. Alternatively, once hands have been cleaned, 10 ml 0.5% chlorhexidine in 95% alcohol can be rubbed into the skin to dryness.

Surgical Gloves. Although handwashing will temporarily remove surface bacteria, "resident" organisms reappear during operation and accumulate in "glove juice". Gloves therefore act as a barrier and should be changed if punctured. Nevertheless, formal proof of the value of wearing gloves has never been obtained.

Theory and Practice of Antimicrobial Therapy

Description of Antimicrobials

In this brief description antimicrobials will be divided into the penicillins, the cephalosporins and others, with particular attention to their role in gynaecological surgical sepsis. The *penicillins* include (a) benzyl penicillin and its oral forms, (b) flucloxacillin, active against most strains of *Staphylococcus aureus*, (c) ampicillin/amoxycillin, which enlarged the penicillin spectrum to Gram-negative bacilli and *Streptococcus faecalis* and (d) the ureido penicillins, with broader Gram-negative cover. Benzyl penicillin is the drug of choice against haemolytic streptococci of group A, *Clostridium welchii* and actinomycosis, being the most potent agent available for them. Only some 10% of *Staphylococcus aureus* are sensitive to penicillin; for the remainder flucloxacillin or cloxacillin are the drugs of choice. In recent years strains of this organism resistant to flucloxacillin (methicillin-resistant *Staphylococcus aureus*, MRSA) have appeared mainly in urban teaching hospitals but in other hospitals too. These strains are also resistant to many other antibiotics and they require some form of isolation nursing for the patient. Amoxycillin retains a slowly decreasing spectrum of activity against coliforms; in combination with clavulanic acid as augmentin, the spectrum is enlarged to many otherwise resistant Gram-negatives and to anaerobes. The ureidopenicillins are suitable for treating abdominal sepsis arising in hospital patients.

The *cephalosporins* have a similar molecule to the penicillins and side chain substitution provides for many variations with but slightly varying properties. Modern secondary and tertiary forms are active against streptococci (except *Streptococcus faecalis*), *Staphylococcus aureus* and a wide range of Gram-negative bacilli. Thus cephalosporins possess the safety of penicillins, with probably fewer hypersensitivity reactions, together with a broad spectrum. They are expensive, and heavy use may encourage resistant secondary invaders. In particular they more often cause pseudomembranous colitis than other antibiotics (except clindamycin).

Metronidazole is a safe, well-absorbed and potent agent whose activity, while being limited to the obligate anaerobes, is almost complete against them. It has assumed considerable importance with the recognition of the role of anaerobes in abdominal, pelvic and postoperative infection.

Erythromycin is active against most strains of haemolytic streptococci and *Staphylococcus aureus*.

It should remain as second choice to the appropriate penicillins for these organisms. It is active against chlamydia, some anaerobes and gonococci. *Co-trimoxazole* retains wide activity against coliforms and is useful in urinary infection with these organisms as is trimethoprim, one of its components. *Tetracyclines* have a reduced role; many haemolytic streptococci and *Staphylococcus aureus* strains are resistant. They are, however, active against chlamydiae. The *aminoglycosides*, i.e. gentamicin, tobramycin, netilmicin and amikacin, are active against Gram-negative bacilli and *Staphylococcus aureus* but not against streptococci or anaerobes. They are ototoxic and nephrotoxic and require monitoring of serum levels. Gentamicin remains the most commonly used, with amikacin as reserve.

Use of Antimicrobials

Taking Specimens

Accurate use of antimicrobials demands isolation of the causative organism(s) and reliable sensitivity testing. Organisms will survive better in pus or tissue, rather than on swabs, and such specimens are preferred by the laboratory. It is important to give clinical information, date of operation and current antibiotics. Not infrequently microbiology laboratory staff exercise judgement in deciding whether to investigate certain cultures and this is influenced by clinical data. The operation date will help decide whether the infection is early or late after operation, i.e. originating at operation or later, and, if the former, whether it is related to postoperative infections in other patients. If antibiotics are present in the specimen, these can be diluted out or neutralised if appropriate. Obviously, specimens must be taken before starting treatment.

Specimens are best taken by medical staff, and a discussion with a microbiologist in unusual or difficult cases may be helpful in obtaining appropriate specimens and diagnosis.

High vaginal and endocervical swabs must be taken with the aid of a speculum, to avoid contamination with the vaginal flora. In the diagnosis of pelvic infection, needle aspiration of the pouch of Douglas is valuable; a vaginal swab is unlikely to yield the pathogen and may be misleading if a potential, but irrelevant, pathogen is temporarily and harmlessly residing in the vaginal flora. Urine specimens in catheterised patients are best taken by syringe and needle from a sleeve over the catheter placed close to the patient. A few millilitres are sufficient. Specimens taken from the urine reservoir bag are liable to contamination from handling the tap and from delay during accumulation in the bag. Sputum specimens benefit from chest physiotherapy by loosening deep lung secretions. Anaerobic organisms are killed by exposure to air and survive better in pus and tissue, or in transport medium or evacuated containers.

General Principles

The decision to give antibiotics is usually a clinical one. There are few instances where bacteriology dictates their use—the isolation of haemolytic streptococci of group A is the most common in gynaecology. The isolation of *Clostridium welchii*, of other haemolytic streptococci, *Staphylococcus aureus* or a heavy pure growth of a coliform from an operation wound or from an incision in the vagina warrant inspection of the wound and assessment of the patient.

Once antibiotics have been prescribed delay should not be tolerated—ward stocks of the commonly used antibiotics should be available. Initially, doses at the higher range suggested in the British National Formulary should be used. Ill patients and patients with moderate renal dysfunction will tolerate these doses of penicillins and cephalosporins, as well as of metronidazole.

Antibiotics in general are poorly absorbed from the gut; when given by mouth the oral forms should be used, e.g. flucloxacillin rather than cloxacillin, phenoxymethyl penicillin (penicillin V) rather than benzyl penicillin, amoxycillin rather than ampicillin, although increasing the dose of the latter may be cheaper. Absorption is improved by giving drugs $\frac{1}{2}$–1 h before meals. In an ill patient i.v. or i.m. administration ensures rapid and total input; the technique of choice is by bolus injection of the penicillins, cephalosporins and aminoglycosides. Erythromycin, co-trimoxazole and very high doses of penicillins require infusion over 1 h. Aminoglycoside, co-trimoxazole and tetracycline dosage must be adjusted for renal dysfunction and serum levels of aminoglucosides monitored on the 2nd day treatment by taking clotted blood just before and 1 h after a dose by either the i.m. or i.v. route.

The antibiotics in use, dosages and routes of administration should be reviewed at 2 days and again at 5 days—most acute surgical infections will respond quickly and longer treatment is rarely required. Optimal antibiotic regimens have not been investigated, but in terms of selecting resistant bacteria high-dose/short duration treatment is less dangerous than longer durations, and it is known that in certain infections the first few doses eliminate viable bacteria.

Combinations and Interactions

In general, combinations of antibiotics are safe, but narrow-spectrum agents or single drugs are preferable. Broad-spectrum agents are more likely to destroy the normal bacterial flora of the gut, vagina and mouth, leading to pseudomembranous colitis and secondary invasion. Some combinations, e.g. ticarcillin or piperacillin with gentamicin, are synergistic against some coliforms and *Pseudomonas* and therefore valuable in abdominal infection. Interaction with other drugs and between antibiotics may occur, e.g. gentamicin with cephalosporins in the presence of diuretics may lead to increasing creatinine levels. Very high serum concentrations of penicillins can lead to blood-clotting disorders and platelet dysfunction. Erythromycin given i.v. frequently produces thrombophlebitis, and co-trimoxazole may occasionally depress the bone marrow in patients with poor nutrition.

Prophylaxis of Infection in Gynaecological Surgery

General Principles

Prevention of surgical sepsis involves measures aimed at reducing the potential sources of infection in the theatre, staff and in the patient herself. These have been discussed earlier in terms of providing clean theatre surroundings and air, protection against dispersal of bacteria by staff and disinfection of the patient's own skin and vaginal flora.

Inevitably, however, some bacteria will enter the operation field from these sources. As already described, many of these organisms will be of low pathogenicity, being the normal flora of the skin or vagina. Occasionally, pathogens from a *Staphylococcus aureus* disperser or from some untoward incident, such as a contaminated instrument or a perforation of the bowel, will occur. The use of antimicrobials for prophylaxis provides a means of eliminating these organisms in the patient.

Antibiotic prophylaxis against surgical sepsis has improved in efficacy with better understanding of (a) timing of administration of doses, (b) the type of organisms causing sepsis with different forms of surgery and (c) because of improved antimicrobial agents.

Dosage Regimens

Experimental work in laboratory animals demonstrated that within 1 h of inoculating organisms into a wound the effect of giving antibiotic was reduced, and after 4 h had disappeared (Burke 1961). This result matched the logical conclusion that in order to protect an operation field from contaminating bacteria, antibacterial activity in the tissues and blood of the patient should be at their height during the operation, when contamination of the operation site occurs.

The complication of selecting resistant organisms in the patient's bacterial flora is reduced by avoiding antibiotics before operation. It has been shown, for example, that increasing numbers of resistant bacteria and decreasing numbers of the normal flora of the mouth appear within a few hours of giving antimicrobials. Consequently, prophylactic regimens should begin 1 h before operation or start at the time of operation by intravenous bolus injection or infusion. In some procedures it is best to give an antibiotic bolus at the time of a critical procedure, such as the insertion of an arterial graft. In a prolonged operation antibiotic serum concentrations should be maintained by reinjection at 2-h intervals.

Antibiotics will kill organisms within 2 h or quicker if present at or above the minimal bactericidal concentration. Normal doses will provide such levels in blood for perhaps as long as 4 h for most antibiotics and peak levels occur immediately following i.v. and after 1 h following i.m. administration. Logically therefore a single dose will cover an operation and this has been confirmed for patients undergoing cholecystectomy and in high-risk patients undergoing Caesarian section (Hawrylyshyn et al. 1983). Commonly, however, two further doses are given postoperatively at 6- or 8-h intervals, and these may eliminate surviving organisms or haematogenous deposition of organisms in the immediate postoperative period. In gynaecological surgery further doses are not required and are contraindicated as they may select for resistant organisms in the bowel or in postoperative urinary infection.

Causative Organisms

Postoperative infections in the wound after abdominal and vaginal hysterectomy involve both aerobes, e.g. staphylococci and less often coliforms, and anaerobes, mainly *Bacteroides* species. In pelvic sepsis after operation, *Bacteroides* is probably the predominant organism isolated, but usually in mixed infection with other organisms. Although this organism alone may not be as pathogenic as haemolytic streptococci, *Staphylococcus aureus* or *Escherichia coli*, there is experimental evidence that an inoculum of *E. coli* with *Bacteroides fragilis* is more virulent than either alone (Kelly 1980). Indeed, anaerobes may hinder phagocytic activity against aerobes, and the latter provide conditions for growth of anaerobes by lowering the redox potential in tissue. Improved culture methods for anaerobes and recent experiments in animal models of infection have shown the importance of anaerobes in surgical sepsis in gynaecology. The role of chlamydiae in postoperative pelvic inflammation is debatable, and further research is required.

Indications for Prophylaxis

The clinical benefits of prophylaxis must outweigh the dangers; this balance may vary for different gynaecological operations. The potential advantages of prophylaxis are a reduced incidence of postoperative infection in the wound or vaginal cuff, and of pelvic cellulitis and urinary infection. This will lead to reduced febrile morbidity and length of stay in hospital and less long-term damage to the reproductive organs due to infection. However, the incidence of infection in many gynaecological operations is low and the consequences often not serious. On the other hand, antimicrobials have a generally low incidence of side effects, although there will always be some effect on the bacterial flora of the patient. Antibiotic-induced diarrhoea and pseudomembranous colitis may be more common than is appreciated clinically. Nevertheless prophylactic regimens of short duration, i.e. single doses or three doses over 1 day, are accepted as less dangerous from this point of view, and had no overall effect on bacterial resistance rates in one study (Grossman et al. 1979).

Resistance rates among bacteria from a surgical unit or hospital match the extent of use of antibiotics. The undoubted clinical success and cost benefits of prophylaxis in abdominal and implant surgery have fuelled its use in other forms of surgery. This trend has been accompanied, luckily, by the realisation that shorter courses of prophylaxis and modern antimicrobials are safer than longer courses and previous antibiotics.

Prophylactic Antimicrobials for Gynaecological Operations

The value of prophylaxis for vaginal and abdominal hysterectomy is established (Allen et al. 1972). Both operations involve incision of the vagina, with subsequent possible contamination of the operation site with bacteria surviving local vaginal antisepsis. Prophylaxis for Caesarian section during labour is accepted. At present it is uncertain whether tubal surgery, vaginal repair, termination of pregnancy and insertion of IUCDs justify prophylaxis. Dilatation and curettage does not.

The problem of postoperative urinary infection will also influence prophylaxis. This is caused mainly by urinary catheterisation, which should be carried out preferably in theatre and the catheter retained for as short a time as possible. Another cause is pre-existing bacteriuria, which in females rises with age and may reach 10% by age 60; it should be treated before operation. Postoperative bacteriuria or urinary infection in patients not given prophylaxis may be substantial, but many cases will respond to removal of the catheter. It is appropriate, however, to use agents for surgical prophylaxis that cover the bacteria commonly causing urinary infection (see below).

Antimicrobials for Prophylaxis

The requirements of the agents for use in antimicrobial prophylaxis in gynaecology are (1) appropriate spectrum, i.e. against *Bacteroides* spp. and coliforms for vaginal surgery; against *Staphylococcus aureus*, coliforms and anaerobes for the abdominal approach and against coliforms for prevention of postoperative urinary infection and (2) the attributes of safety, both clinical and bacteriological, potency, penetration of tissues and bactericidal activity. Tetracyclines and chloramphenicol have inappropriate spectrum or serious side effects; erythromycin is better reserved for patients hypersensitive to penicillins and is less potent and bacteriostatic; clindamycin is the antibiotic most associated with pseudomembranous colitis.

Antimicrobial Regimens

Vaginal and Abdominal Hysterectomy. The presence of anaerobes, particularly *Bacteroides fragilis*, in the vaginal flora and their importance as a cause of postoperative sepsis demand prophylaxis against them for both these operations. The Study Group (Luton and Dunstable Hospital 1974) clearly showed the effectiveness of metronidazole and this remains an agent of choice. It is well absorbed by suppository and gives good blood levels although maximum absorption may be delayed and it is advisable to give a 1-g suppository 2 h before operation. Metronidazole is not active against *Staphylococcus aureus*, streptococci or coliforms. Clindamycin has been used previously to provide anaerobic and *Staphylococcus aureus* cover, but its association with pseudomembranous colitis prevents such use. The spectrum of cephalosporins is inadequate for anaerobes in this context, and chloramphenicol and tetracyclines have both potentially dangerous side effects and inadequate cover. It remains possible that augmentin (amoxycillin plus clavulanic acid) will prove to have efficient anaerobic activity in clinical trials; if so this agent may be appropriate for prophylaxis.

It is advisable to use an additional antimicrobial for organisms not covered by metronidazole. This was confirmed in a trial by Giles et al. (1984), who found significantly reduced postoperative wound infection and urinary infection rates in patients given cephradine with metronidazole compared with metronidazole alone. The former group also had lower postoperative temperatures, white cell counts and excess days in hospital.

The spectrum of activity required by the additional agent to partner metronidazole is less clear. There are three aspects to consider: (a) the role of the aerobic vaginal flora in causing infection in a suture line haematoma; (b) the importance of *Staphylococcus aureus*, coliforms and aerobic streptococci in abdominal wound infection and (c) the sensitivities of *E. coli* and other coliforms in urinary tract infection. Ampicillin or amoxycillin are effective against streptococci and many coliforms, and are safe; their efficacy is reduced if the patient has been in hospital some time and thereby acquired more resistant strains in her bowel flora. Ninety per cent or so of *Staphylococcus aureus* strains are resistant. A cephalosporin, common choices being cephradine or cefuroxime, will cover more coliforms than amoxycillin and also *Staphylococcus aureus*, but is more expensive. Cephalosporins are associated with pseudomembranous colitis more frequently than other types of antibiotics (except clindamycin); this potentially dangerous infection is caused by toxins of *Clostridium difficile* and is a cross-infection hazard. However, the use of a single-dose or three-dose regimen reduces this risk.

Alternative choices of agents for combination with metronidazole are benzyl penicillin, with no action against coliforms and most *Staphylococcus aureus*, but good streptococcal activity; tetracyclines with reduced streptococcal activity but effective against chlamydiae; sulphonamides with variable activity against the bacterial pathogens mentioned; and co-trimoxazole with enlarged spectrum but involving three agents (with metronidazole) when two should be sufficient.

In patients with penicillin hypersensitivity the cephalosporins will usually be safe unless the patient suffered an anaphylactic reaction. Erthyromycin, which can be used as an alternative in these cases, will provide streptococcal and *Staphylococcus aureus* cover, but none against coliforms.

Caesarian Section in Labour. There is less evidence of the value of prophylaxis in this operation; the operation field should be sterile although the potential for contamination of the uterine contents increases with the duration of labour. Antibiotics should be aimed at the vaginal and bowel flora and be safe for the baby; ampicillin or amoxycillin and metronidazole are appropriate. Ampicillin is also active against *Listeria*, haemolytic streptococci and clostridia which may infect the uterus on rare occasions.

Other Gynaecological Operations. It is undecided whether prophylaxis is of value in other gynaecological operations. All operations and procedures involving the female genital tract above the cervix take place in a potentially contaminated field, and if undertaken through the vagina, involve the vaginal flora. This is particularly relevant for IUCD insertion, where organisms will be frequently deposited in the uterine cavity but later disappear, probably via the menses. If prophylaxis is contemplated, ampicillin or amoxycillin with metronidazole, for a single or for triple doses only, are appropriate.

Catheter Management. In patients who have indwelling catheters there is a high probability that the urine will be permanently infected, usually with several organisms. Estimates of the rate urine becomes infected once a catheter is inserted vary: a measurable increase occurs with each day of catheterisation and about half will be infected within 2 weeks. Treatment of infected urine in postoperative patients without symptoms or signs of urinary infection or renal damage should be avoided and the catheter removed as soon as possible. In patients who have long-term indwelling catheters there is a high probability that the urine will be permanently infected, usually with several organisms. Here emphasis should be placed on adequate drainage, prevention of renal damage and adequate treatment of symptomatic episodes.

In the presence of symptoms, a specimen of urine should be cultured and an antibiotic given according to the combined sensitivities of the organisms present. If initial therapy is required before results are available, a broad-spectrum antibiotic should be started. Trimethoprim, ampicillin or augmentin are appropriate. When resistant organisms are present, e.g. *Proteus* spp., enterobacters or pseudo-

monads, gentamicin or ceftazidime will be required. When renal damage is present, blood cultures should be taken and antibiotics should be given for 10 or 14 days.

The value of regular urine culture in the presence of long-term catheters is doubtful. They may indicate the advent of a resistant organism contaminating the urine, but this should be ignored unless symptoms are present, when fresh cultures should be obtained. Few laboratories undertake a full investigation of mixed cultures from such patients.

Patients at Risk. The list of patients who require prophylaxis for medical reasons for any surgical procedure is lengthening: heart valve deformities and artificial heart valves; joint implants and organ transplants; immunosuppressed and immunodeficient patients require prophylaxis for all gynaecological surgical procedures, probably including dilatation and curettage, but not vaginal examination. Again, ampicillin or amoxycillin or cefuroxime together with metronidazole are appropriate, in a single or triple dose.

Postoperative Sepsis

Causes

Deep sepsis in the wound or at the site of operation originates from organisms deposited in the tissues during operation. Their sources will be exogenous, i.e. outside the patient, or the patient's own bacteria of the skin, vagina or gut. Precautions taken in theatre will help to exclude exogenous sources, but a septic lesion due to *Staphylococcus aureus* in a member of staff will overwhelm the usual barriers, as may an unrecognised disperser of skin organisms who is otherwise well. Improperly sterilized instruments and procedures whose implicit dangers are unappreciated may also introduce bacteria.

Superficial wound infection found more than 7 days after operation is more likely to have originated from a source in the ward. Abdominal wounds are best left covered for some days postoperatively unless there is specific reason to examine them.

Postoperative urinary infection results from undiagnosed preoperative bacteriuria or from the effects of catheterisation. Urinary catheters inevitably carry into the bladder organisms residing in the urethra, the distal third of which is usually colonised by bacteria and the middle third frequently so. In addition, the periurethral opening is often colonised by bowel coliforms and these too, unless the catheterization technique and preparation of the vulva is sufficient, may be transported via the catheter into the bladder. However, the return of bladder function will wash out organisms in the bladder urine and frequently aborts infection. Catheters should therefore be removed as soon as possible.

Investigation

A postoperative pyrexia should be investigated by examination of the abdominal or vaginal wound, the abdomen, the chest and urine. If a vaginal vault haematoma is aspirated or released some of the contents, rather than a swab, should be sent to the laboratory. Pelvic abscess or cellulitis should be sampled, if possible, by needle aspiration through the vaginal wall. If an abscess is operated upon, some of the contents and a sample of the abscess wall should be cultured. Swabs are inefficient at picking up, retaining and releasing bacteria. An endocervical swab taken with a speculum and blood cultures will often be worthwhile.

Urine for culture in a catheterised patient should be taken by syringe and needle aspiration from the catheter lumen, close to the patient. This avoids contamination of the urine from the reservoir and handling of the tap.

Treatment

A deep abdominal wound abscess with pyrexia, occurring within 7 days of operation, may be assumed to be due to *Staphylococcus aureus* as the most common organism. This organism should be treated with cloxacillin or flucloxacillin, or in penicillin-sensitive patients with erythromycin. If there is surrounding erythema and evidence of septicaemia and toxaemia, haemolytic streptococci group A may be involved, or a mixed infection with anaerobes and coliforms. Here, initial therapy should be by a second generation cephalosporin (cefuroxime, cefoxitin, cefamandole) with metronidazole. Benzyl penicillin is the drug of choice for haemolytic streptococci. Suitable specimens should be taken before treatment; a Gram film of the pus or swab may help direct the appropriate antibiotics. Antibiotics should be avoided in superficial wound infection without cellulitis since removal of stitches or probing will probably be sufficient.

Vaginal vault infection in a haematoma, without evidence of surrounding or deep infection, will respond to drainage alone. More serious infection is usually due to streptococci, anaerobes and coliforms; pending culture results amoxycillin with metronidazole are appropriate. Suspicion of *Staphylococcus aureus* or more resistant coliforms requires cefuroxime and metronidazole.

Pelvic infection, such as abscess formation or pelvic cellulitis, requires cefuroxime and metronidazole. In seriously ill patients gentamicin (for coliforms) with ticar-, azlo- or piperacillin (for streptococci and coliforms) and metronidazole will be justified, particularly if *Pseudomonas* is suspected.

These recommendations may require modification once culture results and sensitivities of the isolates are available. However, in pelvic infection with parametritis, abscess formation or infective thrombophlebitis it is wise always to use metronidazole whether anaerobes are cultured or not. Delayed specimens or overgrowth by aerobes on culture media may prevent their isolation. The incidence of anaerobes in pelvic infection is high and their pathogenic role is well established. The growth of *Staphylococcus aureus* from these sources demands a specific agent, i.e. flucloxacillin or erythromycin. Vancomycin (in future perhaps teicoplanin) is appropriate for *Staphylococcus aureus*, resistant to flucloxacillin (i.e. methicillin-resistant strains). A positive blood culture may indicate overspill into the blood stream, i.e. a bacteraemia, rather than necessarily a septicaemia. Most pelvic infections will be due to mixed organisms and in this case broad cover should be continued, while taking into account the bacteraemic organism.

Urinary Infection

Clinical indication for treatment of postoperative urinary infection is guided by the response of the patient to the removal of the catheter. Culture results will determine the appropriate antibiotic and are usually available next day. In general, first-line antibacterials should be used, e.g. trimethoprim ampicillin, nitrofurantoin or nalidixic acid. Resistant organisms are treated with cefuroxime, *Pseudomonas* by gentamicin or by reserve aminoglycosides if resistant to this agent.

The most common causative organism in both domiciliary and hospital practice is *E. coli*; in the former it may account for 80% of isolates. In hospital, more resistant organisms, including *Klebsiellas* and *Enterobacters* are more common. Strains of *Proteus* spp. are not infrequently associated with stones in the urinary tract, while *Micrococcus* type III (sometimes reported as staphylococci) are found in young women. Strains obtained in domiciliary practice are more likely to be fully sensitive to antibiotics; hospital isolates are more likely both to be resistant and to belong to more resistant genera. Co-trimoxazole has retained wide activity against urinary isolates and remains a satisfactory first-line choice of treatment. The increasing use of trimethoprim has led to a recorded increase in resistance to it in some areas; at the present time its spectrum is nearly as wide as that of co-trimoxazole. Resistance to ampicillin and its better absorbed esters has slowly increased, but these drugs are appropriate when indicated by antibiogram. Both nitrofurantoin and nalidixic acid remain useful urinary antiseptics for lower tract infection. Augmentin has enlarged the spectrum of amoxycillin significantly, but in treating urinary infection single drugs would usually be preferable if they are appropriate.

Interpretation of Urine Reports

In urine infection the diagnostic finding is a culture of a single bacterium at a concentration of $>10^5$ organisms/ml. A count less than this will not be classified as "significant" by the laboratory but may nevertheless be relevant in some patients; e.g. in high fluid intake, if death of the organism occurs during transit of the specimen, in partial antibiotic treatment or where low excretion of the organism occurs. Pyuria is not required for a positive result since polymorph excretion may be irregular and these cells may lyse in the specimen. A bacterial count of $<10^4$ organisms/ml is indicative of probable contamination of the specimen by organisms in the periurethral area, on the labia or perineum; organisms present in the bladder urine will usually occur in large numbers. In view of the inconsistency of excretion for both bacteria and inflammatory cells, and in the collection and transport of samples, a repeat specimen is useful. A bacterial count between 10^4 and 10^5 organisms/ml lies in the "doubtful" category; again a repeat specimen should be obtained.

Intermittent Self-Catheterisation

Antibiotic prophylaxis for intermittent self-catheterisation is not required. Good technique and adequate care of the catheter between catheterisations will avoid urinary infection. As in the case of patients with indwelling catheters, antibiotics are given when symptoms of infection appear. An established infection requires an early specimen and antibiotics chosen according to the sensitivities of the isolate obtained.

Bladder Washouts

Reports in the literature vary as to the effect of bladder washouts for the treatment and prophylaxis of bladder infection (Warren et al. 1978). Their appeal lies in the high local concentration of antibacterial obtained in the bladder. However, in lower tract infection, the site of infection is the wall of the bladder and adequate blood concentrations will give both good excretion of antibiotic in the urine itself and in the blood supply to the bladder. In addition, the nursing time required and the risk of contamination to the urine drainage system are disadvantages of washout. In the presence of local structural changes which may be difficult to treat, e.g. bladder diverticula or bladder stone, bladder washouts may have a temporary value.

References

Allen JL, Rampone JF, Wheeless CR (1972) Use of a prophylactic antibiotic in elective major gynaecologic operations. Obstet and Gynecol 39: 218–224

Burke JF (1961) The effective period of preventative antibiotic action in experimental incisions and dermal lesions. Surgery 50: 161–165

Cruse PJ, Foord R (1973) A five year prospective study of 23,649 surgical wounds. Archives of Surgery 107: 206–210

George JW, Ansbacher R, Otterson WN, Rabey F (1975) Prospective bacteriologic study of women undergoing hysterectomy. Obstet Gynecol 45: 60–63

Giles JA, Ashe RG, Heap JND, Hey Fiona M, Maloney MD, Newman Mercy J, Pomeroy Louise, Scane TM, Smith JH, Wathen CG, Hawkins DF (1984) A prospective controlled trial of cephradine and metronidazole as prophylaxis with abdominal hysterectomy. J Obstet Gynaecol 5 (Suppl 1): 513–517

Grossman JH, Greco TP, Minkin MJ, Adams RL, Hierholzer WJ, Andriole VT (1979) Prophylactic antibiotics in gynaecological surgery. Obstet Gynecol 53: 53–544

Hawrylyshyn PA, Bernstein P, Papsin FR (1983) Short term antibiotic prophylaxis in high risk patients following Caesarian section. Am J Obstet Gynecol 145: 285–289

Kelly MJ (1980) Wound infection: a controlled clinical and experimental demonstration of synergy between aerobic (Escherichia coli) and anaerobic (Bacteroides fragilis) bacteria. Ann R Coll Surg 62: 52–58

Lidwell OM, Lowbury EJL, Whyte W, Blowers R, Stanley SJ, Lowe D (1982) Effect of ultraclean air in operating rooms on deep sepsis in the joint after total or knee replacement: a randomised study. Br Med J 285: 10–14

Seropian R, Reynolds BM (1971) Wound infections after pre-operative depilatory versus razor preparation. Am J Surg 121: 251–254

Study Group (1974) Metronidazole in the prevention and treatment of Bacteroides infections in gynaecological patients. Lancet 2: 1540–1543

Vorherr H, Vorherr UF, Mehta P, Ulrich JA, Messer RH (1980) Vaginal absorption of povidone-iodine. J Am Med Assoc 244: 2628–2629

Warren JW, Platt R, Thomas RJ, Rosner B, Kass EH (1978) Antibiotic irrigation and catheter-associated urinary tract infections. N Engl J Med 299: 570

5 · Recent Advances in Imaging

David Cosgrove, Elizabeth Bellamy and Malcolm Pearce

Introduction

Recent developments in imaging techniques have improved the diagnosis and management of gynaecological problems. Some techniques may be used intraoperatively to guide surgery. Most of the newer techniques present their images in the form of tomographs. Interpretation therefore requires an appreciation of pelvic anatomy and the ability to perceive three dimensions from two-dimensional sections.

In this chapter the principles and gynaecological applications of ultrasound, computerised X-ray tomography, advances in isotope imaging techniques (tomography and the application of monoclonal antibodies) and magnetic resonance imaging will be reviewed.

Ultrasound

Principles

Ultrasound imaging depends on detecting the echoes returning from interfaces within tissues. The interrogating ultrasound pulse is formed into a narrow beam by a lens-like focussing process at the transmitting transducer which also serves as a receiver. The beam is then swept by mechanical or electronic means through a plane to produce a tomographic slice which may take the form of a rectangle (linear scan) or a triangle (sector scan). Because the image is formed in a fraction of a second it may be quickly updated to display movement.

This approach is analogous to a cine film and is known as realtime ultrasound. It allows the operator total flexibility to take tomograms in any plane so that the image can be aligned for optimal display of the significant anatomy.

Ultrasound cannot penetrate gas or bone so that bowel loops in the pelvis interfere with the examination, as do stomas and surgical dressings. Resolution is somewhat variable, being worse in the very obese, but in the average patient structures down to approximately 1 mm can be defined. Ultrasound is fraught with artefacts, mostly due to the ultrasound beam being deviated from the simple straight line path assumed by the operator. The presence of these artefacts, together with the use of realtime ultrasound, make this a very operator-dependent technique. Machines are now relatively cheap and therefore widely available. Many are mobile so that bedside and interoperative applications are possible.

An ultrasound scan is simple for the patient, a full bladder being the only preparation or cooperation required. This is needed to displace the bowel loops out of the pelvis and because urine hardly attenuates the ultrasound beam so that structures posterior to the bladder are better visualised. A coupling gel is placed on the skin and the transducer is applied to generate a realtime image on the screen. Searching movements of the probe allow the whole pelvis to be scanned and immediately viewed in realtime. Sample freeze frame images are then recorded. A typical examination takes 15 min and is usually well tolerated by the patient.

Special procedures may be added. Contrast in the form of a water enema is occasionally required to define the position of a confusing lobe of cut. Fine

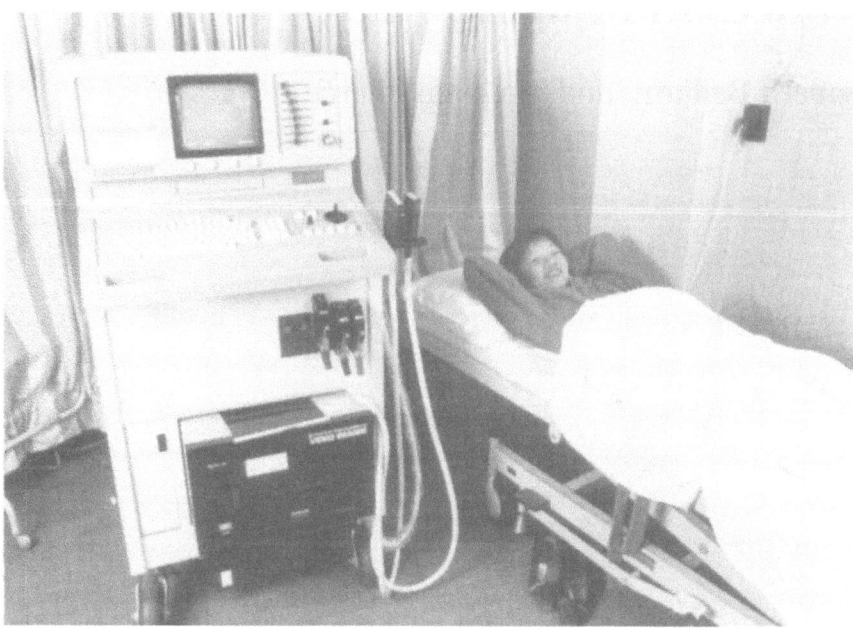

Fig. 5.1. A realtime ultrasound machine (Acuson 128)

needle aspiration of mass lesions may be guided under direct ultrasound vision for cytological samples or for harvesting ova.

Ultrasound machines are portable (Fig. 5.1) compared with other forms of imaging equipment. They are cheaper and generally require less maintenance.

Normal Findings

The uterus is seen to lie behind the bladder and in front of the rectum in both cross and longitudinal sections (Fig. 5.2). The ovaries are usually easily visualised as they lie in their position against the muscles of the pelvic side wall. In longitudinal section the posterior border of the ovary is marked by the internal iliac vessels (Fig. 5.3). In the presence of pelvic pathology or adhesions or in patients who have undergone hysterectomy the anatomy may be markedly disturbed in which case it is necessary to locate the ovarian vessels entering the ovary from their lateral aspect to confirm that the structure under examination is indeed the ovary. In about 2% of patients one ovary cannot be visualised, usually the left as it is covered by the sigmoid colon. Loops of bowel lying in the pelvis may be most confusing since their echo pattern can be the same as that of normal or pathological soft tissue. The presence of gas, however, usually gives them a distinctive appearance but otherwise it is necessary to wait until peristaltic movement is detected to aid

in differentiation. The Fallopian tubes are usually too tortuous and narrow to be seen, but if there is pelvic ascites their margins, together with those of the broad ligament, may be defined. Although both external and internal iliac vascular bundles are normally visualised, lymph nodes of normal size cannot be detected.

Demonstrating Follicular Growth and Ovulation

The physiological changes of the normally cycling ovary are readily demonstrated on ultrasound. Ovarian follicles are seen as rounded echo-poor spaces within the ovary (Fig. 5.4). Most workers have reported the growth of ovarian follicles in the terms of a mean diameter. The internal follicular diameter is measured in three planes (longitudinal, transverse and sagittal) and the average diameter is then calculated and reported.

In spontaneous 28-day cycles, two to three small follicles (3–5 mm in diameter) can be visualised in each ovary on the 4th day after the last menstrual period (day 4). On day 9 it is usual to find that one follicle dominates and has a mean diameter of about 10 mm. Follicular growth is then linear at a rate of about 2 mm/day until ovulation (Hackeloer and Sallam 1983). There is high correlation between the size of the developing follicle and plasma oestradiol levels (Hackeloer 1985).

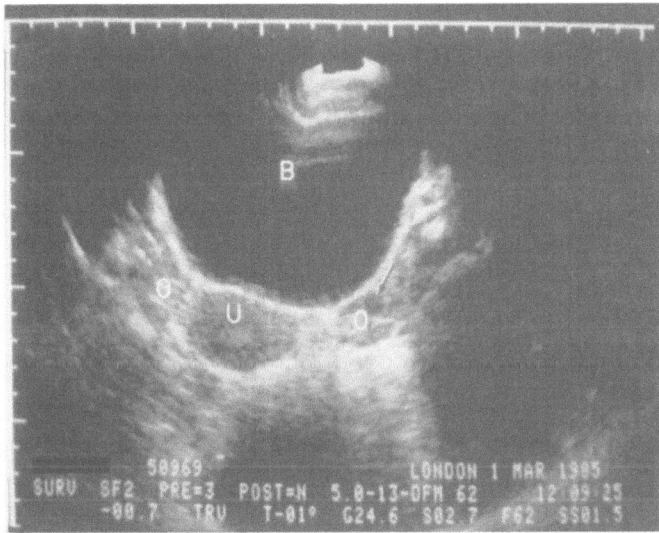
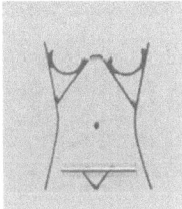

a

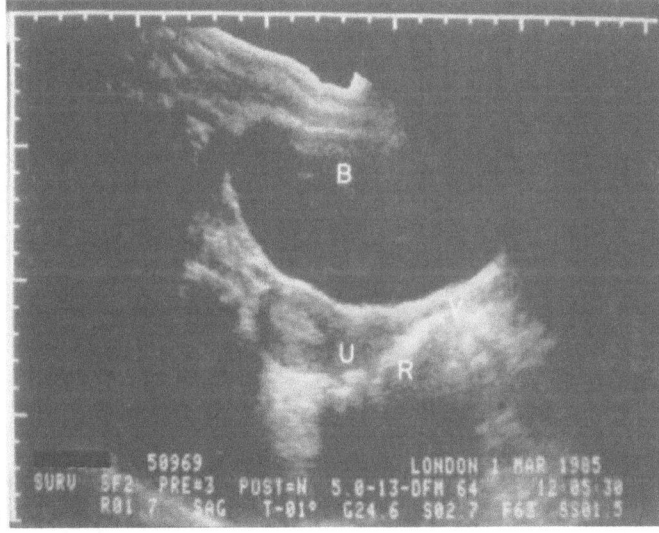
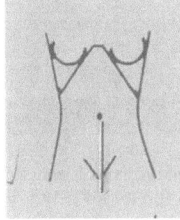

b

Fig. 5.2a, b. Ultrasound of the normal pelvis. **a** Transverse and **b** longitudinal section though a normal pelvis in the proliferative phase of the menstrual cycle showing the prominent endometrial line and a developing follicle (*arrowed* in the left ovary). *B*, bladder; *O*, ovaries; *U*, uterus; *V*, vagina

Ovulation occurs at a mean diameter of 21 mm (18–24 mm). With the latest generation of ultrasound equipment resolution is such that the cumulus oophorus may occasionally be visualised within the growing follicles.

Ovulation is usually diagnosed ultrasonically when one or more of the following has occurred:

1. Disappearance of the follicle
2. The appearance of internal echoes within the follicle or collapse of the follicle with crenation of the edges
3. The appearance of free fluid in the pouch of Douglas

Commonly the corpus luteum is difficult to visualise in spontaneous cycles but is occasionally seen as a target-like structure with an echo-free central area. It is more commonly seen in stimulated cycles which may also result in a cyst of the corpus luteum. Stimulated cycles may also result in multiple follicles (Fig. 5.5).

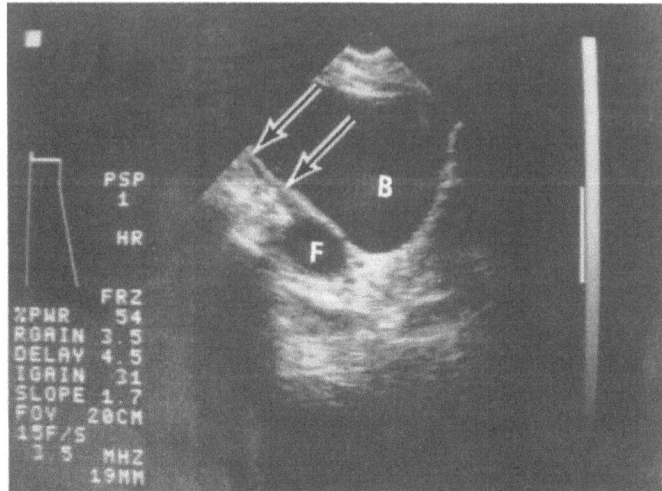
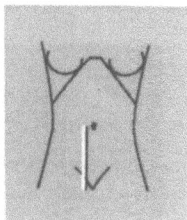

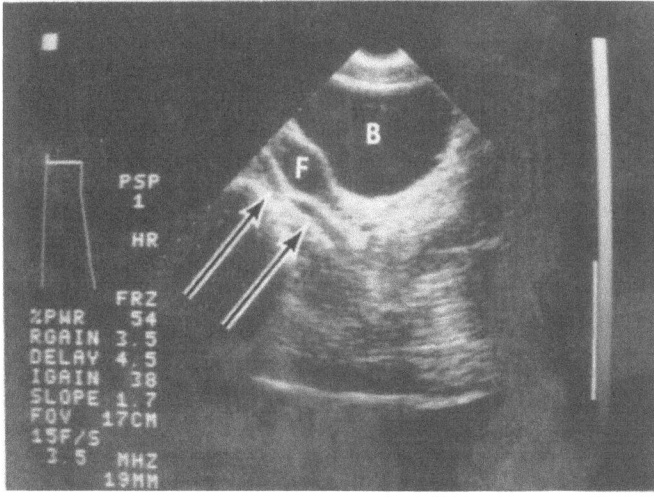
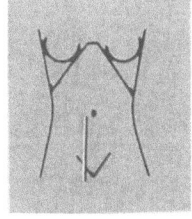

Fig. 5.3a, b. The anatomical relations of the normal ovaries. **a** In longitudinal section the ovarian vessels (*arrowed*) can be seen entering the ovary laterally via the mesovarium. **b** A segment of the internal iliac artery (*arrowed*) can be seen beneath the ovary. *B*, bladder; *F*, follicle

Failure of ovulation may be diagnosed when (Hackeloer 1985):

1. No follicles develop
2. Internal echoes develop before the follicle reaches critical size (a minimum of 18 mm)

3. Continuing cystic enlargement occurs beyond 30 mm

To date no pregnancies have been reported from follicles of less than 18 mm or more than 30 mm in size (Hackeloer 1985).

Fig. 5.4a–c. The development of the growing follicle and ovulation. The longitudinal scan illustrated in **a** was performed on day 12 of a normal menstrual cycle and shows a follicle (*arrowed*) within the right ovary that had a mean diameter of 16 mm. **b** A transverse scan of the same patient taken on day 14 and now illustrates that the follicle in the right ovary has achieved 19 mm mean diameter and that there is also a smaller follicle developing in the left ovary. The transverse scan illustrated in **c** taken on day 15 shows that the right ovary now does not demonstrate follicular activity and that there is a small collection of fluid (*arrow*) posterior to the uterus; this indicates that the patient has ovulated. Note that the follicle (*F*) in the left ovary has continued to grow and now has a mean diameter of 30 mm, indicating that ovulation will not occur from this follicle and that this may persist as a follicular cyst. *B*, bladder; *U*, uterus; *F*, follicle; *R*, right.

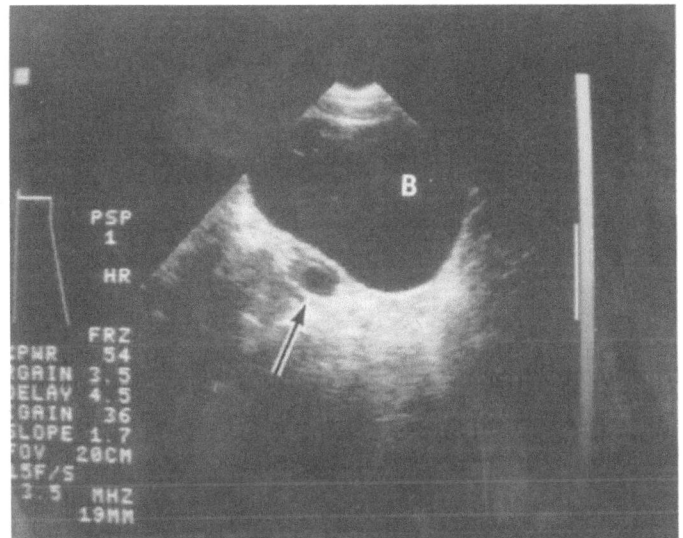
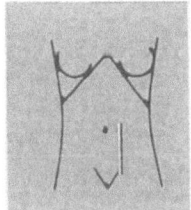

a

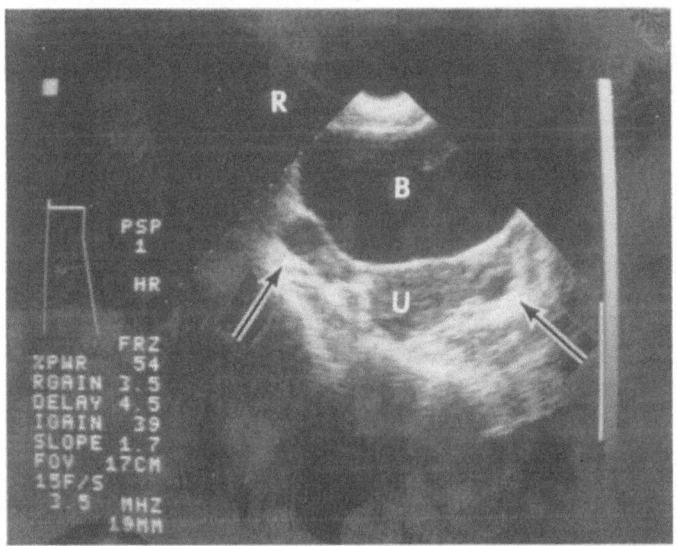
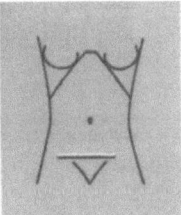

b

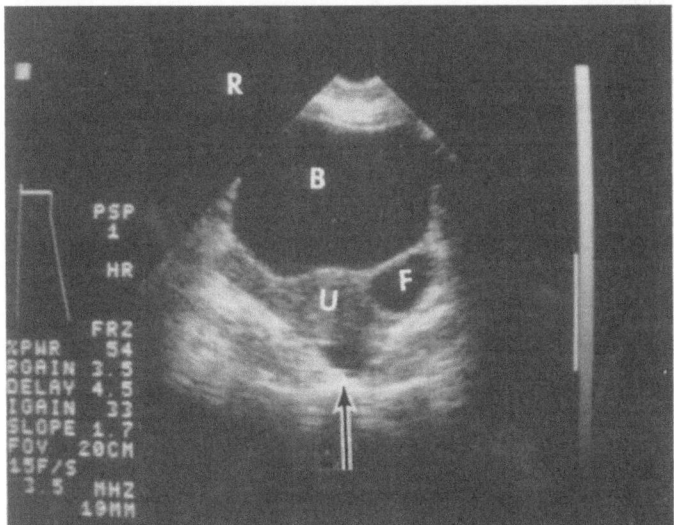
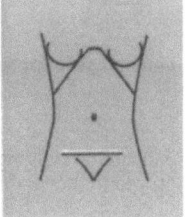

c

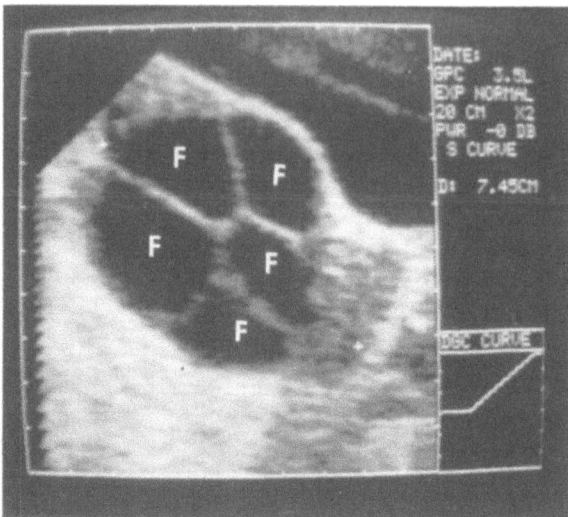
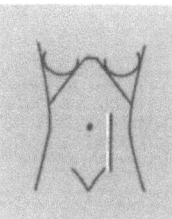

Fig. 5.5. A Pergonal-stimulated ovary. In response to the gonadotrophins contained in Perganol five follicles have developed in this ovary. As this appearance may result in a multiple pregnancy and/or the hyperstimuation syndrome the HCG should be withheld in this patient. If, however, the patient was undergoing ovulation induction as part of IV fertilisation this situation would be ideal. In the latter case it is preferable to remove two or more oocytes from the ovary in order to increase the patient's chances of pregnancy.

Endometrial Changes

Cyclic changes in the endometrium can also be seen on ultrasound. In the early stage the endometrium is thin and gradually thickens until the time of ovulation. Thereafter the endometrium decreases in thickness probably due to a loss of oedema in the superficial layer of endometrium. This commonly produces the ring sign (Fig. 5.6), which many observers believe does not occur in the absence of ovulation (Hackeloer 1985). Recently endometrial appearances have been related to the success of embryo transfer at the time of in vitro fertilisation.

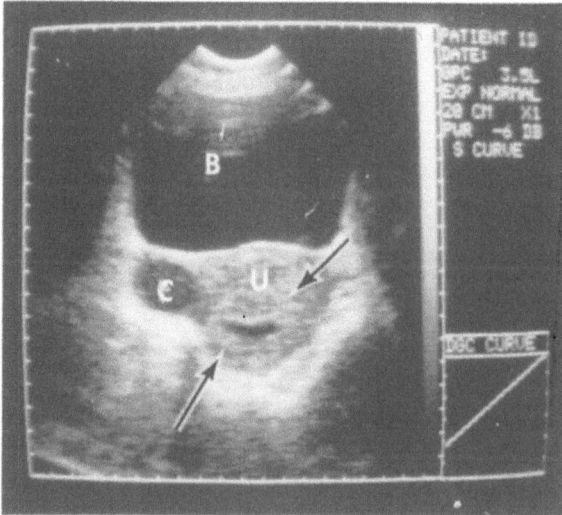
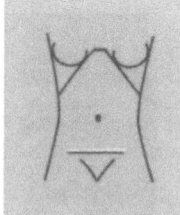

Fig. 5.6. The ovulation ring. This transverse scan shows a collapsed follicle with internal echoes in the left ovary together with an obvious ovulation ring. The ovulation ring (*arrowed*) is an area of brighter echoes containing a central area devoid of echoes representing a small fluid collection within the uterus. *U*, uterus; *B*, bladder; *C*, corpus luteum.

Other Applications

Pelvic Inflammatory Disease

Abscesses can be detected with about 90% accuracy by ultrasound (Arger and Colman 1983; Saunders and James 1985). They appear as fluid-filled spaces with irregular margins (Fig. 5.7a). The distortion of the anatomical boundaries may obscure their exact location, a tubal abscess being indistinguishable from an ovarian abscess or even an abscess within the pouch of Douglas. The facility with which ultrasound can be repeated makes it especially useful in following patients with acute pelvic sepsis to monitor resolution (Arger and Colman 1983). It cannot, however, distinguish between infections of different aetiologies, and collections that are overlaid by bowel loops are likely to be missed. In this circumstance CT is more helpful. Chronic pelvic inflammatory disease cannot be seen as the affected normal boundaries often mimic the poor-quality scans that are sometimes seen in such patients.

Endometriosis (Saunders and James 1985)

Ultrasonically endometriosis can easily be confused with pelvic inflammatory disease (PID) (Figs. 5.7a, b) although the clinical presentation is usually different.

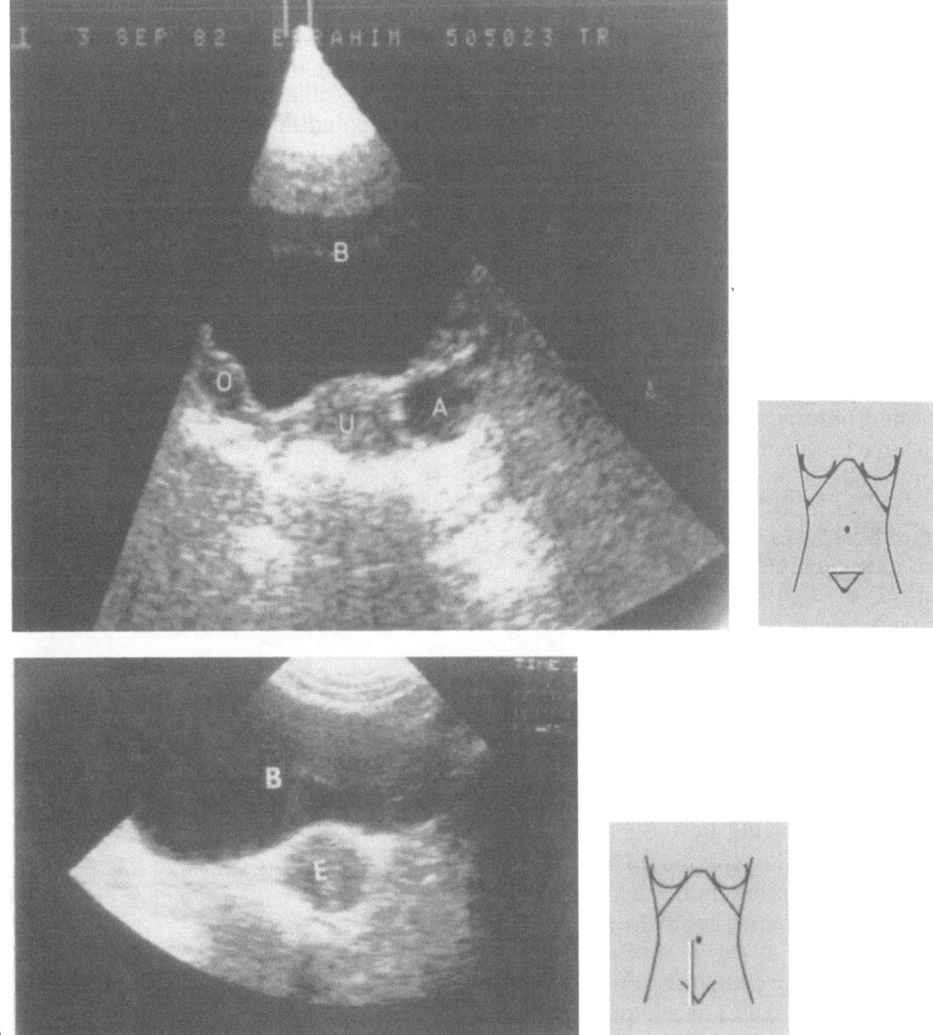

a

b

Fig. 5.7a. Tubal abscess. **b** Endometriotic cyst. It can be difficult on ultrasound to distinguish between a tubal abscess and an endometriotic cyst of the ovary as can be seen above. The complex internal echoes within the cyst may represent either blood or pus. *B*, bladder; *O*, ovary; *A*, abscess; *E*, endometriotic cyst; *U*, uterus.

The chocolate cysts of endometriosis appear as echo-free space which may be rounded or irregular (Fig. 5.7b). They often show less distal acoustic enhancement than ovarian cysts but cannot be reliably diagnosed. Small foci and extra pelvic foci are extremely difficult to detect. If lesions are seen (and confirmed by laparoscopy) then serial ultrasound may allow the evaluation of the progress during hormone therapy.

Problems of Early Pregnancy (Chudleigh and Pearce 1986)

The two most common complaints in early pregnancy are vaginal bleeding and abdominal pain. The sensible use of ultrasound may be very reassuring to the patient: if the pregnancy is not viable it may save her a long stay in hospital waiting for the pregnancy test to become negative.

With modern mechanical sector scanners, a gestation sac may be seen within the uterus from about 5 weeks of amenorrhoea. Fetal heart activity can usually be observed from 6 weeks and the fetus can be measured from about 7 weeks amenorrhoea.

The clinical finding of an open cervix after a recent vaginal bleed in the first trimester of pregnancy is indicative of an incomplete or inevitable abortion. This is a clinical diagnosis and ultrasound has no role to play aside from the very occasional patient who wishes to have the diagnosis confirmed before evacuation of retained products of conception.

The demonstration of fetal heart activity after a recent vaginal bleed is extremely reassuring to the patient. It is the most reliable sign of a continuing pregnancy and approximately 80% of such pregnancies (Robinson 1975) will continue. The finding of an empty gestational sac needs care in interpretation. This may represent an early pregnancy or it may represent a blighted ovum or a missed abortion. The sac volume is calculated by measuring the anterior and posterior, transverse and longitudinal diameter and multiplying by 0·5233 (derived from the formula for the volume of a sphere). If the volume of the sac is more than 2·5 ml then a fetal heart should be seen. It must be stressed, however, that fetal heart activity at this gestation can only be seen with good-quality equipment and if there is any doubt it is better to wait a week and rescan the patient. Failure to demonstrate growth of the sac and to visualise the fetal heart will allow the confident diagnosis of a blighted ovum to be made.

Ectopic Gestation (Robinson and De Crespigny 1983)

This remains one of the more difficult diagnostic problems in gynaecology but ultrasound can now prove to be a useful adjunct. The primary role of ultrasound is the demonstration of an intrauterine pregnancy or of any empty uterus. With modern equipment and a careful observer it may also be possible to assess the presence or absence of adnexal mass and to determine whether or not there is free fluid in the pouch of Douglas.

In patients suspected of having an ectopic pregnancy the demonstration of an intrauterine sac together with a live fetus effectively precludes the diagnosis. Only 1 in 30 000 pregnancies (Winer et al. 1957) demonstrate a coexistent intra- and extrauterine pregnancy (Fig. 5.8). Having demonstrated an intrauterine pregnancy it is important, however, to examine the adnexa for a twisted ovarian cyst or a possible ruptured corpus luteum. A well-described potential source of error is the pseudogestational sac formed by the decidual cast that may accompany ectopic gestation (Winer 1981). Decidual casts may be seen from about 5–9 weeks gestation. The larger sacs do not pose a

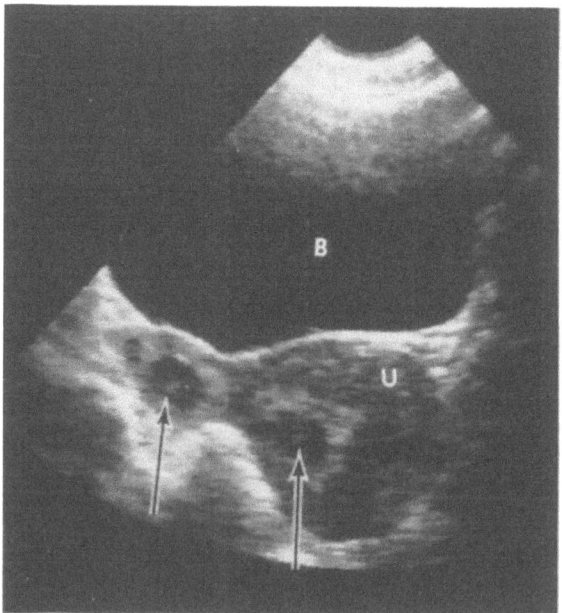

Fig. 5.8. A combined intrauterine and ectopic gestation. This is a very rare example and is the result of a clomiphene-induced pregnancy. A gestation sac can clearly be seen both within the uterus and in an extrauterine site. The fetal poles (*arrowed*) both showed fetal heart activity. The ectopic pregnancy was removed by means of linear salpingostomy and the intrauterine pregnancy continued to term and resulted in a healthy infant. *B*, bladder; *U*, uterus.

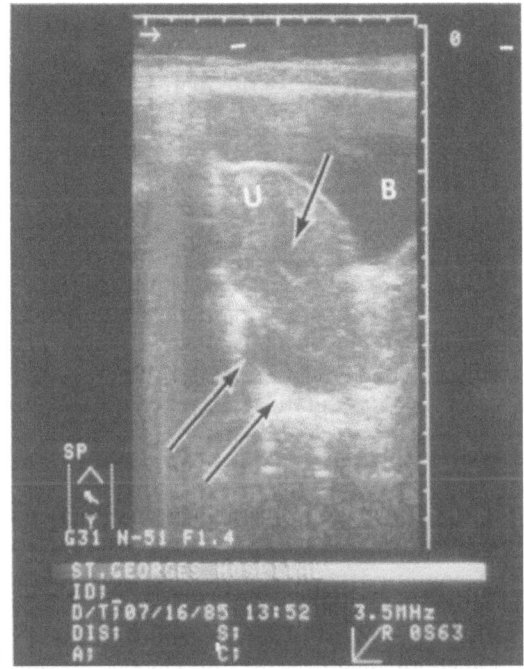
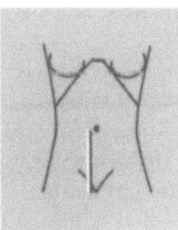
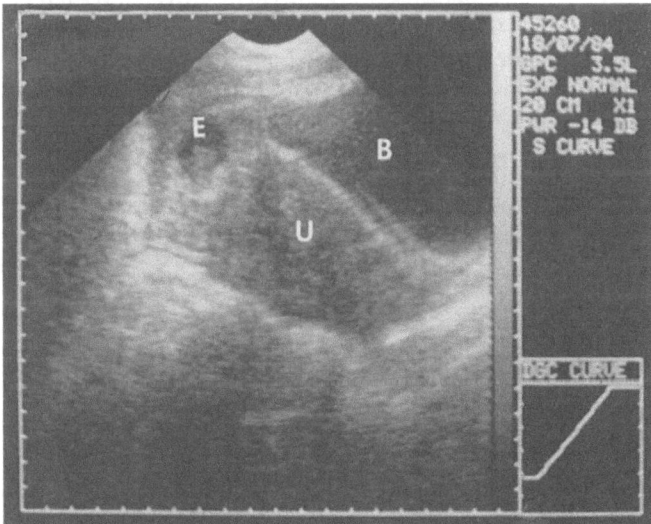
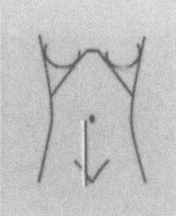

Fig. 5.9a, b. Ectopic pregnancy. **a** demonstrates the pseudogestational sac (*single arrow*) that may be a catch as it may be mistaken for an intrauterine pregnancy. A further clue to the presence of an ectopic gestation is the free fluid (*double arrow*) in the pouch of Douglas. **b** illustrates an extrauterine gestation sac and embryo which is only seen in about 6% of ectopic gestations. *U*, uterus; *B*, bladder; *E*, ectopic gestation.

problem in diagnosis in that careful examination will show low-level echoes and blood clot within the sac rather than the clear sonolucent appearance that is seen with a true gestation sac (Fig. 5.9). It must be said, however, that small pseudogestational sacs are difficult to distinguish from the 5-week gestational sac or an early blighted ovum. In such cases the presence or absence of an adnexal mass and of free fluid in the pouch of Douglas may aid diagnosis.

The demonstration of a gestational sac together with fetal heart activity in an extrauterine site (Fig. 5.9b) confirms the diagnosis of ectopic pregnancy but is only seen in about 6% of ectopic gestations

(Robinson and De Crespigny 1983). Even with careful observers and modern equipment, adnexal masses are probably only seen in less than half of ectopic gestations, so absence of such a mass does not preclude the diagnosis of ectopic gestation.

Many causes of adnexal masses demonstrated by ultrasound mimic ectopic pregnancy, for instance, a ruptured corpus luteal cyst, an accident to an ovarian cyst or endometriosis. The maximum efficiency of ultrasound in the diagnosis of ectopic gestation is gained by combining it with an assay for the beta-subunit of human chorionic gonadotrophin (HCG). HCG assays are usually reported as positive or negative, the test becoming positive approximately 10 days after conception. The two tests are interpreted as follows (Robinson and De Crespigny 1983):

1. A negative HCG effectively excludes an ectopic pregnancy.

2. An empty uterus with an adnexal mass and/or free fluid together with a positive HCG indicates the need for laparoscopy.

3. Demonstration of a living fetus outside the uterus whilst uncommon provides an absolute diagnosis of ectopic pregnancy.

4. An empty uterus in the absence of adnexal mass or free fluid but with a positive HCG is not a reliable guide to the presence of an ectopic pregnancy.

If it is possible to have quantitative results of beta HCG, Kadar et al. (1981) have demonstrated that at levels of more than 6500 milli-international units/litre an intrauterine sac should be visible on ultrasound. The findings of an empty uterus combined with a high HCG level therefore are indicative of ectopic gestation.

Ovarian Neoplasms

Ovarian cysts are very obvious on ultrasound as echo-free areas with posterior acoustic enhancement. Follicular and luteal cysts are common and may reach a diameter of 6 cm. If the cyst is entirely cystic and unilocular all that is required is to rescan the patient in 6 weeks time as most will involute spontaneously (Berland et al. 1982).

Ultrasound is not reliable in differentiating between benign and malignant ovarian cysts (Meire et al. 1984; Saunders and James 1985). Size, irregularity of contour, the presence of solid areas or septae (Fig. 5.10), ascites and thickness of the cyst wall are all suspicious features but as with CT scanning a definite diagnosis is not always possible unless metastases are also demonstrated (Deland et al. 1979). Ultrasound is used to confirm that a pelvic mass is cystic and has proved especially useful in postoperative follow-up for pelvic recurrences or liver metastases in carcinoma of the ovary (Meire et al. 1984). Laparoscopy, however, is required to evaluate the abdominal peritoneum.

Solid ovarian tumours are seen as parametrial masses with low-level echoes. Again the pattern is not specific for malignancy (Fig. 5.11). Dermoid

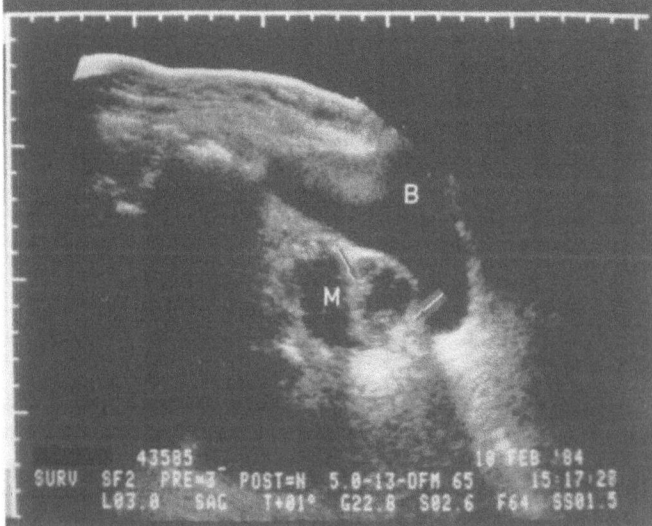
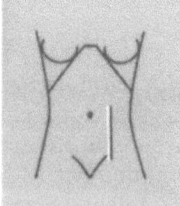

Fig. 5.10. Cystadenocarcinoma of the ovary. The parametrial mass though predominantly cystic has thick septi and solid components (*arrow*). These features suggest its malignant nature. *B*, bladder; *M*, mass.

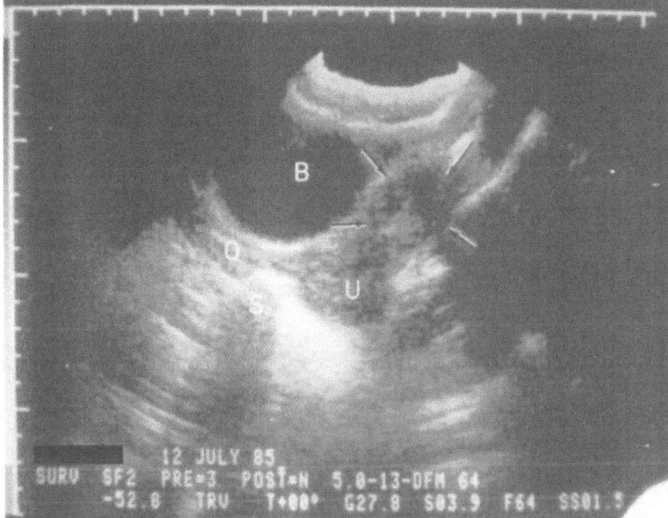
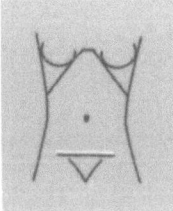

Fig. 5.11. Ovarian teratoma. A solid mass (*arrows*) replaces the left ovary. At laparotomy this proved to be a teratoma although the ultrasound appearances are non-specific. *B*, bladder; *O*, right ovary; *S*, sigmoid colon; *U*, uterus.

cysts have a spectrum of appearances (Jones et al. 1980). They may be indistinguishable from simple cysts but more typically have a complex pattern of echoes due to their heterogeneous content. Sebaceous material and hair give very strong echoes with marked attenuation of the sound beam so that the full extent of the lesion may not be appreciated (tip of the iceberg sign, Fig. 5.12). Indeed the pattern is easily mistaken for a gas-containing loop of bowel. It is wise to consider a dermoid whenever

a palpable mass cannot be demonstrated on ultrasound. A plain X-ray after excluding pregnancy on ultrasound will often reveal tell-tale tooth or bone formation.

Screening for Ovarian Cancer

More than 75% of patients with an ovarian cancer present with advanced disease (FIGO stage III or

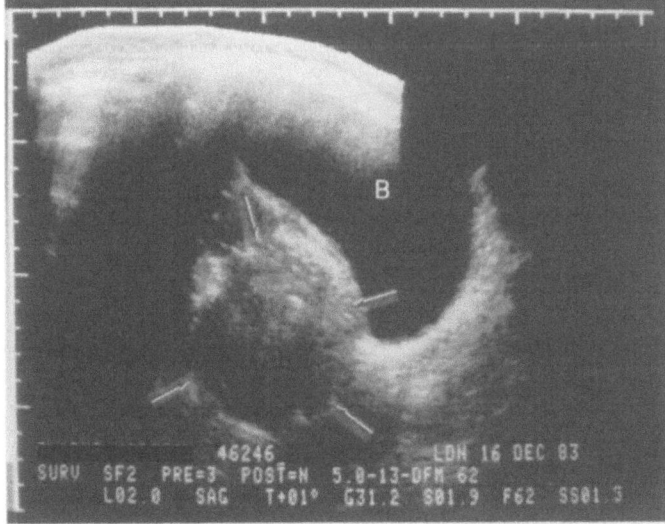
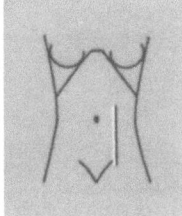

Fig. 5.12. A dermoid. Only the anterior margin of the mass (*arrows*) was clearly discernible on the sonogram of this dermoid. Ultrasound often underestimates the size of dermoids and may miss them because the pattern may be indistinguishable from a bowel loop. *B*, bowel.

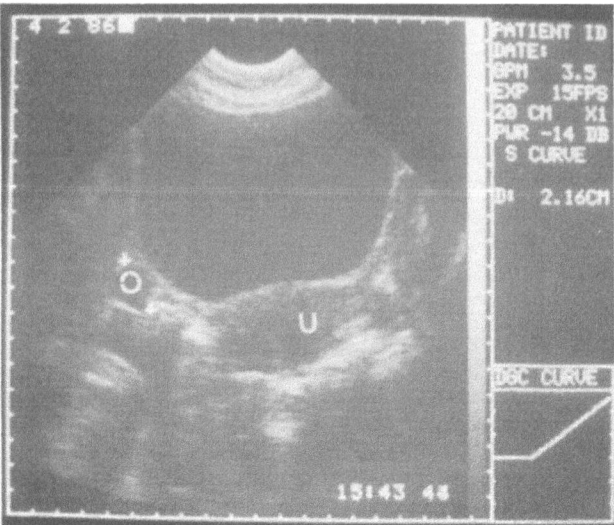 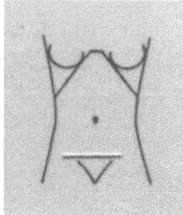

Fig. 5.13. Postmenopausal uterus and ovary. Note that the ovary is similar in echo pattern to the uterus. *U*, uterus; *O*, ovary.

IV). This means that whilst ovarian cancer is only responsible for a quarter of all gynaecological malignancies it kills more women than both cervical and endometrial cancer combined. The mean survival time for women who present with advanced ovarian cancer is 6 months, whereas the 5-year survival rate for stage 1 carcinoma of the ovary is approximately 85%.

There is need therefore for a simple and reliable screening test to detect early ovarian cancer. Screening by regular pelvic examination and by tumour markers has proved to have a low sensitivity and specificity.

Since 1982 King's College Hospital have been evaluating the use of a mechanical sector scanner as a means of screening for ovarian cancer. They (Campbell et al. 1982) initially demonstrated that the volume of normal ovaries as measured by ultrasound correlated well with direct measurements made at the time of laparotomy.

The screening programme was then initiated along the following lines (Campbell 1983):

Table 5.1. Results from King's College Hospital screening programme for ovarian cancer

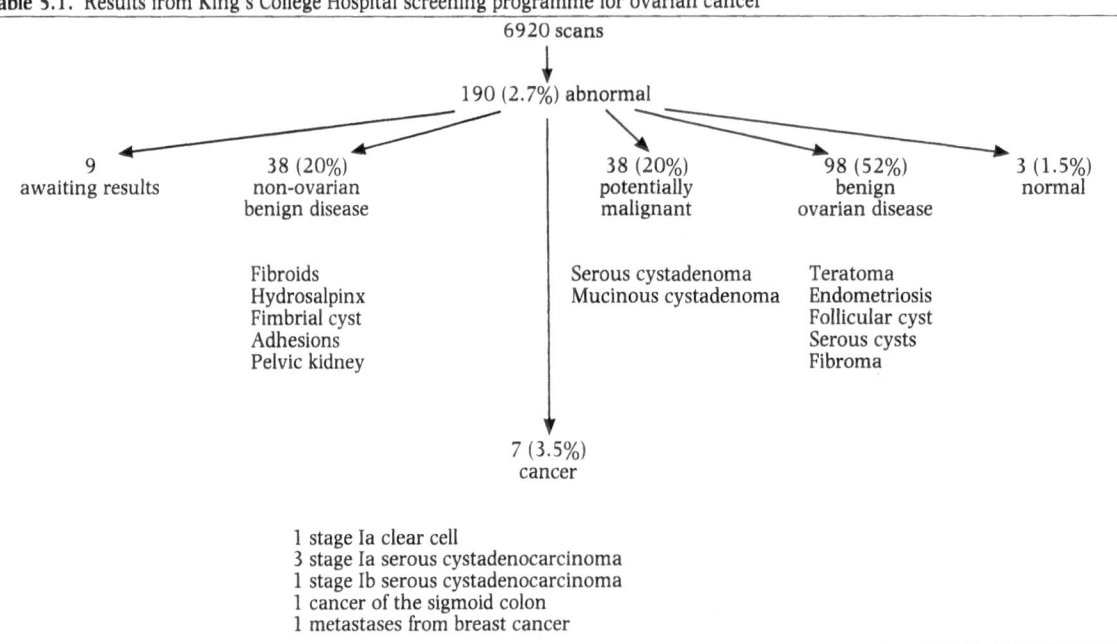

1. Postmenopausal women of more than 45 years of age were recruited by advertising in the popular press.

2. Each patient had both ovaries scanned and the volumes were calculated. A volume of more than 10 cm (Berland et al. 1982) was considered to be abnormal. In addition if one ovary was more than twice the volume of the other ovary this was also considered to be abnormal.

3. Morphology was also assessed. The postmenopausal ovary has approximately the same echo pattern as the uterus (Fig. 5.13). The appearance of cystic areas or solid areas within the ovary that had differing echo patterns was considered to be abnormal, even if the ovarian volume was within normal limits.

If the ovary was considered to be abnormal the patient was recalled for a scan in 6 weeks time. If the abnormality was still present the patient underwent a laparoscopy or laparotomy as determined by the referring gynaecologist. Table 5.1 illustrates the results so far.

Uterine Pathology

Congenital uterine anomalies such as bicornate uterus can be detected by ultrasound (Jones et al.

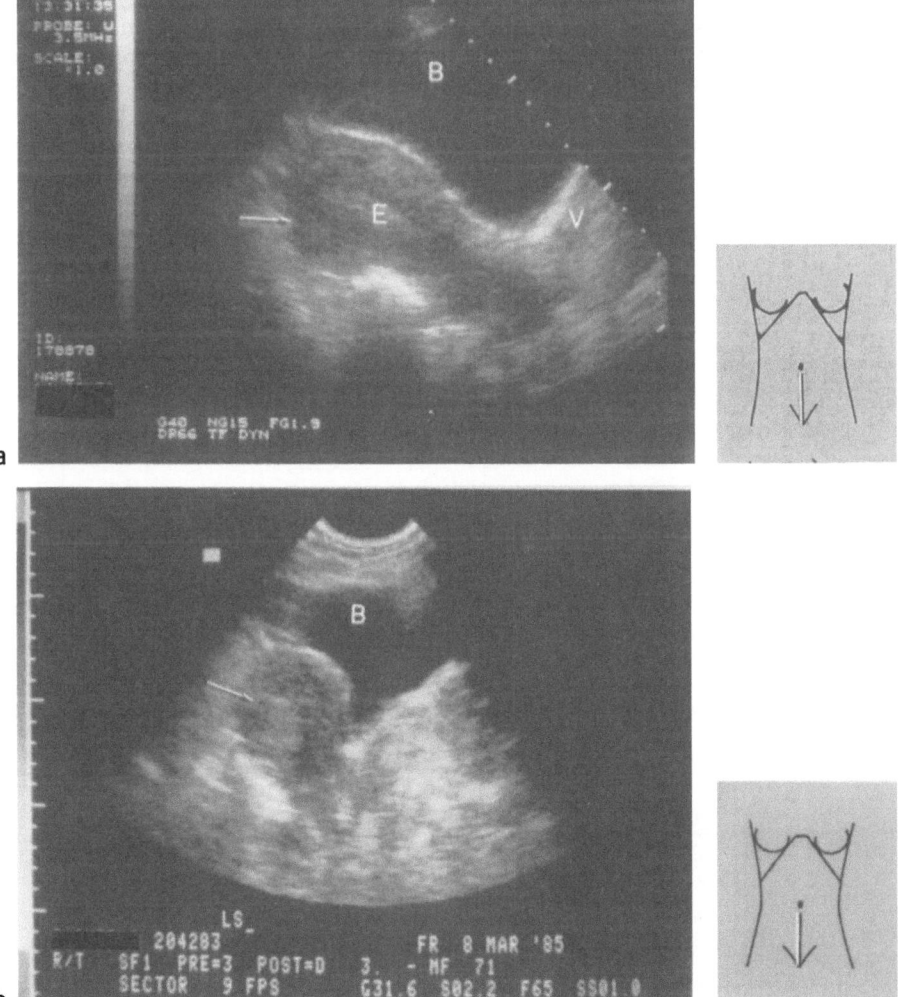

Fig. 5.14a, b. Fibroids. The varying patterns of fibroids are illustrated in these two patients. **a** demonstrates an echo-poor mass (*arrow*) that disturbs the normal outline of the uterus. **b** demonstrates a mass with high-level echoes (*arrow*) due to calcification within the fibroids. *B,* bladder; *V,* vagina; *E,* endometrium.

1980). Haematometra and haematocolpos, whether congenital or acquired, are readily identified as echo-free areas within the uterus, although the site of obstruction cannot usually be demonstrated and the difference between blood and pus may be difficult.

Fibroids are easily demonstrated by ultrasound but present a bewildering variety of patterns depending upon the histology and position. Commonly they are seen as relatively echogenic masses within the uterus but if there is necrosis, hyaline or fatty degeneration they become echo poor (Fig. 5.14). Calcification gives a characteristic appearance that is specific for fibroids with intense focal echoes and distal shadowing. Only with this pattern can fibroids be distinguished readily from other pathology such as sarcoma or carcinoma. When pedunculated, fibroids may simulate parametrial masses. Sarcoma degeneration of a fibroid has no characteristic ultrasound findings. Submucus fibroids are not readily demonstrated with ultrasound, especially if they are small. Salpingography or hysteroscopy is therefore necessary if submucus fibroids are suspected as the cause for infertility or recurrent early first trimester abortion.

The ease with which intrauterine contraceptive devices can be visualised makes ultrasound the ideal technique for ascertaining their position (Fig. 5.15). If the intrauterine device is not found within the uterus and a gestation sac has not been demonstrated a plain abdominal X-ray is required as bowel gas makes ultrasound unreliable for detecting intrauterine devices lying within the abdominal cavity.

Carcinoma of the endometrium, although visible on ultrasound, when of sufficient size is better diagnosed by conventional curettage. Ultrasound can be helpful in evaluating pelvic extension, although this is more reliably done using CT scanning. Lymph node involvement may be shown with ultrasound but lymphangiography remains the most sensitive technique. Similarly for carcinoma of the cervix, ultrasound has no place in making the diagnosis but may improve on clinical staging (Fig. 5.16) although again CT scanning is more reliable (van Doorn et al. 1985).

New ways to use ultrasound can extend its applications in gynaecology. The value of introducing contrast into the rectosigmoid by water enema to provide positive identification of gut loops has already been mentioned. The ultrasound equivalent of a salpingogram is a simple method of establishing tubal patency but cannot as yet be recommended as a replacement for traditional methods. Intracavity

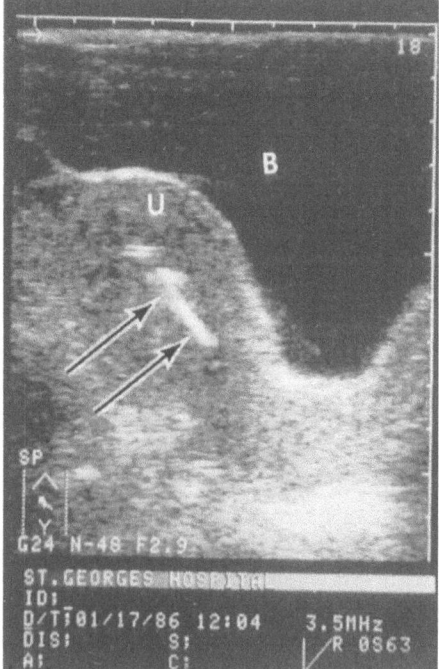
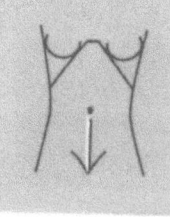

Fig. 5.15. An intrauterine contraceptive device. The very bright echoes (*arrowed*) are produced from the interface between the stem of the Copper 7 and the uterine fluid. *U*, uterus; *B*, bladder.

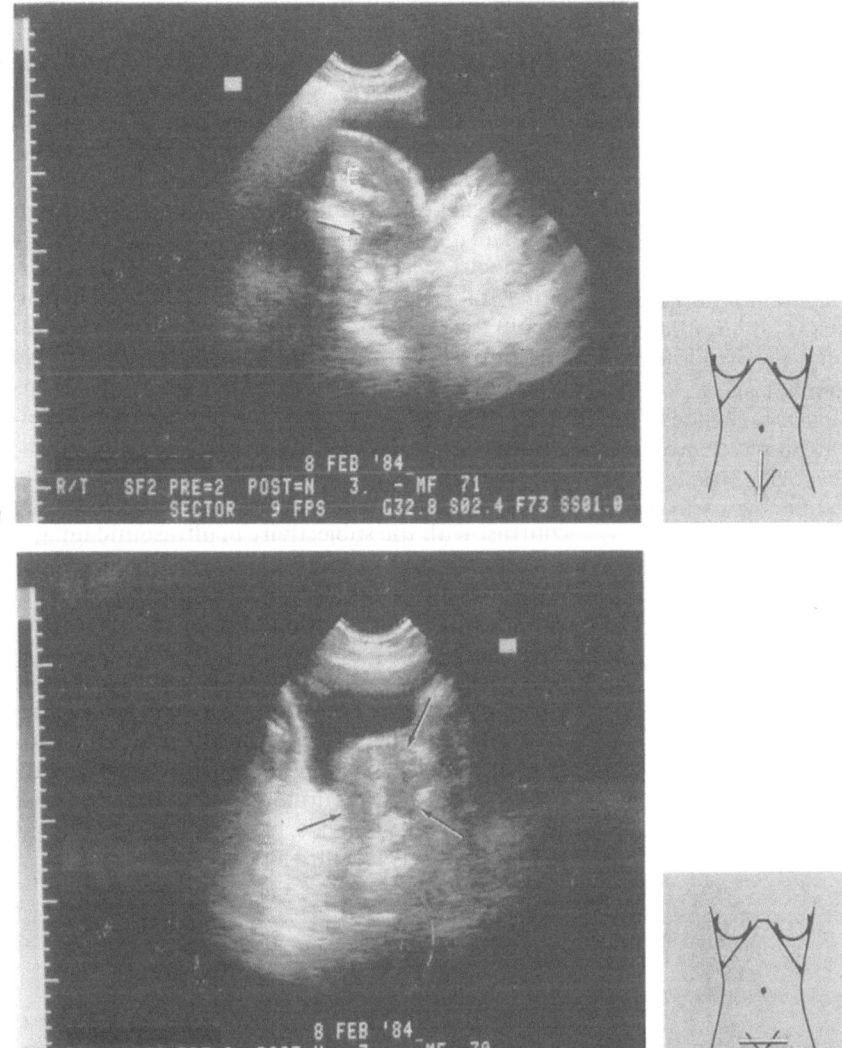

Fig. 5.16a, b. The ultrasound appearances of carcinoma of the cervix. Expansion of the cervix by a heterogeneous, lobulated mass (*arrows*) is apparent in this patient with an extensive carcinoma of the cervix. Involvement of the left pelvic side wall is obvious. There is a fluid accumulation in the endometrium. **a** Longitudinal view; **b** transverse view. *E*, endometrium; *R*, rectum; *V*, vagina.

probes allow the transducer to be inserted into the rectum or via the cystoscope into the bladder for better evaluation of deep anatomy. This application may also be used to control the placement of radium or caesium. Finally, interesting attempts are being made to extract more information from the ultrasound echoes to provide quantitative indices that may improve differential diagnostic limitations and allow a better assessment of the progress of malignancy than just simple gross anatomical changes. This research field is known as tissue characterisation.

Computerised X-Ray Tomography

Principles

Computerised X-ray tomography (CT) employs conventional X-rays but used in a novel way to produce tomograms with very high contrast differences in X-ray attenuation as small as 0·5% being detected. The scanner employs an X-ray source mounted on a moving arm, a narrow collimated beam being directed towards a detector on the opposite side of the frame. The whole assembly is progressively rotated through 180°. Multiple measurements are made to give a series of some 180 attenuated readings at different angles. These data are computer analysed to produce a back-projected reconstruction of the attenuated readings within the slice.

The technology is relatively expensive and involves exposure to X-ray. It produces a series of transaxial tomograms which show all types of tissue from bone, soft tissues to gas-containing organs in exquisite detail. Where contrast is high (more than 10%), resolution down to 1 mm is possible in the pelvis. Conventional X-ray contrast agents can be used to delineate structures such as the bladder, gut loops and the vaginal vault. Realtime scanning is not possible but tomographic angiograms can be produced by rapid scans taken after an intravenous bolus of contrast.

To obtain a pelvic CT, the patient is prepared with dilute oral and rectal contrast (2% gastrograffin) to outline gut loops which could otherwise be confused with soft tissue masses. The position of the vagina

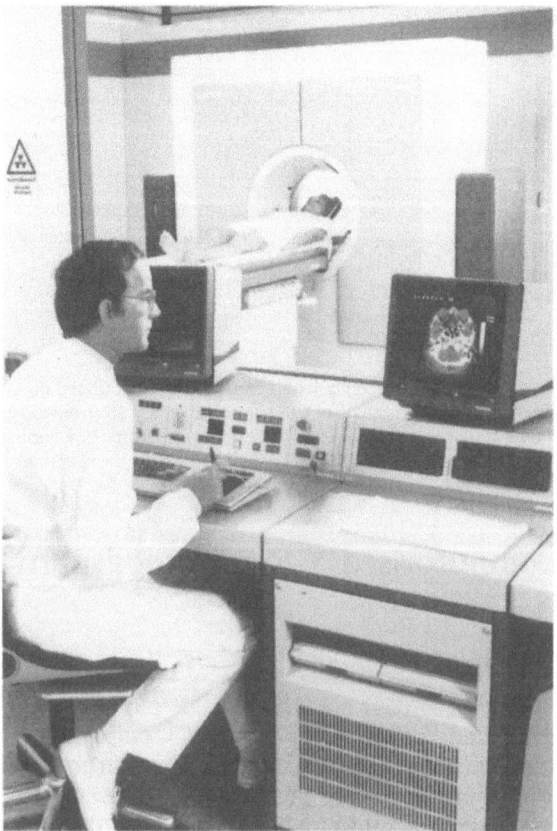

Fig. 5.17. A computerised X-ray tomography scanner (Siemans Somatom DR).

is indicated by the insertion of a tampon (the contained air providing contrast with the surrounding soft tissues). The patient lies on a couch which slides into the scanner (Fig. 5.17). She needs to be able to lie flat and still for about 20–30 min.

The resulting images are viewed on a TV monitor, being presented after a delay of a few seconds. Within each slice a range of densities is present from bone to gas. By altering the window width the radiologist selects the optimum setting to display either soft tissue or bony details. The actual density within the region of interest can be measured (given in Houndsfield units) and allows an accurate distinction between fat, fluid, soft tissue, bone and gas. Each image is recorded on film and the original data can be stored on magnetic tape so that the density information can be recalled subsequently. The quantitative nature of the CT images is in striking contrast with the subjectivity of ultrasound images.

Computerised X-ray tomography images are degraded by patient movement and by metallic objects within the scanning field. This means that examinations in patients with surgical clips can be difficult to interpret and in the patient with a metallic hip prosthesis the whole pelvis can be obscured by artefacts. Otherwise CT can be relied on to give good images even in the obese where ultrasound often fails. Scars and drains do not pose a problem and while a filled bladder is an advantage it is not essential, as it is for ultrasound.

Normal Findings

Normal pelvic anatomy is displayed in a series of cross sections (Walsh 1983). The uterus, cervix and vagina are clearly seen as soft tissue structures lying behind the bladder. The pelvic side walls are well seen and the relationship of the pelvic organs to muscle and bone clearly demonstrated. In general, all soft tissue structures have similar density, bowel loops being identified by the contrast medium that has been administered. The iliac vessels also have soft tissue density and are identified by their characteristic relationship to the psoas and the piriformis muscles. Pelvic lymph nodes are grouped round the vascular bundles and are classified accordingly. Nodes of diameter greater than 1·5 cm are considered to be abnormal. Occasionally difficulty arises in differentiation between a prominent vessel and an enlarged group of lymph nodes. In these instances intravenous injection of contrast is useful to delineate the vascular anatomy. Whereas with ultrasound the normal ovaries are routinely identified this is not possible even with the most recent CT scanners. However, the normal ureters are frequently picked out as they cross the pelvis into the bladder. The outline of the uterus is clearly seen with CT but internal detail is better appreciated following intravenous contrast injection as normal myometrium exhibits intense enhancement due to its high blood flow.

Applications

The special value of CT lies in its ability to demonstrate pelvic soft tissues together with their muscular and bony relations. This is especially useful in evaluating mass lesions particularly in malignancy. In general ultrasound should be the first examination for such patients, with CT reserved for problems where ultrasound is equivocal or unsatisfactory (Oldham 1983; van Doorn et al. 1985).

Pelvic masses are well displayed by CT and it has a particular value in characterising normal structures that may be confused on ultrasound. The pelvic kidney is an example where ultrasound can mislead and bowel loops, though sometimes posing a problem for both techniques, are more easily recognised on CT. A further important example is gas-containing abscesses. These are obvious on CT but on ultrasound they may simulate gas-filled bowel and so be missed (Ott et al. 1983; Arger and Colman 1983).

Malignant Tumours

Computerised X-ray tomography has a useful role in the staging of endometrial carcinoma, primary diagnosis usually being made on curettage (Ott et al. 1983; Arger and Colman 1983). The detection of tumour depends upon the relative lack of perfusion compared with the normal uterus. Intravenous contrast increases the attenuation of the uterus and thus enhances the contrast between it and the tumour. CT has an accuracy of 88% in staging compared with 72% by clinical staging (Balfe et al. 1983), and this is especially reliable in more advanced tumours. Cystoscopy is more accurate in assessing bladder involvement and ultrasound is better suited for determining uterine length which may be underestimated on CT. Pelvic and retroperitoneal lymphadenopathy can also be detected at the same examination. Distant metastases to the liver and lungs can be detected by CT. The sensitivity for detection of lymph node metastases within the pelvis by CT ranges between 73% and 80%, with a specificity of 92%. Lymphangiography is more sensitive (75%–90% with a specificity of 57%–87%). The advantage of lymphangiography

over CT is its ability to detect small deposits in nodes of normal size. The ability of lymphangiography to display the internal nodal structure allows reactive hyperplasia to be distinguished from metastases.

Similar considerations apply to carcinoma of the cervix where conventional methods are best suited to diagnosis but CT is helpful in staging, especially in FIGO stage IIIB and IVB tumours. The CT appearance of tumours comprises enlargement of the cervix with hypodense areas which fail to enhance after intravenous contrast. Occasionally the uterine cavity is seen to be fluid filled due to obstruction of the cervix (Fig. 5.18). Paramedial extension is seen as whispy, soft tissue densities extending into the fat or as soft tissue mass. Spread to the pelvic side walls is best appreciated with CT. The sensitivity of CT in the detection of pelvic lymphadenopathy is about 75% while that of lymphangiography approaches 90%. As with endometrial carcinoma, a negative CT does not exclude metastases and in these instances lymphangiography is required and has the advantage that if a Wertheim's hysterectomy is performed, the surgeon can identify particularly suspicious nodes that should be excised. Intraoperative screening following lymphangiography also allows a more complete lymphadenectomy.

In both endometrial and cervical cancer CT plays a major role in planning radical radiotherapy, since not only does it show the tumour and the sensitive normal tissue in relation to the bony skeleton, it also gives a direct reading of the X-ray attenuation values which can be incorporated into the radiotherapy plan. Furthermore it provides all these data in digital form that allows direct transfer to the planning computer (Walsh 1983). CT is also useful in detecting recurrent tumour, whether local or distant, although the differentiation between radiation fibrosis and recurrence may be difficult. There is a reasonable expectation that nuclear magnetic resonance imaging will allow this distinction to be made.

CT is not reliable in staging early carcinoma of the ovary, although it is very useful in determining spread. Deposits of down to 3 mm in diameter in the liver or lungs are detectable whilst deposits of larger than 2 cm in the peritoneum can also be detected. The typical appearance of the primary tumour, as cystic masses, often septated with thick irregular walls, are similar to those demonstrated on ultrasound (Butler et al. 1984; van Doorn et al. 1985) (Fig. 5.19). Spread to peritoneal surfaces gives plaques of tumours along the anterior abdominal wall (Fig. 5.20). The CT appearance of cystic pelvic masses, ascites, omental disease and liver deposits are so characteristic that a confident diag-

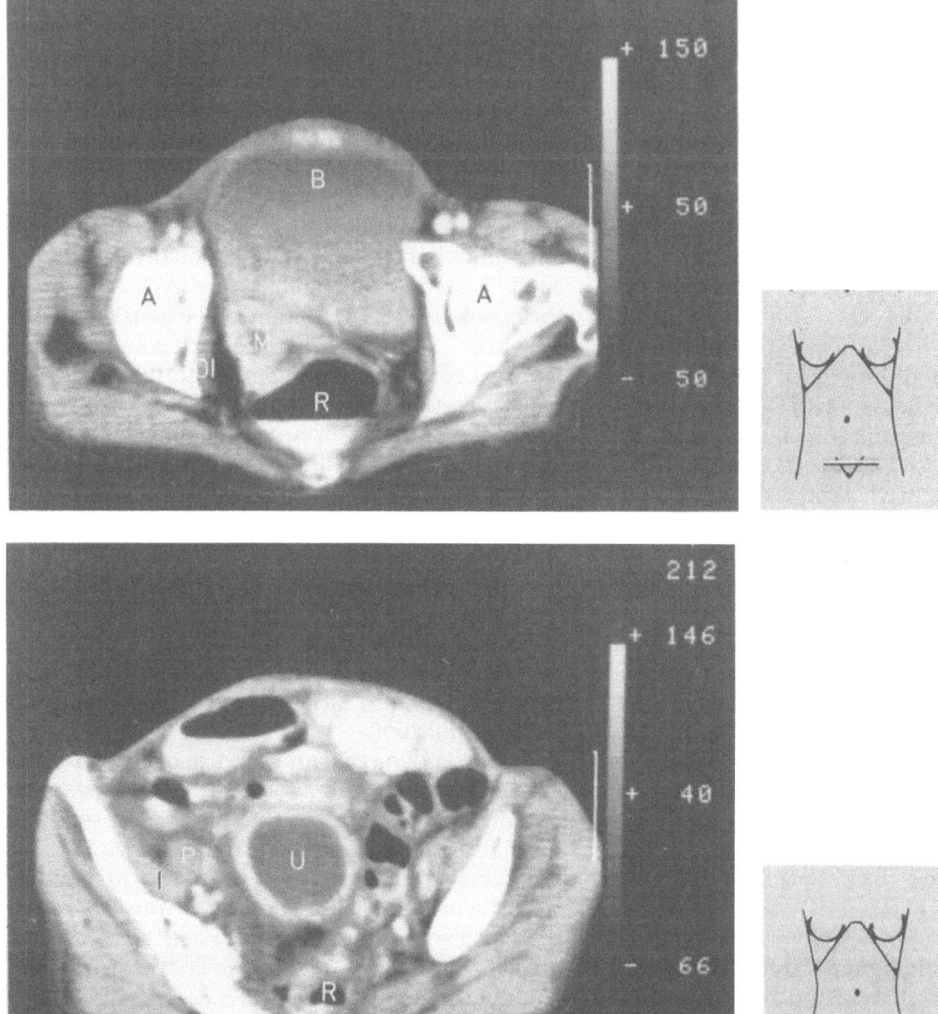

Fig. 5.18a, b. A CT scan of a patient with carcinoma of the cervix. The irregular mass is well seen. The cavity of the uterus is expanded with endometrial fluid **b**. Anterior to the uterus bowel loops containing contrast are seen. *A*, acetabulum; *B*, bladder; *I*, iliacus muscle; *M*, mass; *OI*, obturator internus muscle; *R*, rectum; *U*, uterus.

nosis of ovarian cancer can be made in a patient with unknown primary. A similar appearance is common in recurrences where both ultrasound and CT form a useful complement to laparoscopy.

Benign Disease

Fibroids are the commonest cause of an enlarged uterus (apart from pregnancy) and are frequently detected incidentally. As on ultrasound they produce a confusing range of appearances and may simulate malignancy. Typically they form rounded, well-circumscribed masses either distorting the outline of the uterus or impinging on the uterine cavity (Fig. 5.21). Categorisation into subserous, submucus or intramural can easily be made. On the unenhanced CT scan, fibroids may appear as homogeneous soft tissue densities or may contain high-density flecks due to calcification or low-density lesions due to necrosis or haemorrhage. Following intravenous contrast they may enhance uniformly or show regions of diminished contrast

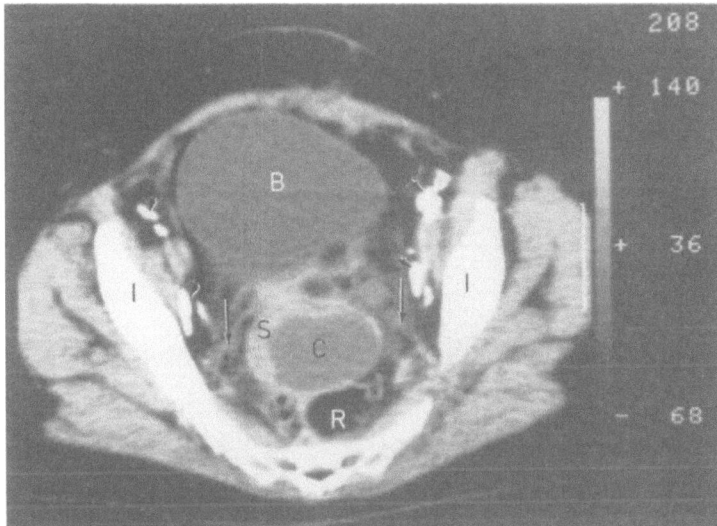
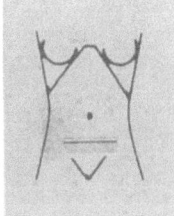

Fig. 5.19. A CT scan of a patient with carcinoma of the ovary. This scan taken through the level of the false pelvis shows the irregular tumour posterior to the bladder with both solid and cystic elements. Note the fine strands of tumour tissue spreading posterolaterally to the pelvic side walls (*arrows*). The *arrowheads* point to the external iliac node groups which are dense due to contrast from a recent lymphogram. The internal iliac nodes are not highlighted in this way because they do not lie in the drainage path of the foot injection site. *B*, bladder; *C*, cystic component of tumour; *I*, iliac bone; *R*, rectum; *S*, solid component of the tumour.

depending on blood flow. Pedunculated fibroids contrast depending on blood flow. Pedunculated fibroids may pose a difficult problem as they simulate extrauterine masses. Sarcomatous degeneration can only be detected if there is frank invasion. Similarly endometrial carcinoma can have the same appearance as fibroids unless there is extension beyond the uterus.

Simple ovarian cysts appear as rounded lesions of near-water density seen in relation to the uterus. Features are similar to those observed on ultrasound, which is the primary imaging technique

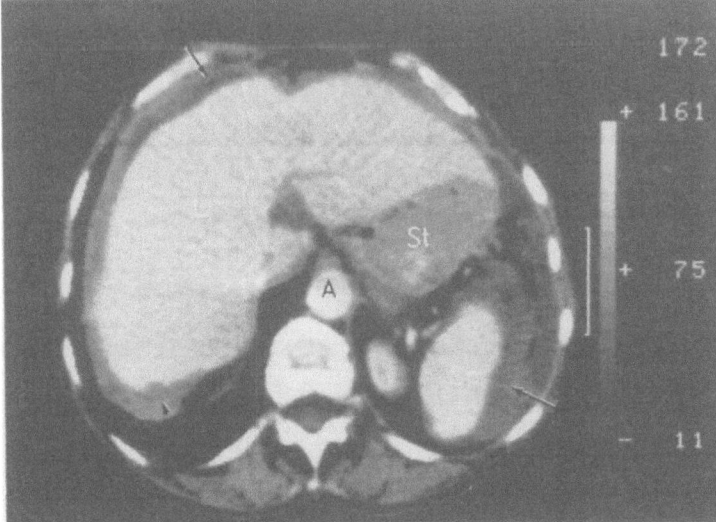
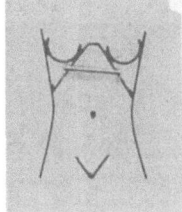

Fig. 5.20. A CT scan illustrating peritoneal spread from carcinoma of the ovary. In this upper abdominal section, ascites is seen around the liver and spleen (*arrows*) but there are also plaques of solid tumour on the parietal peritoneum one of which (*arrowhead*) is eroding the posterior surface of the liver. *A*, aorta; *L*, liver; *Sp*, spleen; *S*, stomach.

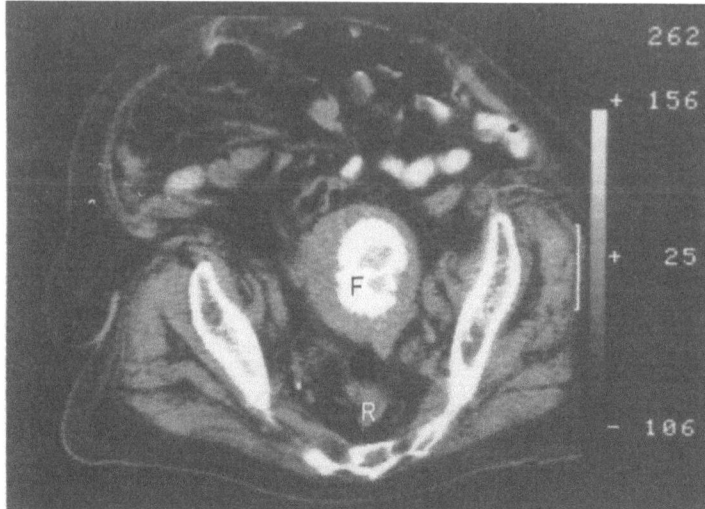

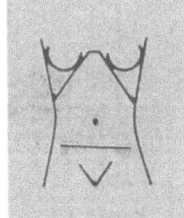

Fig. 5.21. A CT scan of a fibroid uterus. Calcification in a leiomyoma gives high attenuation numbers and a characteristic appearance on CT. In its absence the distinction between benign and malignant uterine masses is more difficult. *F*, fibroid; *R*, rectum.

although they are often encountered incidentally on CT scanning.

Dermoids are particularly well demonstrated on CT. They have a characteristic appearance as their fat components provide striking contrast with the other soft tissue and calcium-containing elements that they often contain (Fig. 5.22). Ultrasound tends to underestimate the size of the lesions as the fatty and calcific components are not readily appreciated and CT is more revealing.

The diagnosis of pelvic inflammatory disease is usually made clinically and if more information is required ultrasound is the method of choice (Arger and Colman 1983). CT has a role in those patients who remain difficult to evaluate with ultrasound where accurate localisation of an abscess is required for drainage. This can be performed under local anaesthesia in the majority of patients. As the whole cross-sectional anatomy is displayed the safest route for drainage can be determined and accurate

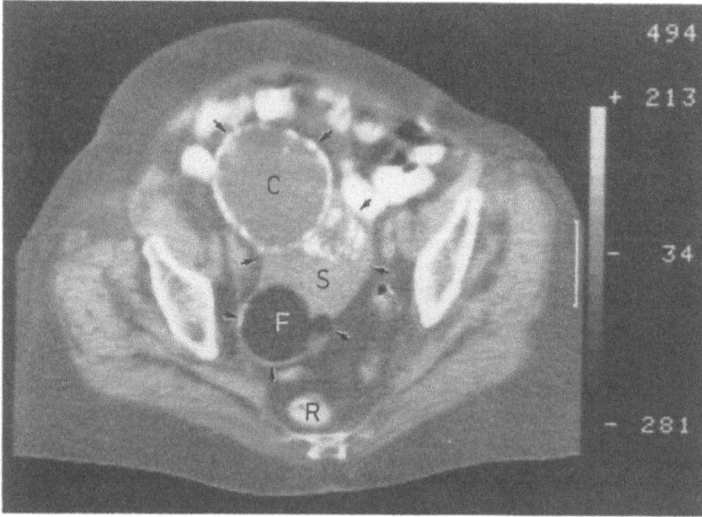

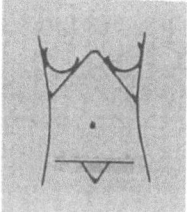

Fig. 5.22. A CT scan of a dermoid. A variety of tissue types is a characteristic feature of a dermoid (*arrowed*). This example contains calcified, solid (*S*), cystic (*C*) and fatty (*F*) elements. *R*, rectum.

measurements of the depth of the lesion are possible. Follow-up studies with either ultrasound or CT can be used to monitor the resolution of the abscess and allow a decision as to the most appropriate time to remove the drainage tube.

Isotope Scanning

Principles

The prime role of isotopes in medicine lies in the functional information they provide in metabolism, the isotope being used as a tracer. Images that display the spatial distribution of these functions can be obtained by scanning the patient after administration of the isotope. A fairly familiar example is thyroid scanning to assess the distribution of radioiodine in nodules. Non-physiological agents can also be exploited, as in lung scanning for pulmonary embolism, where albumin is prepared in particulate form for intravenous injection, the particular size being such as to embolise in lung capillaries and thus provide a perfusion image. The usual isotope for such studies is 99m-technetium, which is also employed in liver scanning. Here another particulate preparation is used, colloidal sulphur, the size being chosen so that reticuloendothelial phagocytosis into the Kupffer cells occurs. As with lung scanning, lesions are indicated by defects in the scan and abnormalities are non-specific although the method is suitable for routine use.

The images are usually formed on a gamma camera rather than a scanner, cameras being much faster. A gamma camera is equipped with an array of gamma photon detectors (usually 37) located behind a drilled lead block (the collimator)—rather in the manner of an insect's eye. Computer processing of the signals from the detector allows the reconstruction of images with resolution of around 1–2 cm using small radiation doses.

These are known as planar images (Fig. 5.23a) because, as with X-ray, all the information in a volume is displayed in one plane as viewed from one direction. Tomograms can be obtained in exactly the same manner as with X-rays for CT scanning, by reconstruction from information obtained from numerous projections. This is known as ECAT (emission computer assisted tomography) scanning. It utilises conventional gamma-emitting isotopes with extra mechanisms to rotate the camera and special computing programs.

Another approach to isotope tomography uses a different class of isotope, the positron emitters, and is known as PET (positron emission tomography) (Bryan et al. 1983). Here the determination of the position of the isotope in the body relies on the curious decay mode of the positron which, on contact with an electron, its antiparticle, disappears by annihilation, leaving only a pair of electrons of closely defined energy that travel away from each other at exactly 180°. A pair of photon detectors is positioned on either side of the patient and linked to a fast timing circuit that signals a count only when a pair of photons is detected at exactly the same time. The detectors are large and the availability of positron-emitting isotopes is restricted because they derive from cyclotrons and have short useful lives (of the order of minutes or a few hours). PET scanning gives remarkable information on the physiology of the living brain, the effects of mental or visual stimulation being readily apparent. Routine application will depend upon on the development of cheaper detectors and of generators for producing positron-emitting isotopes in a more convenient form. There is rapid progress on both of these fronts (Robinson and De Crespigny 1983).

Application

In gynaecology, apart from the use of isotopes to screen the liver for metastases, routine applications have been limited. However, with the development of specific antitumour antibodies that can be labelled, there is the prospect of improved early detection of tumours especially in carcinoma of the ovary. This could be important in the screening, staging and detection of recurrence (Deland and Goldenberg 1985; Light 1985). Preliminary work has used placental alkaline phosphatase (Hricak et al. 1983) and cell surface components of milk (Light 1985) from which monoclonal antibodies are raised. These are radiolabelled and injected. Scanning at 48 h shows uptake in tumour masses, some of which were unsuspected clinically and had not been detected on CT scanning (Fig. 5.24a,b). Improvements in antibody specificity and availability are expected to enhance the usefulness of the technique. Labelled with therapeutic concentrations of isotopes such as ^{131}I they are already showing promise in specific, directed radiotherapy (Saunders et al. 1983). It may also be possible to develop antibodies specific for uterine tumours even perhaps for non-malignant processes.

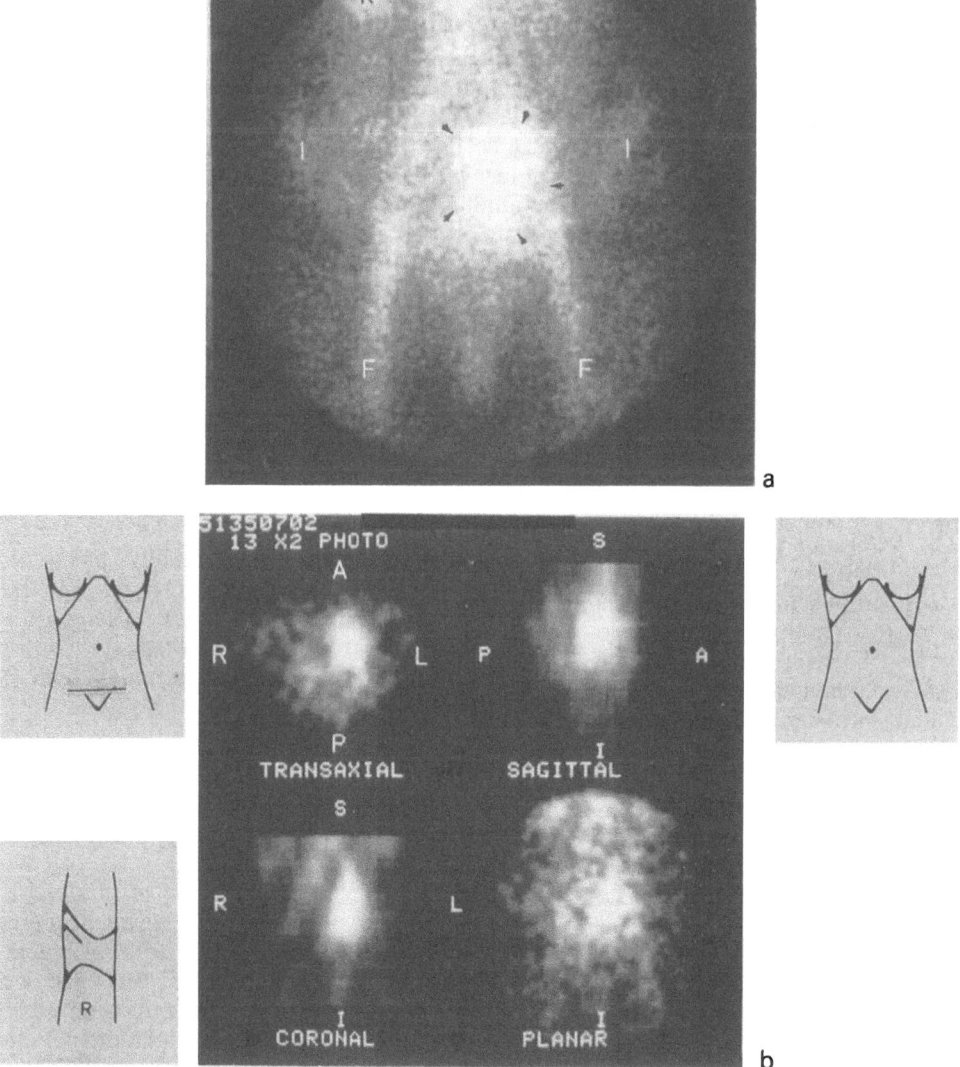

Fig. 5.23a, b. A monoclonal antibody scan of a patient with carcinoma of the ovary. A monoclonal antibody against cell surface markers (M8), tagged with ^{111}In, was injected 14 h before these pelvic scans. The anterior view in **a** shows uptake in the pelvis in the mid-line and to the left (*arrowheads*). The precise distribution is better appreciated in the SPECT tomograms in **b**. *A*, aorta; *F*, femoral arteries; *I*, iliac bones; *K*, kidneys. (Images courtesy of Dr. Bob Ott, Royal Marsden Hospital, London, England.)

Magnetic Resonance Imaging

Principles

The magnetic resonance signal derives from the fact that the atomic nucleus can behave as a minute magnet. In atoms with an even number of protons and neutrons the north and south poles are bal-anced but in those with odd numbers there is a net magnetic force or moment (Balfe et al. 1983). The force varies with the element and its isotopes and it is fortunate that hydrogen, which is abundant in biological tissues, has a particularly large magnetic moment.

If hydrogen is placed in the magnetic field, its nuclei (protons) tend to line up along the field. If energised with an appropriate electromagnetic

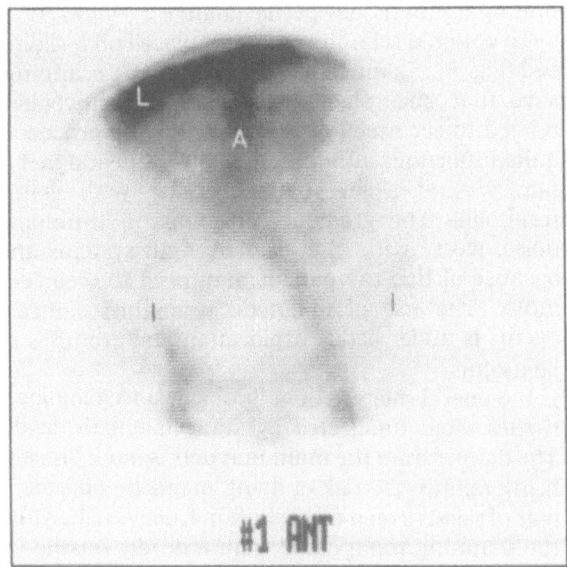

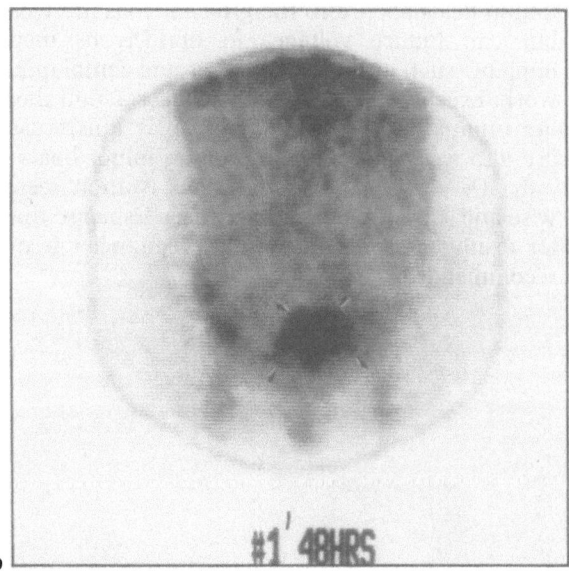

Fig. 5.24a, b. An MABS scan of a patient with carcinoma of the ovary. A monoclonal antibody raised against placental alkaline phosphatase was labelled with ^{123}I for these scans. The blood pool is visualised in the early view soon after injection **a**. By 48 h **b** there is an intense uptake into the pelvic tumour (*arrowheads*). If the diagnostic isotope used here is replaced by ^{131}I, MABS-directed radiotherapy can be performed. *A*, aorta; *I*, iliac bones; *L*, liver. (Images courtesy of Dr. A. Epenetos, Hammersmith Hospital, London.)

impulse, in this case a radio pulse, they can be flipped into reverse orientation. The frequency of the pulse required for a particular atomic nucleus is highly critical and depends on the strength of the applied field.

The energised protons tend to revert to the lower energy orientation (a process called relaxation) and as they do so they release their stored energy as radio waves. This is the magnetic resonance signal. The rate of relaxation is determined by the environment of the protons, that is the physical and chemical state of the tissue containing them. Relaxation constants are measured in two planes, along and across the direction of the magnetic field (T1 and T2 respectively). These principles have formed the basis of sophisticated laboratory techniques over several decades for the physicochemical analysis of biochemical samples. To obtain images a further step must be added in the form of a small biasing magnetic field that alters from negative to positive progressively along or across the body. When the perfectly tuned exciting radio pulse is applied, only those protons that lie in the plane where the biasing magnetic field is zero will be in tune and therefore only these are able to absorb the radiation. These are then energised and will emit the resonance signal while all other regions have been detuned and are silent. Thus the magnetic resonance signal comes from a plane whose thickness is determined by the purity of the radiofrequency pulse used and whose position and orientation can be controlled simply and rapidly by adjusting the biasing or gradient magnetic field which is produced by a set of electromagnetic coils.

To reconstruct a tomogram the magnetic resonance signals from the defined plane are given a spacial tag by applying another magnetic gradient during the relaxation phase. This controls the frequency of the emitted radio signals, protons in a region of the slice with higher field giving a higher frequency signal, those in a lower field giving a lower frequency. Frequency separation of the composite signal allows the spatial position of the protons to be determined along lines of site in the body. The two gradients, one applied with energising pulse the other applied during the reception of the signal, are usually arranged to lie at right angles to each other, so that, for a transverse section the gradient during the pulse cycle would lie along the patient while the relaxation period gradient would lie transversely in the plane to the image. The frequency separation then gives signals in the anteroposterior lines across the planes to be tomographed. Now the entire process is repeated but with the received gradient rotated by a few degrees to yield another set of measurements along lines. Repeating this gives computer sets of projections. By using the same mathematical reconstruction process as for X-ray CT, a tomogram is produced.

In practice the main magnet has to be powerful and of high uniformity. So called low-field magnets have strengths around 1 500 G and are usually electromagnetic coils of the solenoid type. High fields require superconducting coils and operate in the range of 15 000 G (the conventional unit is the Tesla = 10 000 G). At these strengths protons resonate at 6 and 60 million cycles/s respectively. The radio pulses are very short, in the range of microseconds, and the returning signals take between 0·2 and 2 s along the field T1 and 0·05–0·2 s along the field T2 to decrease to half the initial value. This determines the maximum pulsed repetition rate and means that examination times range from 10 min to 1 h. Magnetic resonance scanners are thus very expensive and slow. Their advantage apart from the obvious one of flexibility of imaging planes lies in the differing signals produced by the different normal and pathological tissues. This is due mainly to their different content of unbound water which determines the signal strength. Inflammatory and malignant tissues for example have a higher free water content than normal tissue. Secondly the two relaxation times, T1 and T2, are very sensitive to the physicochemical state of the water and this varies with normal and pathological states. For example, it is possible to distinguish between oxygenated and deoxygenated blood in the two sides of the heart. Magnetic resonance imaging (MRI) offers the prospect of deter-

mining useful tissue-specific changes.

To obtain a scan the patient is placed on a sliding bed (Fig. 5.25), much like that used in CT scanning, save that once she is in position all movement related to slice section is electronic. The process is quite innocuous although the bore of the magnet is narrow and a few patients suffer with claustrophobia. The gradient coils make a thumping noise, worse with high-field strength systems and because of this the patient may need to wear ear muffs. The use of magnetic resonance contrast agents is under active exploration and promises to be useful.

In general safety is not a problem since biological tissues seem unaffected by static magnetic fields. The danger from the main magnets is more prosaic, being mainly the risk of flying magnetic objects. A pair of scissors on a resuscitation trolley rushed into the scanning room could form a deadly missile for the patient lying in a powerful magnet! The fluctuation fields applied to the gradient coils are weak but can induce voltages in non-ferrous metal implants such as pins, pacemaker and dental metal work. Except for upsetting pacemaker action these are unimportant. The radiofrequency pulses used are also weak and seem to produce minor heating only. Despite these considerations caution seems wise and safety guidelines have been issued so that, for example, scanning normal pregnancies is not recommended.

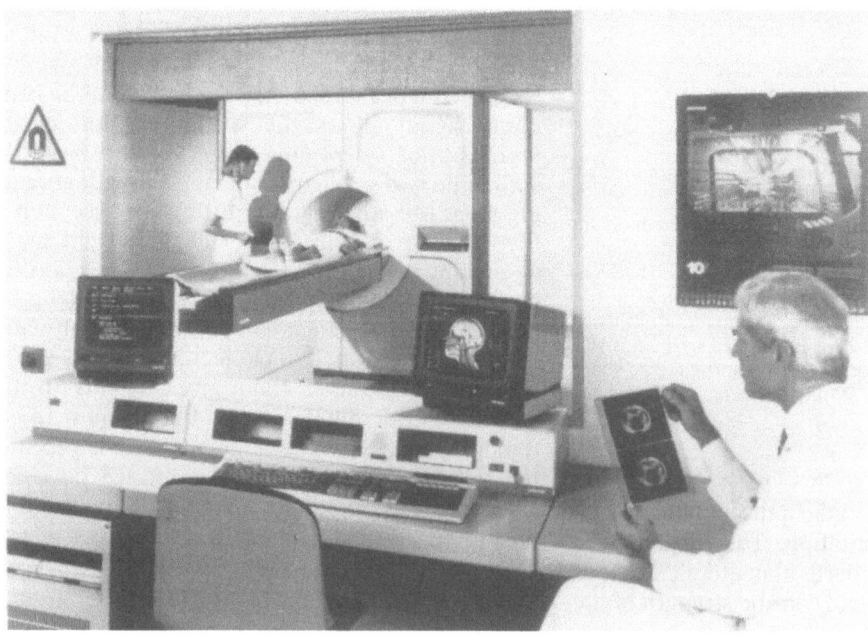

Fig. 5.25. A magnetic resonance imaging scanner (Siemans Magnatom).

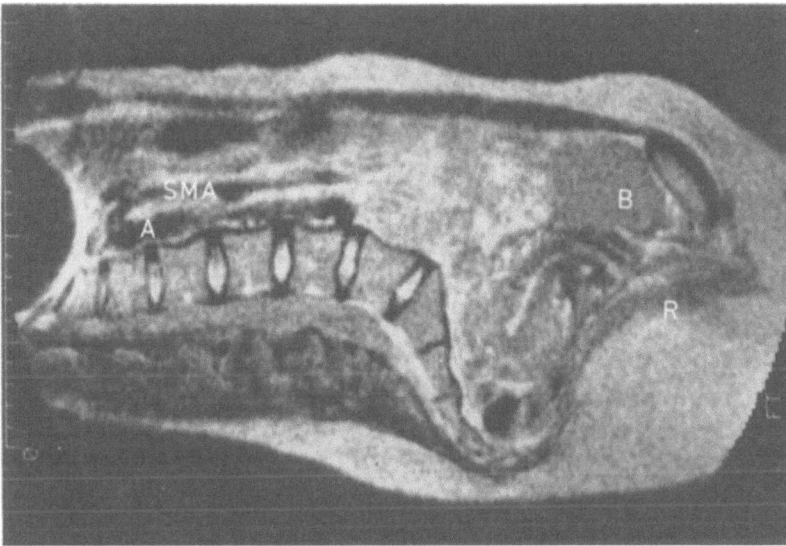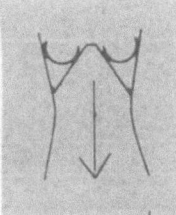

Fig. 5.26. A magnetic resonance scan of a normal pelvis. In this sagittal MRI scan of the pelvis, the retroverted uterus can be seen with a strong signal from the endometrium and a weaker signal from the hyperaemic subendometrial layer. Note the detail displayed in the spine and abdominal soft tissues. *A*, aorta; *B*, bladder; *Cx*, cervix; *P*, pubic symphysis; *R*, rectum; *S*, sacrum; *SMA*, superior mesenteric artery; *U*, uterus; *V*, vagina.

Normal Findings

The flexible tomography planes of MRI allow display of normal organs in their optimal orientation, as with ultrasound (Bryan et al. 1983; Jones et al. 1980; Walsh 1983) (Fig. 5.26). MR images show good differentiation between normal tissues, with fat giving the strongest signal (displayed as white) and bone, with minimal water content giving no signal (displayed as black). Soft tissues span the intermediate shades. The uterus is clearly seen in sagittal section and it is possible to make out the cyclical endometrial changes. The cervix is distinct from the corpus while the vagina, urinary bladder and rectum are clearly imaged. In transverse section the uterus and pelvic wall muscles are displayed as well as the bony framework, which is imaged by virtue of the marrow since bone itself gives no signal. Bowel loops are easily displayed. The ovaries may be imaged as well as the larger blood vessels. In general the images are clear and for the most part free of artefacts. They have a similarity to cadaver sections with a clear differentiation between the tissues of different types.

Application

The range of pelvic disease studied to date is rather limited (Butler et al. 1984). Dermoids and simple ovarian cysts are clearly shown and can be distinguished while fibroids and cervical tumours have been reported as detectable (Fig. 5.27). In a few cases MR images have shown local invasion by tumours more clearly than CT and show promise of being able to distinguish radiation fibrosis from recurrent tumour. Endometriosis has a spectrum of appearances, no doubt corresponding to the state of the contained fluid, with strong signals from blood products being reported. MR images, while superficially resembling CT and ultrasound tomograms, often reveal other features, though at present not enough systematic work has been performed to allow a realistic assessment of its definitive role.

Acknowledgements. Dr. Martin Leach kindly reviewed the section on magnetic resonance imaging. The isotope applications were discussed with Dr. Bob Ott, who also supplied one of the figures.

 We are extremely grateful to Professor Campbell for permission to publish the updated figues on the King's College Hospital ovarian screening programme.

MRI Images were kindly supplied by Mr. MC Powell. They were obtained with the University of Nottingham scanner, which is supported by the Medical Research Council.

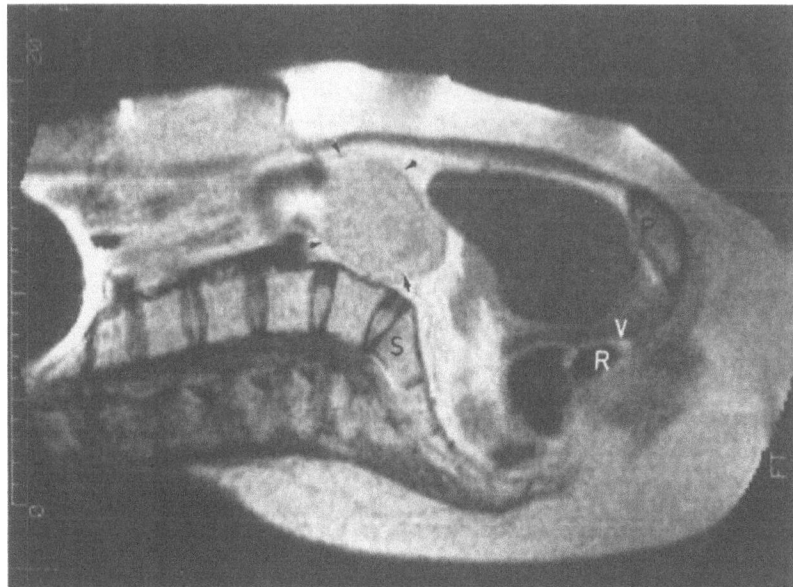

a

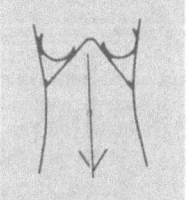

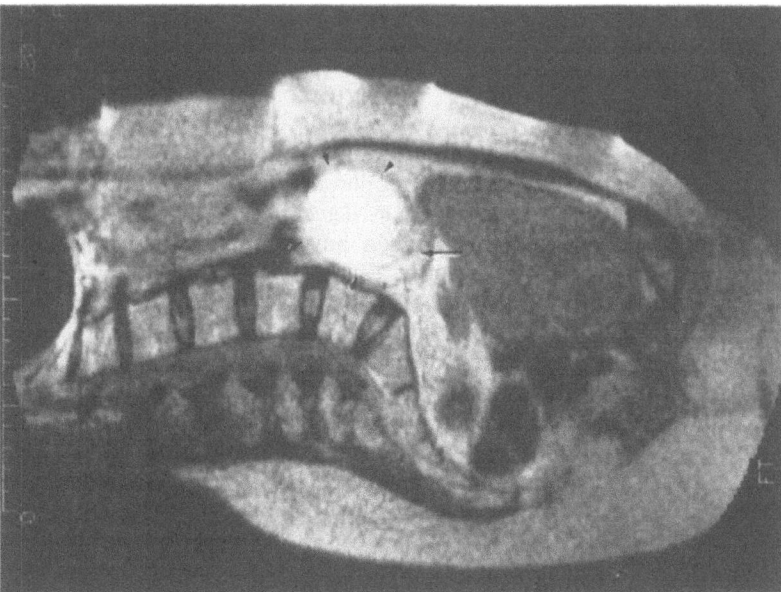

b

Fig. 5.27a, b. MRI scan of an ovarian cyst. This pair of scans in the same sagittal plane were obtained using different pulse sequences. The patient has had a hysterectomy. A cystic mass is shown (*arrowheads*). In scan **a** only slight heterogeneity is apparent but the different imaging parameters in **b** reveal a solid element (*arrow*) in the base of the lesion corresponding with a malignant portion within the cyst. Again note the exquisite display of anatomy throughout the abdomen. *P*, pubic symphysis; *R*, rectum; *S*, sacrum; *V*, vagina.

References

Balfe DM, van Dyke J, Lee JT, Weyman PJ, McLennan BL (1983) Computed tomography in malignant endometrial lesions. J Comp Assist Tomog 7:677–681

Beaney RP (1984) Positron emission tomography in the study of human tumours. Semin Nucl Med 14:324–341

Berland LL, Lawson TL, Albarelli JN, Foley WD (1982) Ultrasonic diagnosis of ovarian and adnexal disease. Semin Ultrasound 1:17–29

Bryan PJ, Butler HE, Li Puma RP, Haaga JR, El Yousef SJ, Resnick MI, Cohen AM, Malviya VK, Nelson AD, Clampitt M, et al. (1983) NMR scanning of the pelvis. Am J Rentgenol 141:1111–1118

Butler H, Bryan PJ, LiPuma JP, Cohen AM, El Yousef S, Andriole JG, Lieberman J (1984) Magnetic resonance imaging in the abnormal female pelvis. Am J Rentgenol 143:1259–1266

Campbell S, Goessens L, Goswamy R, Whitehead, MI (1982) Real time ultrasonography for determination of ovarian morphology and volume: a possible early screening test for ovarian cancer. Lancet 1:425–426

Davies JO, Davies ER, Howe K, Jackson PC, Pitcher EM, Sadowski CS, Stirrat GM, Sunderland CA (1985) Radio-nuclide imaging of ovarian tumours with ^{123}I labelled monoclonal antibodies. Br J Obstet Gynaecol 92:277–286

DeLand FH, Goldenberg DM (1985) Diagnosis and treatment with radio-labelled antibodies. Semin Nucl Med 15:2–12

DeLand M, Fried A, van Nagell JR, Donaldson ES (1979) Ultrasonography in the diagnosis of tumours of the ovaries. Surg Gynecol Obstet 148:346–348

Epenetos AA, Britton K, Mather S, Shepherd J, Granowska M, Taylor-Papadimitriou J, Nimmon OC, Durbin H, Hawkins LR, Malpas JS, Bodmer WF (1982) Targetting of iodine ^{123}I labelled tumour associated monoclonal antibodies to tumour of patients with ovarian, breast and gastrointestinal tumours. Lancet 2:999–1005

Hackeloer BJ, Sallam HN (1983) Ultrasound scanning of ovarian follicles. Clin Obstet Gynaecol 10:603–621

Hackeloer BJ (1985) Follicular size assessment by ultrasound. In: Sanders RC, James AE (eds) The principles and practice of ultrasonography in obstetrics and gynecology, 3rd edn. Appleton-Century-Crofts, Connecticut, pp 517–530

Hricak H, Alpers C, Crooks LE, Sheldon PE (1983) Magnetic resonance imaging of the female pelvis. Am J Rentgenol 141:1119–1128

Jones TB, Fleischer AC, Danell JF, Lindsey AM, James AE Jr (1980) Sonographic characteristics of congenital uterine anomalies and associated pregnancy. J Clin Ultrasound 8:435–437

Kadar N, De Vore G, Romero R (1981) Discriminatory HCG zone: its use in sonographic evaluation of ectopic pregnancy. Obstet Gynaecol 58:156–161

Kerr-Wilson R, Shingleton HM, Orr JW, Hatch KD (1984) The use of ultrasound and computed tomography scanning in the management of gynaecologic cancer patients. Gynaecol Oncol 18:54–61

Levitt RG, Sagel SS, Stanley RJ, Evens RG (1978) Computed tomography of the pelvis. Semin Roentgenol 13:193–200

Meire HB, Farrant P, Suha T (1984) Distinction of benign from malignant ovarian cysts by ultrasound. Br J Surg Gynecol Obstet 148:346–348

Oldham RK (1983) Monoclonal antibodies in cancer therapy. J Clin Oncol 1:582–590

Ott RJ, Bateman JE, Flesher AC, Flower MA, Leach MO, Webb S, Khan O, McCready VR (1983) Preliminary clinical images from a prototype positron camera. Br J Radiol 65:773–776

Robinson H (1975) The diagnosis of early pregnancy failure by sonar. Br J Obstet Gynaecol 82:849–853

Robinson H, De Crespigny LC (1983) Ectopic pregnancy. Clin Obstet Gynaecol 10:407–421

Sanders RC, McNeil BJ, Finberg HJ, Hessel SJ, Siegelman SS, Adams DF, Alderson PO, Abrams HL (1983) A prospective study of computed tomography and ultrasound in the detection and staging of pelvic masses. Radiology 146(2):439–442

Symonds EM, Perkins C, Pimm MV, Baldwin RW, Hardy JG, Williams DA (1985) Clinical implications of immuno-scintigraphy in patients with ovarian malignancy. Br J Obstet Gynaecol 92:270–276

Thickman D, Kressel H, Gussman D, Axel L, Hogan M (1984) Nuclear magnetic resonance imaging in gynaecology. J Obstet Gynaecol 149:835–840

van Doorn GA, Rozenboom AR, Dvorak JJ (1985) Primary diagnosis of gynaecological tumours by ultrasonography and computed tomography. Gynaecol Oncol 21.161–166

Winer CP, Bergman WB, Field C (1957) Combined intra- and extra-uterine pregnancy. Am J Obstet Gynecol 74:170–178

Winer CP (1981) The pseudogestational sac in ectopic pregnancy. Am J Obstet Gynecol 139:959–961

Further Reading

Arger PA, Colman BG (1983) "The pelvis". In: Joseph J, Cosgrove DO (eds) Ultrasound in inflammatory disease. Clinics in diagnostic ultrasound, vol 11. Churchill Livingstone, New York

Campbell S (ed) (1983) Ultrasound in obstetrics and gynaecology: recent advances. Clinical Obstetrics and Gynaecology, vol 10. Saunders, Bournemouth

Chudleigh P, Pearce JMF (1986) Obstetric ultrasound: how, why and when? Churchill Livingstone, Edinburgh

Jensen F (1984) Puncture of gynaecological masses. In: Holm HH, Kristen SEN (eds) Interventional ultrasound, Chap 17. Munksgaard, Copenhagen

Light G (ed) (1985) Monoclonal antibodies in cancer. Marcell Decker, New York

Nuclear Magnetic Resonance Scanning. Semin in Nuclear Medicine. Vol 13, 1983 (special issue)

Saunders RJ, James AE (1985) Principles and practice of ultrasonography in obstetrics and gynecology. 3rd edn. Appleton-Century-Croft, New York

Walsh JW (1983) "Pelvis". In: Greenberg M, Greenberg BM, Greenberg IM (eds) Essentials of body computed tomography. Saunders, Philadelphia

6 · Recent Advances in Anaesthesia and Analgesia

Anthony P. Rubin

Pathophysiology of Pain

Pain is a subjective experience arising from brain activity usually in response to stimulation or damage to body tissues. Impulses are transmitted from the periphery by at least two different types of nerve fibre: the A delta, which are $1-6\,m\mu$ in diameter, fast conducting and transmit the initial sharp pain; and the C, which are $0\cdot2-1\,m\mu$ in diameter, slower conducting and carry the dull, diffuse, more persistent pain which is felt a little later. Both fibres have their cell bodies in the dorsal root ganglion and then enter the dorsal horn of the spinal cord. Most enter via the dorsal root, although some afferent fibres do enter via the ventral route (Jordan 1984a). The A delta system passes through the nucleus proprius directly to the lateral spinothalamic tract, the thalamus and sensory cortex. The C fibre system has many connections in the substantia gelatinosa in the dorsal horn and then passes via an indirect ascending system through the reticular formation and periaqueductal grey matter to the medial nuclei of the thalamus and then to the cortex, hypothalamus and other areas which may be responsible for autonomic activity and emotion. The cortex appears to localise the site of the pain accurately, to judge its quality, to compare the stimulus with past experience, and to determine its emotional qualities.

Autonomic Nervous System and Pain

Autonomic stimuli from visceral and non-visceral structures pass along sympathetic nerves to the dorsal horn of the spinal cord. At that level there is probable interaction between autonomic and somatic input. Referred pain is felt in somatic distribution, probably because the cutaneous somatic innervation is more strongly represented at a cerebral level. This might explain why local anaesthetic infiltration of areas of referred pain and trigger points may control pain by reducing afferent input.

Theories of Pain

The specific theory suggests that each sensory phenomenon has specific receptors and pathways. In the intensity theory, there are not specific receptors, but the intensity of any sensory stimulus may exceed a threshold level and be interpreted as pain. The sensory receptors may be high-threshold mechanoreceptors or polymodal or other nociceptors (Jordan 1984a). The "gate" theory (Melzack and Wall 1965) describes modulation at the level of the substantia gelatinosa of the dorsal horn, depending on the balance of activity in the large and small afferent fibres and in descending pathways. An increase in large fibre activity, which may be produced by rubbing the injured part, transcutaneous nerve stimulation or acupuncture, may close the gate and prevent the onward transmission of pain impulses. Descending control systems modulate the excitability of cells which transmit injury signals (Wall 1978). Focal stimulation of the periaqueductal grey matter produces a profound analgesia in rats without any other sensory or motor deficit (Reynolds 1969). This analgesia can be partially reversed by the opiate antagonist, naloxone (Akil et al. 1976).

Opioid Peptides

Enkephalin (Hughes et al. 1975) is naturally occurring, has morphine-like actions and is antagonised similarly by naloxone. It is one of the endogenous opioid peptides, which are widely distributed in the central nervous system, have a very short half-life and appear to be neurotransmitters (Hughes and Kosterlitz 1983; Akil et al. 1984). There is also a hormone released by the pituitary gland called β-lipotropin and its terminal portion, which has potent opioid activity, is β-endorphin. The latter is only found in the anterior pituitary, the medial thalamus and the central brain stem, and has a longer half-life than enkephalin (Pinnock 1985). There is considerable evidence now for the role of the opioid peptides in pain modulation. Firstly stimulation of the periaqueductal grey matter increases opioid concentration in the cerebrospinal fluid and decreases pain. Secondly, chronic pain patients with a clear diagnosis often have decreased cerebrospinal fluid opioid levels; and thirdly patients with pain of no obvious organic cause often have normal cerebrospinal fluid opioid activity.

Opioid peptides may well be involved in physiological effects other than pain modulation, e.g. on the cardiovascular system and particularly the shock state, the respiratory system, perhaps including sleep apnoea and sudden infant death syndrome, the neuroendocrine system, and possibly the limbic system in relation to behaviour and the temperature-regulating mechanisms (Pinnock 1985).

Opioid Receptors

It is now established that there are opioid receptors in the spinal cord and supraspinal structures, including the thalamus, periaqueductal grey matter and raphe nuclei. There are at least four subtypes of opioid receptors called mu, kappa, delta and sigma. The subject has recently been reviewed extensively (Rance 1983; Jordan 1985). Classical opioid agonist drugs seem to act mainly on mu receptors, but the exact role of each receptor has not been clearly established. The discovery of opioid peptides and receptors has led to the possibility of producing better analgesics with fewer side effects and of new pain therapies, in particular the spinal administration of opioids (Yaksh and Rudy 1976; Behar et al. 1979; Bullingham et al. 1984). Five-hydroxytryptamine, substance P, prostaglandins, gamma-aminobutyric acid (GABA) and several other substances probably also have important functions in the transmission, experience and modulation of pain.

Anaesthesia

Premedication

Certain trends in premedication are apparent. The further development of benzodiazepine anxiolytic drugs, and changing anaesthetic practice whereby analgesia is more often provided during surgery by opiate administration or regional anaesthesia, has resulted in opiate premedication becoming less essential.

The day patient requires rapid recovery from anaesthesia, and therefore premedication is often omitted. If particularly anxious, temazepam 20–30 mg may be administered orally, although this will prolong recovery. Inpatients undergoing procedures without postoperative pain are often premedicated only with an oral benzodiazepine. If postoperative pain is expected, then opiates are administered either as premedication or as part of the anaesthetic technique. The most popular opiates are still papaveretum, morphine or pethidine. Papaveretum and morphine are more effective sedatives and euphoriants, and stronger and longer-lasting analgesics than pethidine. Their main disadvantages are the risk of respiratory depression and the relative high incidence of nausea and vomiting.

Anticholinergic drugs are often included to dry secretions and to ensure some vagal blockade. Hyoscine is often used in patients under 65 years of age as it is sedative and amnesic, and has antiemetic properties. It should not be used in elderly patients in whom it might cause confusion, nor in the presence of pain when it often causes restlessness. Atropine is the most effective anticholinergic and glycopyrrolate is an alternative. Hyoscine is given in a dose of 0·3–0·4 mg, atropine 0·5–0·6 mg and glycopyrrolate 0·2–0·4 mg.

General Anaesthesia

General anaesthesia is usually induced with a rapidly acting intravenous agent. Thiopentone or methohexitone, which are barbiturates, remain the most popular. In some centres etomidate is preferred, or occasionally the combination of a benzodiazepine such as midazolam or diazepam and a short-acting analgesic such as fentanyl or alfentanil. The maintenance of anaesthesia depends on the length and nature of the operation. Minor gynaecological surgery usually requires only light inhalational anaesthesia with nitrous oxide supplemented by halothane, enflurane or isoflurane. Alternatively the nitrous oxide may be supplemented by intravenous opiate analgesia or by intermittent injections of the induction agent. Termination of pregnancy is usually performed under general anaesthesia. Inhalational agents above a certain concentration may produce excessive relaxation of the pregnant uterus. Occasionally regional anaesthesia may be used with a paracervical block of 10 ml 1% lignocaine or prilocaine injected into the base of the broad ligament on each side. Careful technique is essential as the area is vascular and there is a risk of high blood levels of local anaesthetic which may be associated with inadequate analgesia and potential systemic toxicity. No local technique should be used in the absence of full facilities for resuscitation, and the presence of a doctor conversant with the pharmacology and toxicity of local anaesthetics and appropriate methods of resuscitation.

Anaesthesia for laparoscopy raises particular problems. Considerable muscular relaxation is required, the abdomen is distended with carbon dioxide and the patient is placed in a steep headdown position. These three factors necessitate endotracheal intubation and positive pressure ventilation in order to assure adequate oxygenation and carbon dioxide elimination, and also to prevent any risk of aspiration of gastric contents into the lungs. The muscular relaxation is usually achieved with a medium duration non-depolarising muscle relaxant, such as alcuronium, vecuronium or atracurium. Unconsciousness is maintained with nitrous oxide which should be supplemented by a low concentration of an inhalational agent, or an adequate dose of an opiate. At the end of the procedure the muscle relaxant will be reversed by neostigmine, the muscarinic effects (bradycardia,

increased secretions, bronchoconstriction, increased intestinal motility) being prevented by atropine. Suxamethonium, which is a short-acting depolarising muscle relaxant drug, produces intense relaxation and optimal conditions for endotracheal intubation, but is associated with a high incidence of muscle pains, and should be avoided wherever possible in patients undergoing minor and intermediate gynaecological procedures.

For major surgery, the surgeon requires an anaesthetised patient with adequate muscle relaxation and ideally a reduction in bleeding. The choice is between a balanced general anaesthetic including hypnosis (sleep), analgesia, and muscular relaxation or a lighter general anaesthetic supplemented by a regional block, most commonly a lumbar epidural. The balanced general anaesthetic is very similar to that described for laparoscopy, although a more long-acting muscle relaxant such as pancuronium or d-tubocurarine may be chosen. Anaesthesia is maintained with nitrous oxide supplemented by an inhalational anaesthetic agent, or an intravenous analgesic, or a combination of the two.

Certain advantages can be claimed for the combination of a light general anaesthetic with a regional block. Afferent input from the operation site is abolished and this prevents the early development of the stress response to surgery. When the body is injured it responds both locally and generally. The local response is important for healing and defence against infection. The general response is an endocrine metabolic reaction leading to hypermetabolism and substrate mobilisation. Endocrine responses are associated with increased secretion of catabolic hormones and decreased secretion of the anabolic ones. There is an increase in liver glucose production, lipid and protein turnover and a slight reduction in protein synthesis. There is suppression of immune function. It is not known whether the stress response is useful or harmful, but considerable efforts have been based on the hypothesis that its suppression, and the avoidance of its nutritional and immunological consequences, may indeed reduce postoperative morbidity. Many studies have confirmed that spinal and epidural anaesthesia reduce the blood loss during surgery. Moir (1968) studying pelvic floor repairs showed a decrease in blood loss from about 250 ml to 85 ml. This is probably explained by a lower mean arterial pressure, and a diminishing local blood flow in the small vessels of the wound, combined with a lower venous pressure resulting in less venous oozing. Regional anaesthesia with light general anaesthesia allows early awakening and good immediate postoperative analgesia.

Controlled studies on postoperative morbidity suggest that various aspects may be reduced by the use of epidural blockade. There is a reduction in many of the minor sequelae of general anaesthesia including nausea and vomiting, sore throats, and muscle spasm and pains. Gastrointestinal function is improved. Nimmo et al. (1978) showed better gastric emptying, and Aitkenhead et al. (1978) demonstrated a reduction in the incidence of ileus and in the rate of dehiscence of intestinal anastomoses when regional anaesthesia was compared with general anaesthesia and opiates.

The incidence of deep venous thrombosis is reduced by spinal and epidural anaesthesia for hip replacement surgery (Thorburn et al. 1980; Modig et al. 1981), and it is probably also reduced in gynaecology. The thromboprophylactic effects are explained by a beneficial influence on all the factors of the triad of Virchow, on blood flow, rheological factors and the vessel wall (see Chap. 3). A hyperkinetic flow occurs in the major vessels of the lower limb. There is better fibrinolytic function and a lower tendency to blood coagulation, and an inhibitory effect of local anaesthetics on platelet aggregation. Local anaesthetics also have a stabilising effect on the leucocytes and endothelial cells, which might protect the venous endothelium from injury. The use of epidural or spinal anaesthesia is contraindicated in patients with a bleeding dyscrasia or who are on anticoagulant therapy, including low-dose heparin. However, as epidural anaesthesia reduces the incidence of deep venous thrombosis, it can be considered as a suitable prophylaxis, and may be combined with other measures such as the use of dextran solutions or stockings. The disadvantages of regional anaesthesia are that some patients and surgeons fear complications, the procedure is relatively time-consuming, and it has a small failure rate even in the most skilled hands. Most patients and indeed surgeons prefer the patient to be asleep during the operation. This may be achieved easily with sedation with benzodiazepines or with a light general anaesthetic. Epidural anaesthesia may be associated with a number of complications, including excessive hypotension, headache associated with dural puncture, and minor neurological sequelae, all of which are probably preventable by skilled administration and good technique.

Spinal Anaesthesia

Spinal anaesthesia is easier and quicker to perform than epidural anaesthesia, and there is no other technique which produces such excellent and exten-sive anaesthesia with such a small volume of agent (Atkinson 1985). It may be particularly indicated for the elderly with pulmonary and some types of cardiovascular disease. Younger patients will get a rather high incidence of postdural puncture headache even when fine needles are used, and therefore spinal anaesthesia in gynaecology should be restricted to the elderly.

Advances in Analgesia

It is surprising that while the problems of relieving pain during operation and labour are largely solved, we are relatively unsuccessful at relieving it postoperatively. Testimony to this is found in the words of Donald (1976), who described his experiences after cardiac surgery by saying that "I would be a liar if I did not straight away admit the pain defies description!" It is treated inadequately because the drugs are often prescribed by relatively inexperienced doctors and administered by nurses who are often unable to recognise pain, thinking that the patient lying motionless with their eyes closed is comfortable, whereas in fact they are in such pain that they are too frightened to move. Nurses are also governed by misconceptions about the dangers of opiate analgesics, particularly in relation to hypotension, respiratory depression and drug dependence. They are slaves to the need for minimal intervals between administration, and handicapped by the fact that powerful analgesics are controlled drugs and have to be checked by another senior nurse who may not be readily available, particularly at night. The patients often accept pain as an inevitable consequence of surgery and are reluctant to complain for fear of being thought difficult, cowardly or unappreciative of what has been done for them. Failure to treat postoperative pain effectively may lead to an increased incidence of complications and the fear of it may cause delay in patients presenting for urgent surgery.

Postoperative pain is made up of a sharp, well-localised often burning cutaneous pain, a deep somatic diffuse aching local or referred pain, and a visceral pain, often associated with peritoneal irritation or distension or contraction of smooth muscle, which may be dull, diffuse, aching and colicky. Pain initiates muscle spasm which causes more pain. There are also cortical effects: pain and immobility produces fear and this may increase the pain. There are important cultural and personality differences as well as a definite influence of motivation on pain perception and tolerance.

In interpreting the results of trials of postoperative analgesics it should be appreciated that a third of patients will respond to placebo, and that the environment and attention given will influence the quality of pain relief. The usual management is by systemic analgesic drugs. Among the many narcotics, papaveretum, morphine and methadone are particularly useful. They appear to act at multiple sites, but particularly the brain stem and spinal cord. The basis of the analgesia appears to be the activation of endogenous control systems which have a filtering effect on sensory inputs (Jordan 1984b). Pethidine is less effective due to its very short duration of action, relatively poor pain relief and a high incidence of nausea and vomiting. Traditionally the drugs are given by intramuscular injection by the nursing staff, but there is enormous variation in the dose requirements of the individual patient, and the optimal dose and frequency for each patient should be found.

Because of the relative failure of intermittent intramuscular injections, interest has been shown in continuous or intermittent intravenous administration. Intravenous drugs may be given by drip, syringe pump or in special apparatus such as the Cardiff palliator (Evans et al. 1976). This can be set so that the patient can receive exact doses of any drug at set intervals. To achieve the dose the patient has to press a button twice in rapid succession so that they require to be practised and alert to obtain the dose. All powerful analgesics run the risk of respiratory depression in susceptible patients, or if given in overdose, and have a relatively high incidence of nausea and vomiting, as well as increasing the incidence of urinary retention, ileus and constipation.

Newer analgesics such as buprenorphine, meptazinol and nalbuphine have all been the subject of extensive clinical investigation in the past few years. Buprenorphine is attractive as it can be administered sublingually, and they have the advantage of being drugs not bound by the Misuse of Drugs Act, but it is doubtful if they are as effective as the established drugs. The finding that there are different opioid receptors offers the prospect in the future of introducing more selective agonists as analgesics (Jordan 1985).

Less severe pain can be treated with intermediate analgesics such as intramuscular codeine phosphate or dihydrocodeine, or tablets of codeine or omnopon and aspirin. Simple analgesics such as aspirin or paracetamol are very effective for milder pain when given regularly. Inhalational analgesics such as entonox have a small role. They are useful for short periods to enable the patient to cooperate with a physiotherapist, or during short painful procedures such as the removal of packs, drains or buried sutures.

Over the past few years there has been increasing use of regional anaesthesia, particularly continuous lumbar epidural and the possibilities of administering opiate drugs directly into the subarachnoid or epidural space have broadened the horizons. Epidural local anaesthetics can provide complete pain relief with relatively little motor block if used in very dilute concentrations, such as 0·125% bupivacaine by infusion. However, the patient has to remain in bed, and unless the patient is catheterised there is an unacceptable incidence of urinary retention. However, there is little doubt that postoperative morbidity including chest infections, gastrointestinal complications and deep venous thrombosis are reduced. The method is time consuming, and requires the patient to be nursed in a high-dependency nursing area, so that complications such as extensive blockade or hypotension can be readily recognised and managed.

It is hoped that the epidural administration of suitable opioid drugs will produce adequate analgesia without motor or sympathetic blockade. To do this the drug must diffuse across the dura and enter the spinal cord to act on specific opioid receptors before a large part is absorbed by the epidural veins. However, at present neither the ideal drug nor dose has been established, and there is an incidence of complications such as urinary retention, pruritus and respiratory depression which may occur many hours after the administration of the drug. Rostral spread of the drug in the cerebrospinal fluid to the brain stem (the likely cause of respiratory depression) is particularly liable to occur with drugs of low molecular weight and poor lipophilicity, such as morphine. Unfortunately this is one of the drugs which is likely to produce effective analgesia of long duration. It is doubtful whether research has progressed to an extent that should allow spinal opiates to be a routine clinical method, but if they are used the patient must be under close nursing supervision so that serious side effects such as respiratory depression can be rapidly noticed and corrected.

Transcutaneous Electrical Nerve Stimulation (TENS) (Fig. 6.1)

Good results may be obtained by the application of electrodes on either side of surgical incisions, and using low-intensity currents of frequencies of 50–100 Hz continuously (Tyler et al. 1982). The

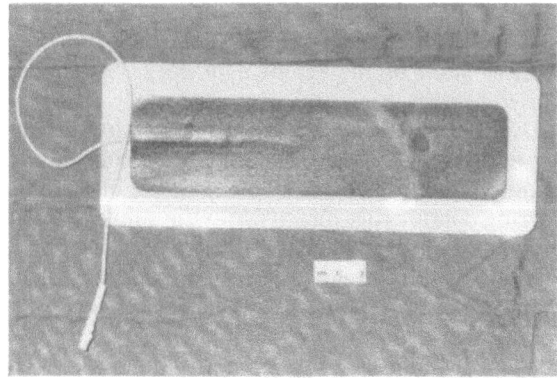

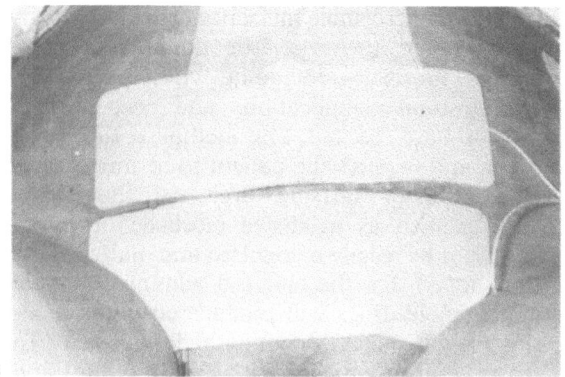

Fig. 6.1.a Underface of one TENS electrode before placement.
b TENS electrodes in place.

Non-steroidal Anti-inflammatory Drugs

Non-steroidal anti-inflammatory drugs have analgesic as well as anti-inflammatory properties. Analgesia may be potentiated by the combination of opiates and anti-inflammatory drugs. Most of them require oral administration, and there is a risk of gastrointestinal side effects, both factors making them unsuitable in the early postoperative period. Indomethacin may be the preferred drug, as its rectal absorption is good, and this route reduces the chance of gastrointestinal complications.

It is apparent that doctors are becoming much more aware of the need to provide better postoperative analgesia. One might consider developing analgesia teams of nurses and anaesthetists as in obstetrics. The patients could be better prepared for postoperative pain as they are for obstetric pain, and there is a need to use a wider range of drugs, dosages and techniques and tailor the analgesia to the requirements of the individual. The management would be made much more effective, easier and safer if postoperative patients could be grouped together in areas of high-dependency nursing, and if epidural administration of drugs could be performed by ward sisters in the same way as it is by midwives. Regrettably shortage of facilities and medical and nursing staff are likely to inhibit the widespread provision of effective analgesia for several years to come.

amount of opiate required is reduced, and the incidence of pulmonary complications may be less. It may work by activating mechanisms in the midbrain reticular formation, which, in turn, exert powerful inhibitory effects on pain and transmitting pathways (Melzack 1985). It seems to be more effective for somatic than visceral pain.

Cryoanalgesia

It has been shown that freezing nerves produces a reversible blockade lasting about 2–3 weeks (Lloyd et al. 1976), and therefore is very attractive as a means of relieving postoperative pain. However, at the present time it is really only applicable where the nerves can be readily exposed, as for example the intercostal nerves at thoracotomy (Glynn et al. 1980). The complex innervation of gynaecological wounds makes it impractical, but it may have a place in the treatment of painful gynaecological scars.

Control of Postoperative Vomiting

Nausea, retching and vomiting may occur in up to 35% of patients after anaesthesia, particularly when opiates have been used. Opiate analgesics should be combined therefore with an antiemetic. Those giving a history of motion sickness or bad anaesthetic experiences and the anxious are particularly liable to it. The site of operation is important and dilatation of the cervix particularly combined with ergometrine-containing drugs increases the incidence. Any operative or postoperative hypoxia, early mobilisation or the premature resumption of oral intake may be additional factors. It is a particularly distressing complication, causing loss of personal dignity as well as increasing pain. Antiemetic drugs may act by depressing the chemoreceptor trigger zone in the floor of the fourth ventricle or by increasing gastrointestinal motility (Clarke 1984). The most effective are probably the phenothiazines, which block dopamine receptors in the chemoreceptor trigger zone. There is a whole range available, with perphenazine 5 mg or prochlorperazine 12·5 mg the most popular. They have mild sedative effects, a small risk of hypotension if the patient is hypovolaemic and occasional dystonic extrapyramidal reactions. Metoclopramide 10 mg has a dual action via dopamine blockade centrally, and increased gastrointestinal motility as well as increased lower oesophageal sphincter tone. It may also produce extrapyramidal reactions occasionally. Domperidone 10 mg has similar actions to metoclopramide, but with less central effects. Hyoscine may be combined with papaveretum in premedication to reduce the incidence of emetic effects.

Management of Chronic Pain

Chronic pain in the gynaecological patient requires full assessment in an attempt to reach a definitive diagnosis. Pain arising from the pelvic organs is usually felt in the lower abdomen, lower back, perineum and occasionally the lower limbs. It is unlikely to rise above the level of the iliac crest unless there is blood in the peritoneal cavity or peritonitis. Gynaecological back pain is usually felt in the lower sacral and gluteal regions, although it may radiate to the anterior thigh. Sciatica-type pain in the posterior thigh usually implies skeletal involvement. This is most usually non-gynaecological, although may be associated with invasion by tumour. Pain arising from the pelvic organs often has a premenstrual accentuation, increases as the day goes on and is often described as a diffuse and aching sensation. A cause such as prolapse, retroverted uterus, endometriosis, neoplasm, adhesions or a cervical infection may be found.

Only after full investigation, including normal findings at laparoscopy, is it possible to conclude that the pain is of unknown origin and can be treated symptomatically. Patients suffering from pelvic pain of unknown origin are mostly introverted subjects, prone to anxiety and to periodic depression, often show hysterical elements, and there is often evidence of unsatisfactory social, marital and sexual relationships. They should be strongly reassured regarding the lack of organic disease. They may require psychological and psychosexual investigation so that the true nature of the condition can be elucidated. It is hoped that many of these patients would respond to psychosexual counselling, psychotherapy or the judicious use of psychotropic drugs, although it must be admitted that many are unwilling to acknowledge the true nature of their problem.

Transcutaneous nerve stimulation may help to alleviate diffuse pain. Pain arising from localised areas, such as trigger points, may respond to injections of local anaesthetic or cryotherapy. There is no place for complex local anaesthetic blocks, and destructive blocks with neurolytic solutions are contraindicated for chronic pain of unknown origin.

Management of Cancer Pain

Patients with pain due to a neoplasm are worthy of energetic treatment. The diagnosis is apparent. Psychological features are much less relevant and often the patient's life expectancy is relatively short. If the pain covers a relatively wide area it is usually necessary to use systemic analgesic drugs. The use of morphine-like analgesics should be dictated by the severity of the pain alone and not just by the brevity of the prognosis. Analgesic should be administered in adequate doses, orally if possible, and at frequent enough intervals to keep the patient pain-free throughout the 24-h period. The effectiveness of the analgesic drugs may be improved by the concomitant use of antiemetic drugs such as phenothiazines, or by combining their use with that of antidepressants, non-steroidal or steroid anti-inflammatory drugs.

If the pain is localised it may well respond to local nerve-blocking procedures. It is usually wise to do diagnostic blocks with local anaesthetic before undertaking a destructive procedure. The diagnostic block enables the patient and the doctor to assess the likely effectiveness of the procedure and also the side effects such as weakness or sphincter disturbance which might accompany it. If appropriate a phenol or alcohol neurolytic block may be carried out carefully. These blocks are particularly indicated for unilateral pain covering only a few dermatomes, and the most common technique is the subarachnoid injection of small amounts of hyperbaric phenol. The spread can be controlled accurately by appropriate posturing of the patient.

More widespread unilateral pain may respond to cordotomy, in which the spinothalamic tract is sectioned. This may be done by open operation or by a percutaneous method in the cervical region. Ipsilateral weakness or sphincter disturbances may follow. Occasionally patients with chronic cancer pain have been managed successfully for a few months with implanted epidural catheters through which regular doses of opiate can be administered. However, this technique requires further investigation with regard to its safety and efficacy.

References

Aitkenhead AR, Wishart HY, Peebles Brown DA (1978) High spinal nerve block for large bowel anastomosis. Br J Anaesth 50:177–183

Akil H, Mayer DJ, Liebeskind JC (1976) Antagonism of stimulation produced analgesia by naloxone, a narcotic antagonist. Science 191:961–962

Akil H, Watson SJ, Young E, Lewis M, Kachaturian H, Walker J (1984) Endogenous opioids: biology and function. Ann Rev Neurosci 7:223–255

Atkinson RS (1985) Spinal intradural analgesia. In: Atkinson RS, Adams AP (eds) Recent advances in anaesthesia and analgesia 15. Chuchill Livingstone, London, pp 79–87

Behar M, Magora F, Olshawang D, Davidson JT (1979) Epidural morphine in treatment of pain. Lancet i:527–529

Bullingham RES, McQuay HJ, Moore RA (1984) Principles of use of extradural and intrathecal narcotics. In: Kaufman L (ed) Anaesthesia review 2. Churchill Livingstone, London, pp 137–147

Clarke RSJ (1984) Nausea and vomiting. Br J Anaesth 56:19–27

Donald I (1976) At the receiving end. Scot Med J 21:49–57

Evans JM, Rosen M, MacCarthy J, Hogg MIJ (1976) Apparatus for patient-controlled administration of intravenous narcotics during labour. Lancet i:17–18

Glynn CJ, Lloyd JW, Barnard JDW (1980) Cryoanalgesia in the management of pain after thoracotomy. Thorax 35:325–327

Hughes J, Smith TW, Kosterlitz HW, Fothergill LA, Morgan BA, Morris HR (1975) Identification of two related pentapeptides from the brain with potent opiate agonist activity. Nature 258:577–579

Hughes J, Kosterlitz HW (1983) Introduction to opioid peptides. Br Med Bull 39:1–3

Jordan CC (1984a) Anatomical and physiological aspects of pain perception. In: Kaufman L (ed) Anaesthesia review, vol 2. Churchill Livingstone, London, pp 87–107

Jordan CC (1984b) Current views on the mechanism of opiate analgesia and some novel approaches to analgesic drugs. In: Kaufman L (ed) Anaesthesia review, vol 2. Churchill Livingstone, London, pp 108–136

Jordan CC (1985) Opioid receptors. In: Kaufman L (ed) Anaesthetic review vol 3. Churchill Livingstone, London, pp 36–48

Lloyd JW, Barnard JDW, Glynn CJ (1976) Cryoanalgesia–a new approach to pain relief. Lancet ii: 932–934

Melzack R, Wall PD (1965) Pain mechanisms: a new theory. Science 150:971–979

Melzack R (1985) Hyperstimulation analgesia. In: Brena S, Chapman SB (eds) Clinics in anaesthesiology. Saunders, Philadelphia, vol 3 pp 81–92

Modig J, Hjelmstedt A, Sahlstedt B, Maripuu E (1981) Comparative influences of epidural and general anaesthesia on deep venous thrombosis and pulmonary embolism after total hip replacement. Acta Chir Scand 147:125:-130

Moir DD (1968) Blood loss during major vaginal surgery. Br J Anaesth 40:233–240

Nimmo WS, Littlewood DG, Scott DB, Prescott LF (1978) Gastric emptying following hysterectomy with extradural analgesia. Br J Anaesth 50:559–561

Pinnock CA (1985) Endorphins. In: Kaufman L (ed) Anaesthesia Review, vol 3. Churchill Livingstone, London, pp 49–62

Rance MJ (1983) Multiple opiate receptors—their occurrence and significance. In: Bullingham R (ed) Clinics in anaesthesiology, vol 1. Saunders, Philadelphia pp 183–199

Reynolds DV (1969) Surgery in the rat during electrical analgesia induced by focal brain stimulation. Science 164:444–445

Thorburn J, Louden JR, Vallance R (1980) Spinal and general anaesthesia in total hip replacement: frequency of deep vein thrombosis. Br J Anaesth 52:1117–1121

Tyler E, Caldwell C, Ghia JN (1982) Transcutaneous electrical nerve stimulation: an alternative approach to the management of postoperative pain. Anaesthesia and Analgesia 61:449–456

Yaksh JL, Rudy TA (1976) Analgesia mediated by a direct spinal action of narcotics. Science 192:1357–1358

Wall PD (1978) The gate control theory of pain mechanisms: a re-examination and reassessment. Brain 101:1–18

Section B:

OPERATIVE

7 · Operative Positions, Incisions and Closure

Timothy E. Bucknall and Stuart L. Stanton

Operative Positions

There are a variety of positions in which the patient may be placed for gynaecological surgery: each reflects the needs of the surgical procedure.

Trendelenberg

This is the standard position for abdominopelvic procedures. Some 20° or more head-down tilt will encourage cranial displacement of bowel from out of the pelvis and in addition it will encourage maximal venous return which will minimise the risk of deep vein thrombosis (Fig. 7.1). A non-slip mattress (without canvas or plastic sheet) is essential for steep Trendelenberg tilt: the final degree of tilt may be limited by impairment of diaphragmatic excursion by the increasing pressure of abdominal contents.

Lithotomy

This is the standard position for vaginal surgery and laparoscopy and requires little comment, save that care must always be exercised in positioning a patient with either lumbosacral spine or hip disorder. The patient is usually positioned horizontally, but steep Trendelenberg is used for laparoscopy and it is important that a non-slip mattress is used. In this position, it is helpful if the leg stirrups are positioned at 45° rather than 90° to the horizontal, allowing the thighs to be more extended, which will give greater access to the abdomen.

Lloyd-Davies (Fig. 7.2)

Originally designed for synchronous abdominoperineal operations, these complicated but invaluable leg supports are appropriate when a synchronous approach is needed for gynaecological surgery, e.g. colposuspension or the Zacharin pelvic

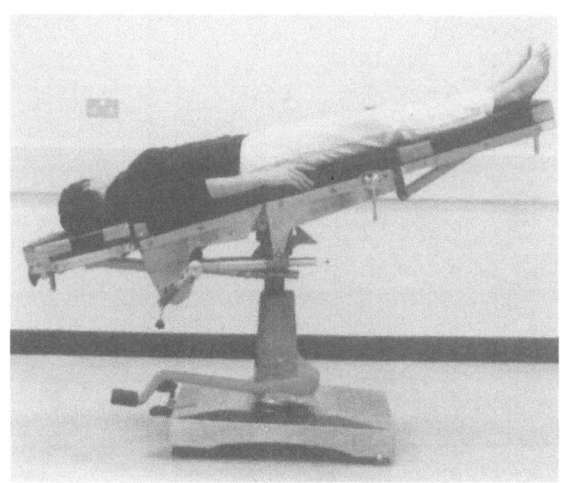

Fig. 7.1. Patient in steep Trendelenberg position. An anti-slip mattress is essential.

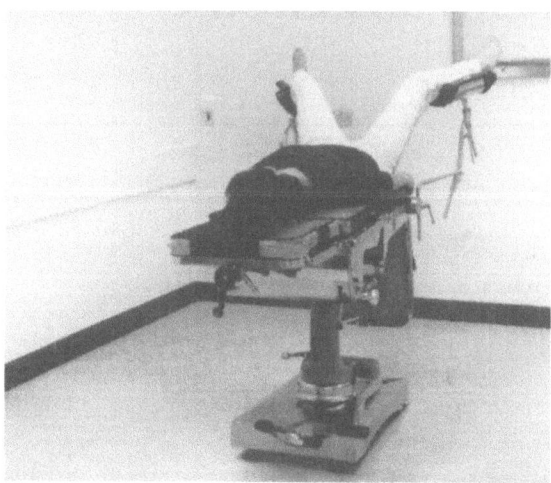

Fig. 7.2. Patient in Lloyd-Davies stirrups and in slight Trendelenberg tilt.

floor repair for recurrent enterocele. Some expertise is required of the operating room attendant to enable the patient to be correctly positioned, including avoidance of pressure in the popliteal fossa by the leg support.

Knee-Chest Position (Fig. 7.3)

This position is ideal for repair of urethrovaginal or vesicovaginal fistulae, which may be invisible in the lithotomy position. It also reduces prolapse of the posterior bladder wall, when there is a massive fistula. Endotracheal anaesthesia with positive pressure ventilation is recommended for this position.

Incisions

Principles of Wound Incisions

It goes without saying that efficient access to the abdominal and pelvic cavities and safe closure of the consequent wounds are two vital, if somewhat neglected, steps in the preformance of every operation. Unfortunately, all too often the choice of access is made without too much thought and closure of the wound, especially at the end of a long and testing operation, may be carried out with less than meticulous care.

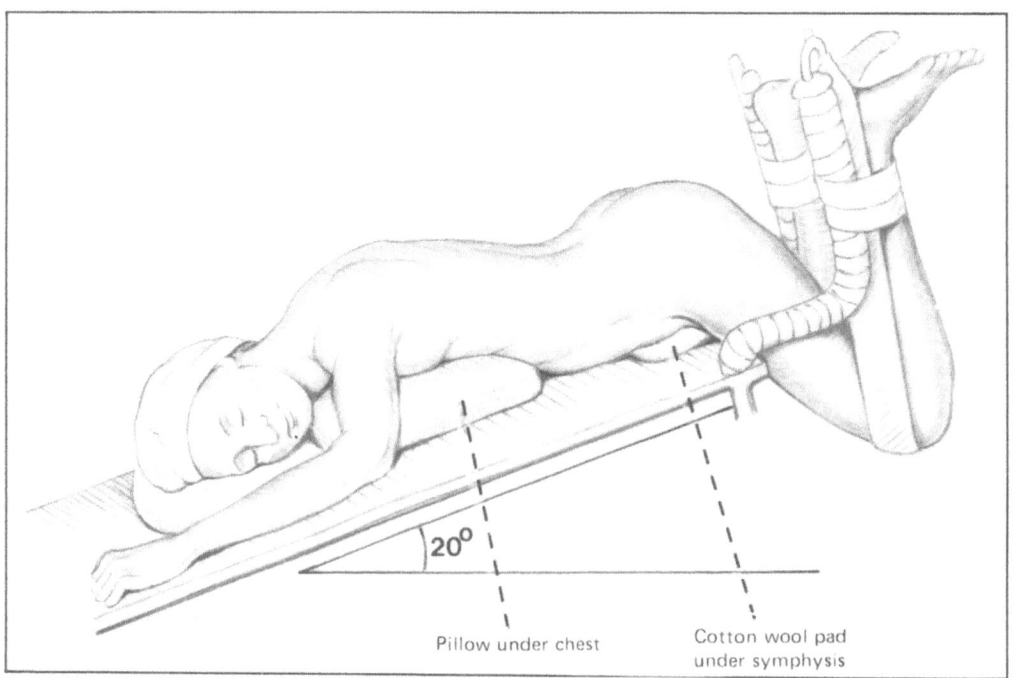

Fig. 7.3. Knee-chest position. The patient's chest and face are positioned according to the anaesthetist.

A well-planned incision allows:

1. Excellent access to the planned field of surgery
2. The possibility of extension of the exposure if some unforeseen problem arises
3. Safe closure to be performed (Ellis et al. 1985)

In turn, effective closure should be a relatively simple and speedy technique but one which is compatible with a low risk of incisional hernia, haematoma, infection and, most serious of all, complete disruption of the operation wound. In addition, the technique should provide a comfortable and reasonably aesthetic scar.

Ideally, the closure of the incision should leave the abdominal wall as strong after surgery as before, and this depends not only on technique of closure but also the choice of suture material and careful planning in placement of drains, should these be necessary.

Therefore in choosing a particular incision, the surgeon requires ready and direct access to the organ requiring investigation or treatment and must also provide sufficient room for the required procedure to be performed. The incision should also be extensible to allow for any enlargement of the scope of operation and needs to interfere as little as possible with abdominal wall function (Ellis 1984).

The incisions most often employed in gynaecology may be classified into vertical (median or paramedian), transverse and oblique.

The choice of the incision depends on numerous factors including the type of surgery to be performed, the organ to be exposed, whether speed is an important consideration, the build of the patient, the degree of obesity and the presence of previous abdominal incisions, which may themselves be the site of wound herniation. Last, but not least, must come the surgeon's individual preference. There is no doubt that in a serious emergency the midline incision gives extremely rapid access and can if necessary be extended for the whole length of the abdomen.

If there has been a previous incision, re-exploration of the abdomen and pelvis should, if possible, be carried out by re-opening the old wound, especially if this is weak or the site of an incisional hernia, since repair can be carried out at the same time. A second incision placed alongside a previous laparotomy wound, especially if heavily undercut, may cut off the blood supply of the skin between the two incisions and result in necrosis of the skin bridge.

Many studies which have been reported in the past and the clinical impressions of a large number of surgeons have indicated that oblique and transverse incisions give stronger wounds, less liable to disruption or herniation, than a midline incision; indeed the same claim is put forward for the paramedian approach. However, such uncontrolled impressions have no science to support them. Often the midline incision is carried out in operations of the greatest urgency, for example, major injury, severe peritonitis or massive haemorrhage, or in the re-opening of previous abdominal incisions, perhaps already the site of herniation. Little wonder that this incision may be followed by a high incidence of complications.

Only carefully conducted controlled trials can give the answer, where the various types of incision are carried out in a randomly allocated manner and where other variables, such as the type of suture material and the technique of closure, are standardised. It is also necessary to go through the tedious procedure of a long-term follow-up, for a minimum of 12 months, before assessing the results of wound healing. When such studies are carried out, there is little if anything to choose between the various incisions. A controlled trial has been carried out in which those patients in whom a vertical incision was desirable were randomised into either median or paramedian incisions. In those patients where the surgeon considered that an oblique or transverse incision could be performed, randomisation was made between this approach and a paramedian incision. All incisions were closed by the same mass nylon technique. The results are shown in Table 7.1 and demonstrate that they could not show any advantage between these three incisions with regard to incisional herniation or dehiscence (Ellis et al. 1984). In a previous study from our Unit (Bucknall et al. 1982) we could find no statistical difference in the incidence of herniation between 544 midline and 558 paramedian incisions performed in the course of a variety of controlled trials.

Table 7.1. Incisional hernias in median, paramedian and transverse incisions (randomised study, 1-year follow-up)

	N	No. hernias	
Paramedian	39	9	NSχ^2
Median	40	7	
Paramedian	46	8	NSχ^2
Transverse	50	7	

Pfannenstiel

This incision is frequently employed for access to the pelvic organs and is used in most Caesarian sections. Provided that the preoperative diagnosis is sound, the Pfannenstiel incision is excellent for local gynaecological conditions, but the exposure is undoubtedly limited and the incision is not yet recommended when a manœuvre outside the pelvis may be required.

The skin incision is usually about 12 cm long, centred above the symphysis pubis and curved along the interspinous skin crease (Fig. 7.4). The incision is deepened through the superficial fascia to expose both anterior rectus sheaths, which are divided along the whole length of the incision. Artery forceps are placed on the upper and lower edges of each rectus sheath, which is then dissected widely both above and below from the underlying sheath, which is then dissected widely both above and below from the underlying rectus muscles (Fig. 7.4b). The sheath is separated in an upwards direction almost to the umbilicus and downwards as far as the pubis. The rectus muscles are then retracted laterally and the peritoneum opened vertically in the midline, commencing in the upper end of the wound, with care being taken caudally not to injure the bladder (Fig. 7.4c, d). When it is intended to employ this incision, it is advisable to catheterise the patient prior to operation, as a full bladder may lend itself to injury and will also limit the exposure of the pelvic organs. The peritoneum can also be opened transversely, just above the bladder and in the same line as the skin incision.

The great advantage of the incision is that because it goes with Langers lines (Fig. 7.5), it leaves an almost invisible scar, which, in any case, is hidden by the pubic hair. The exposure, however, is undoubtedly limited (Fig. 7.4e) and should only be used when the surgeon is quite certain that only pelvic intervention is necessary. The peritoneum is closed with a running stitch. The recti fall together (Fig. 7.4f) and the anterior sheath is approximated with either continuous or interrupted sutures according to the surgeon's preference.

Chest complications are rare after a Pfannenstiel incision, owing to the comparative absence of pain—patients are not afraid to cough and mobilise early.

The Cherney Incision

The Cherney incision may be indicated when a wider exposure of the pelvic organs is imperative in order to simplify certain extensive operations or pelvic exenteration procedures.

The skin incision is made as for a Pfannenstiel incision and then deepened to incise the anterior sheath of rectus muscles and aponeurosis of external and internal oblique muscles (Fig. 7.6a). The tendinous insertions of rectus muscles on the symphysis are exposed and the proposed level for division can be seen in Fig. 7.6b. The recti are then reflected upwards exposing bladder and peritoneum giving good exposure to the pelvic organs (Fig. 7.6c). After peritoneal closure (Fig. 7.6d) the rectus tendons are reattached (Fig. 7.6e).

The Midline Incision

Virtually any operation within the abdominal and pelvic cavities can be performed through this universally applicable incision, which has the advantages of being almost bloodless and quick to make and to close (so that it is of immense value in cases of great urgency). It can be extended the full length of the abdomen by curving the incision around the umbilicus and is made without division of either muscle fibres or nerves.

In the upper abdomen, the incision is placed exactly in the midline and extends downwards from the xiphisternum, usually to end immediately above the umbilicus. Skin, fat, linea alba, extraperitoneal fat and peritoneum are divided—the last best carried out at the lower extremity of the wound, so that the falciform ligament can be seen and avoided. If this ligament interferes with exposure, it should be divided between clamps and ligated. Upward extension of a couple of centimetres can be obtained by running the incision to one or other side of the xiphoid process.

The subumbilical incision differs only in that here the linea alba is usually very narrow so that the rectus sheath on one or other side may be inadvertently opened, although this is not of any consequence. In the lower abdomen the peritoneum should be opened first in its upper part in order to avoid possible injury to the bladder.

Especial care must be taken in opening the peritoneum under two circumstances—and this applies to all laparotomy incisions, not only the midline. In cases of intestinal obstruction, loops of distended bowel immediately deep to peritoneum may be injured and the initial opening into the peritoneal cavity must be made with the greatest care. The second circumstance is when the abdomen is being reopened following previous surgery. In the great majority of cases, there will be underlying adhesions and, if these consist of intestine, the gut may be inadvertently opened. Again, the greatest care must be taken and the peritoneum should be opened at one or other end of the incision, away from the immediate mass of adhesions.

A safe method is to pick up a fold of peritoneum with dissecting forceps, shake it to ensure that no

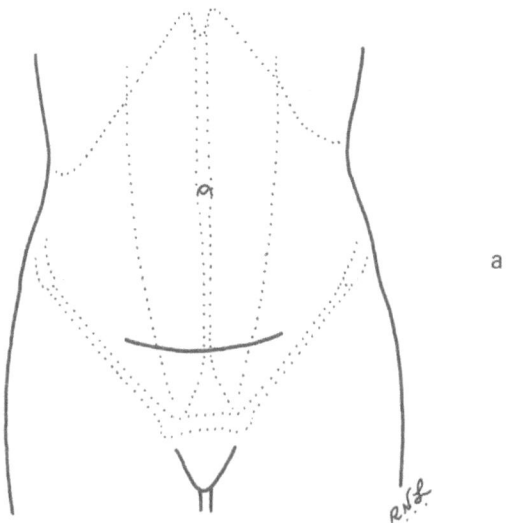

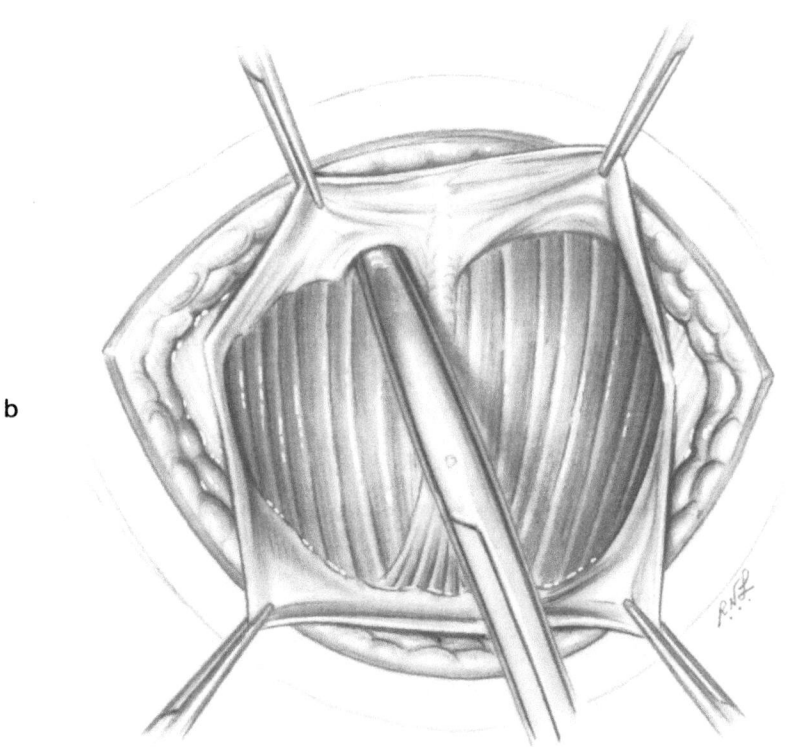

Fig. 7.4a–f. Pfannenstiel's infra-umbilical curved incision: **a** surface marking; **b** dissection of rectus sheath (*continued overleaf*)

Fig. 7.4 (*continued*)

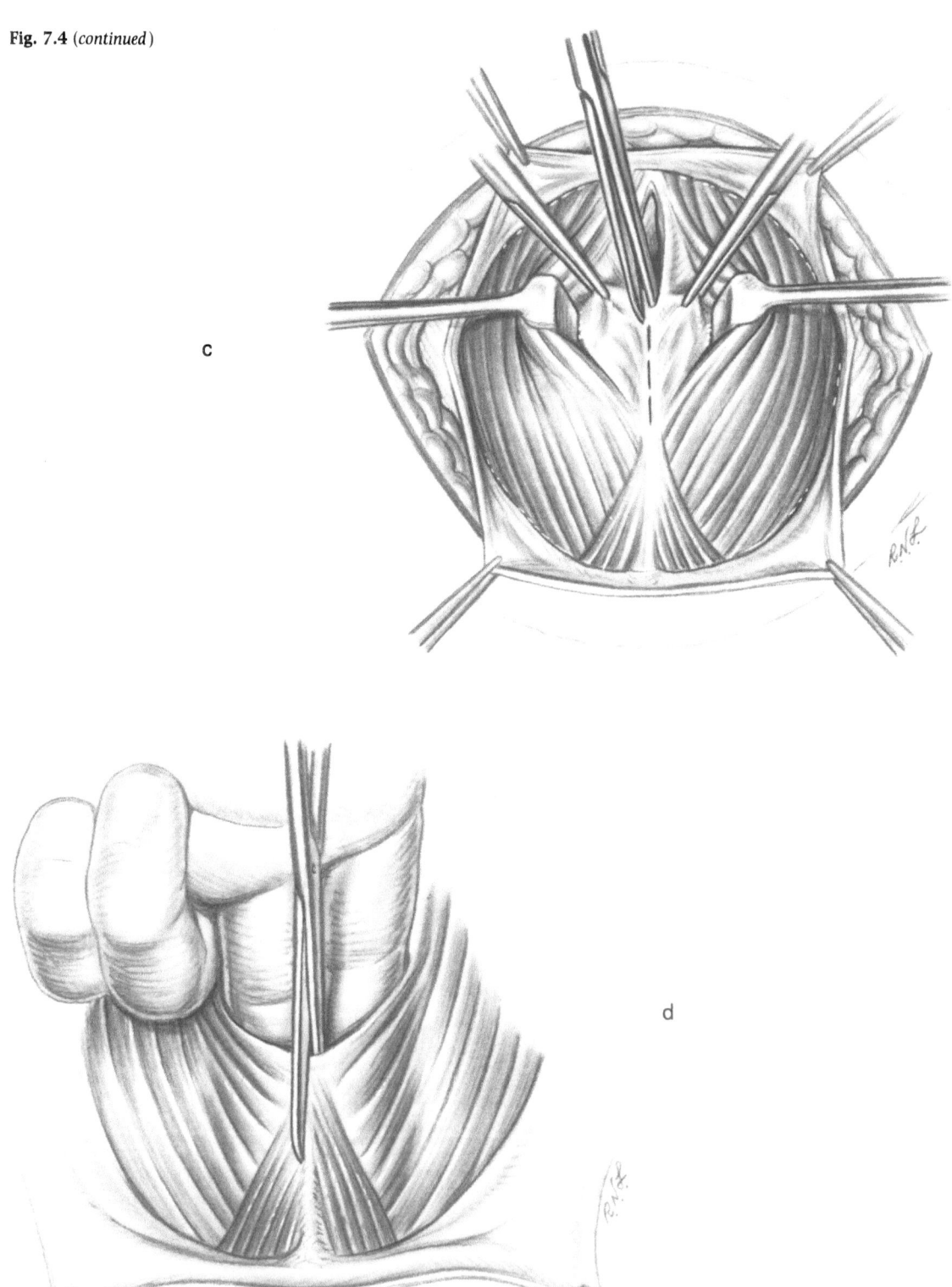

c

d

Fig. 7.4.c peritoneum open; **d** peritoneum opened caudally; care exercised because of bladder; **e** limited exposure may be obtained of pelvic organs; **f** recti come together and are approximated. Anterior rectus sheath is then closed.

Fig. 7.4 (*continued*)

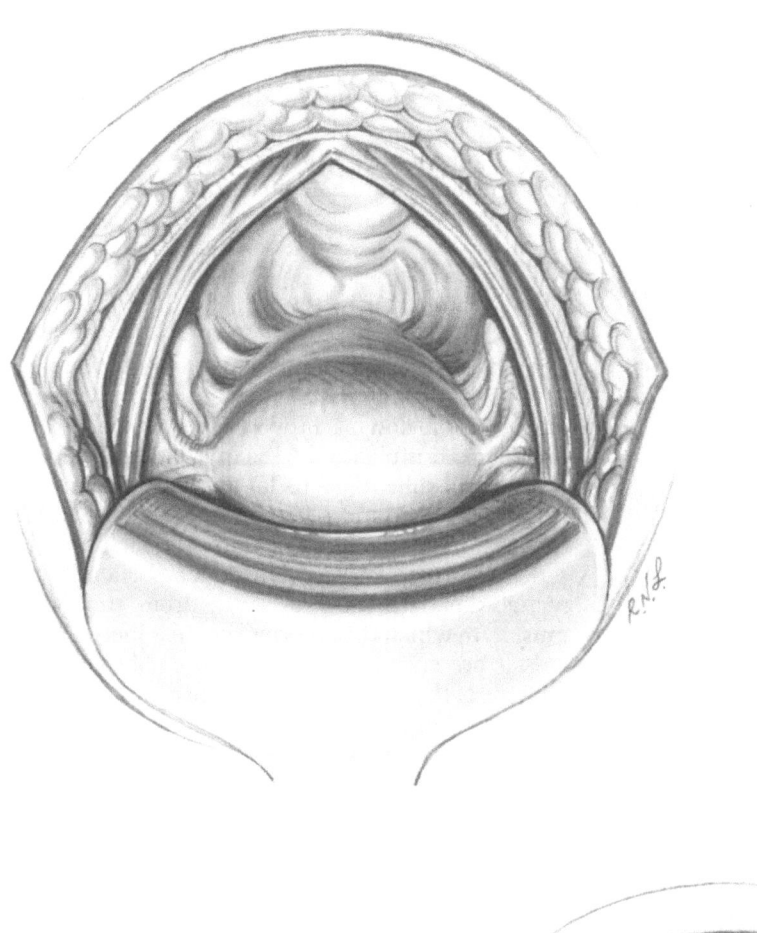

e

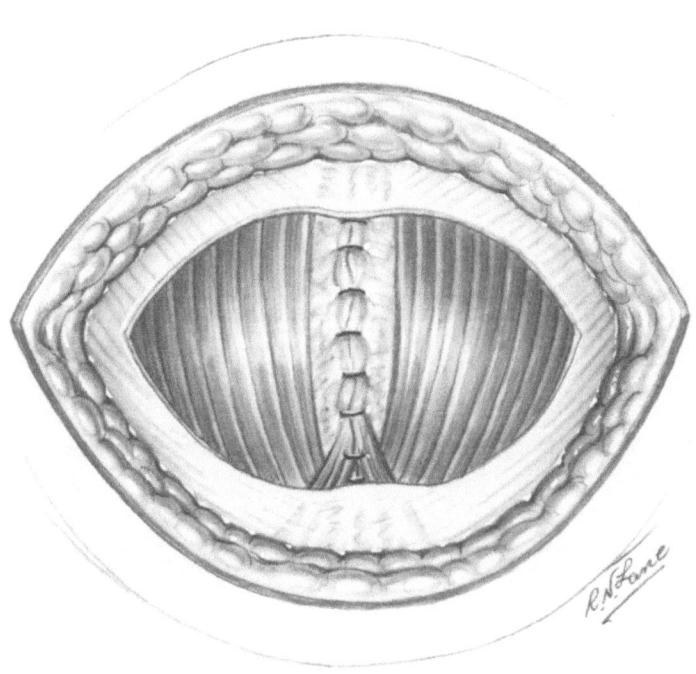

f

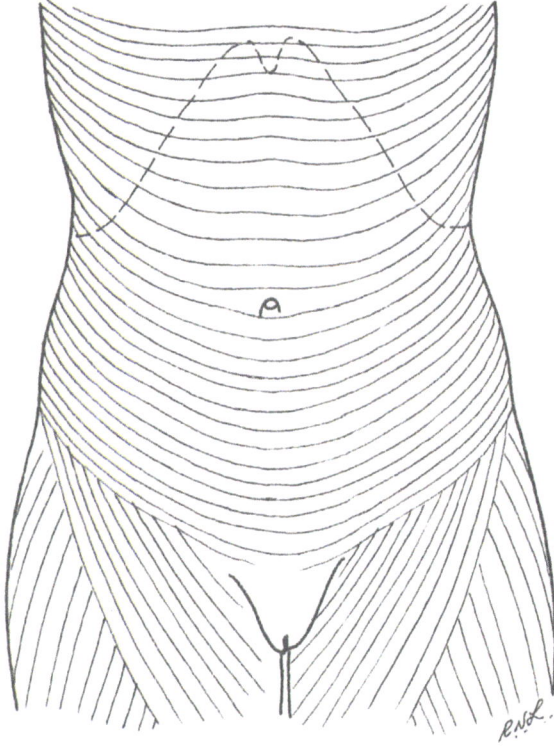

Fig. 7.5. Langer's cleavage lines.

other structure has been caught up with it, clip it with two artery forceps placed slightly apart and then divide this raised fold with the utmost care, using a knife with its blade held almost horizontally. This small opening is then enlarged to admit two fingers, which are then used to protect the underlying viscera while the peritoneum is being divided throughout the whole length of the wound. Once the peritoneal cavity has been safely entered, the peritoneal edges are held up with artery forceps and the adhesions detached under direct vision.

The Conventional Paramedian

The upper paramedian incision, on either the right or left side, usually commences at the costal margin and is taken down to the level of, or below, the umbilicus. It is placed 2·5–5 cm from the midline.

Skin and subcutaneous fat are divided along the length of the wound. The anterior rectus sheath is exposed, incised, and its medial edge lifted up in a series of artery forceps. The inner portion of the rectus sheath is now dissected from the rectus muscle, to which the anterior sheath adheres. Blood vessels are encountered at the three fibrous intersections of the rectus, placed just below the xiphoid, at the level of the umbilicus and halfway between.

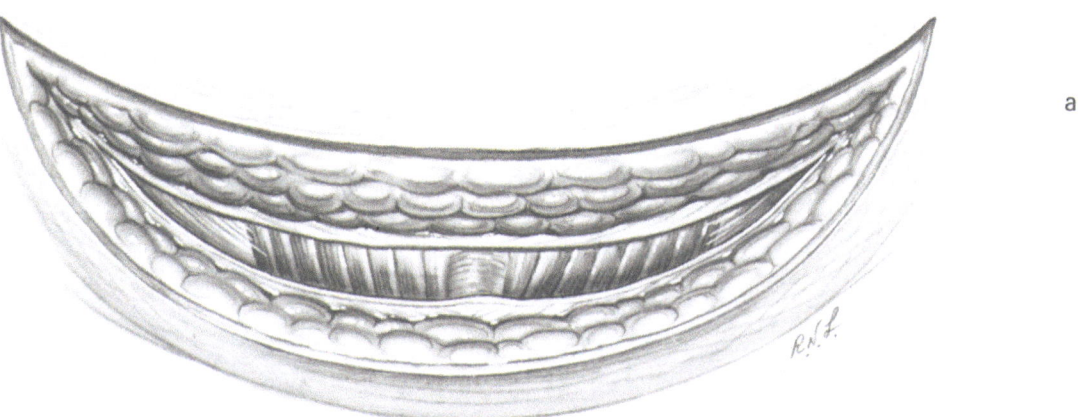

a

Fig. 7.6a–e. Cherney incision: **a** incision of anterior sheath of rectus muscle and aponeurosis of external and internal oblique muscles; **b** proposed level for division of tendons; **c** recti reflected upwards (*continued overleaf*)

Fig. 7.6 (*continued*)

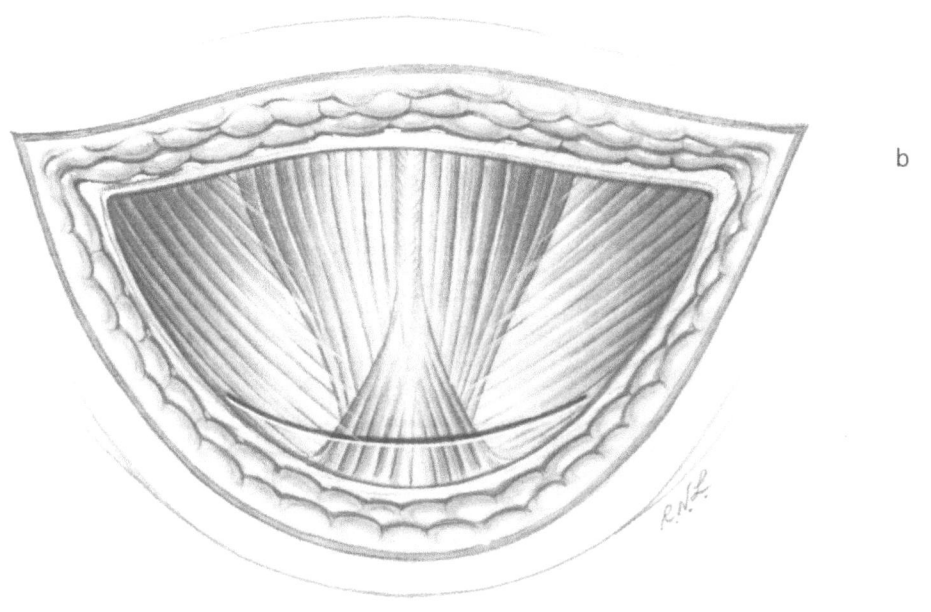

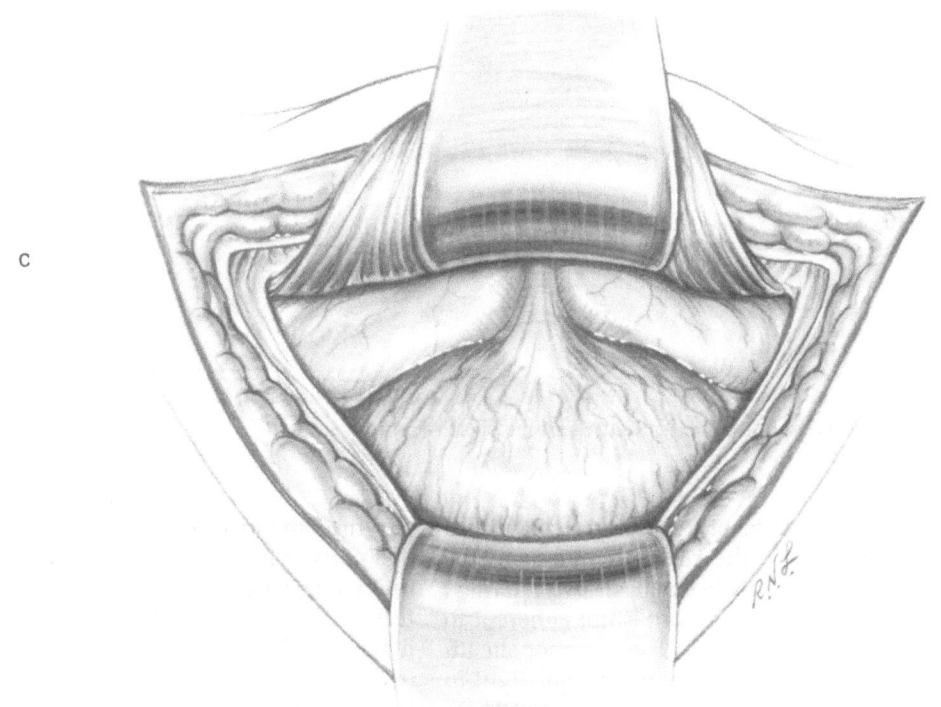

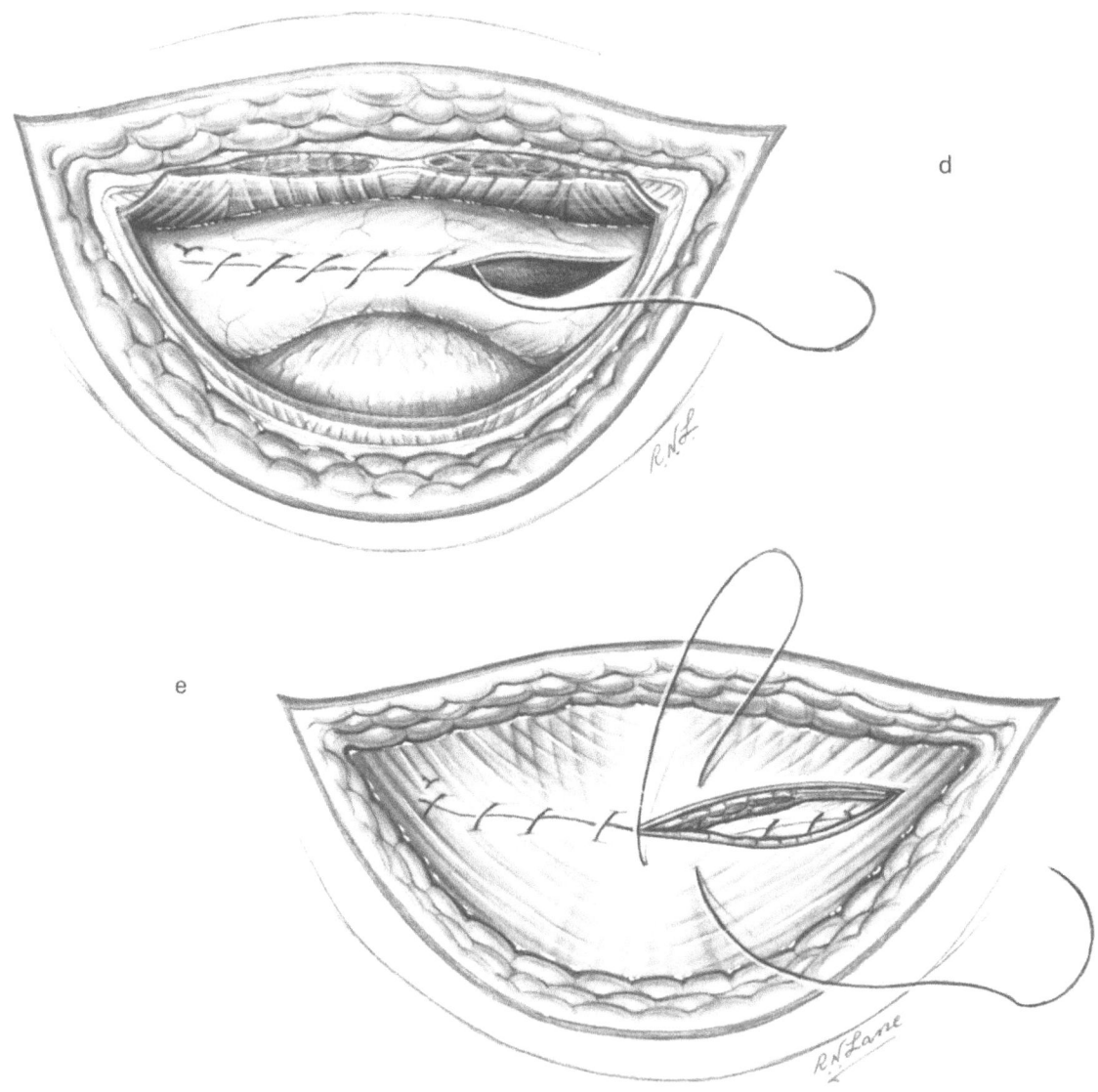

Fig. 7.6d peritoneal closure; **e** muscle and anterior rectus sheath closure.

These vessels should be picked up and coagulated before dividing. Once the rectus is free from the anterior sheath, the muscle can be drawn laterally, since the posterior rectus sheath is not adherent to the back of the rectus muscle. The posterior sheath and peritoneum, which are intimately adherent to each other, are picked up and incised vertically for the whole length of the incision.

The lower paramedian incision is very similar (Fig. 7.7a–e) and in fact can continue the upper paramedian incision the whole length of the abdomen. The only slight difference is that the inferior epigastric vessels are exposed in the posterior compartment of the rectus sheath and require ligation and division. Moreover, the posterior layer of the rectus sheath is deficient below the semilunar fold of Douglas in the lower half of the incision. The lower paramedian incision is, of course, used for exploring the pelvic organs, the caecal region and the lower reaches of the large intestine.

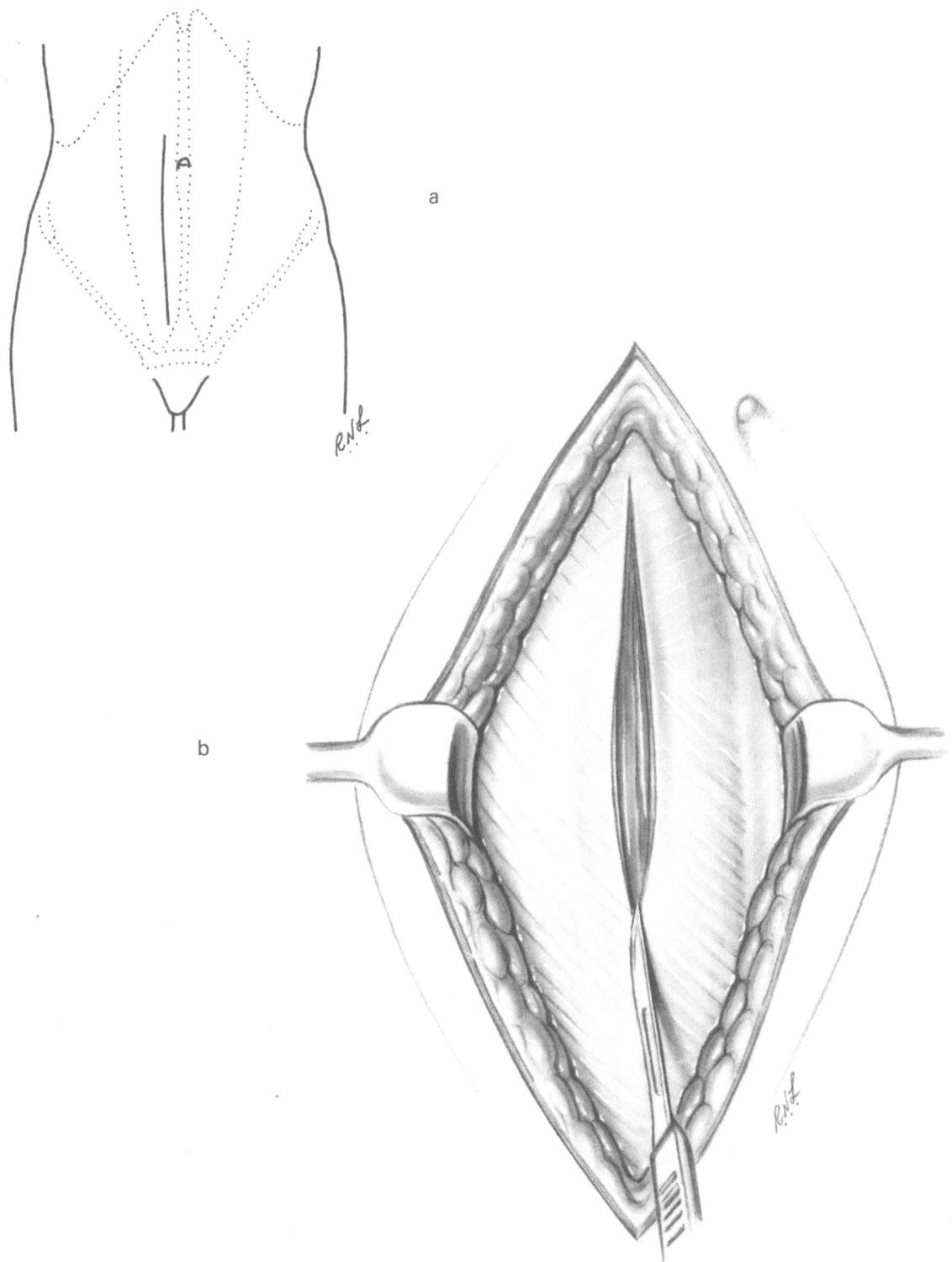

Fig. 7.7a–e. Lower paramedian incision: **a** surface markings; **b** incision of anterior rectus sheath (*continued overleaf*)

Fig. 7.7 (*continued*)

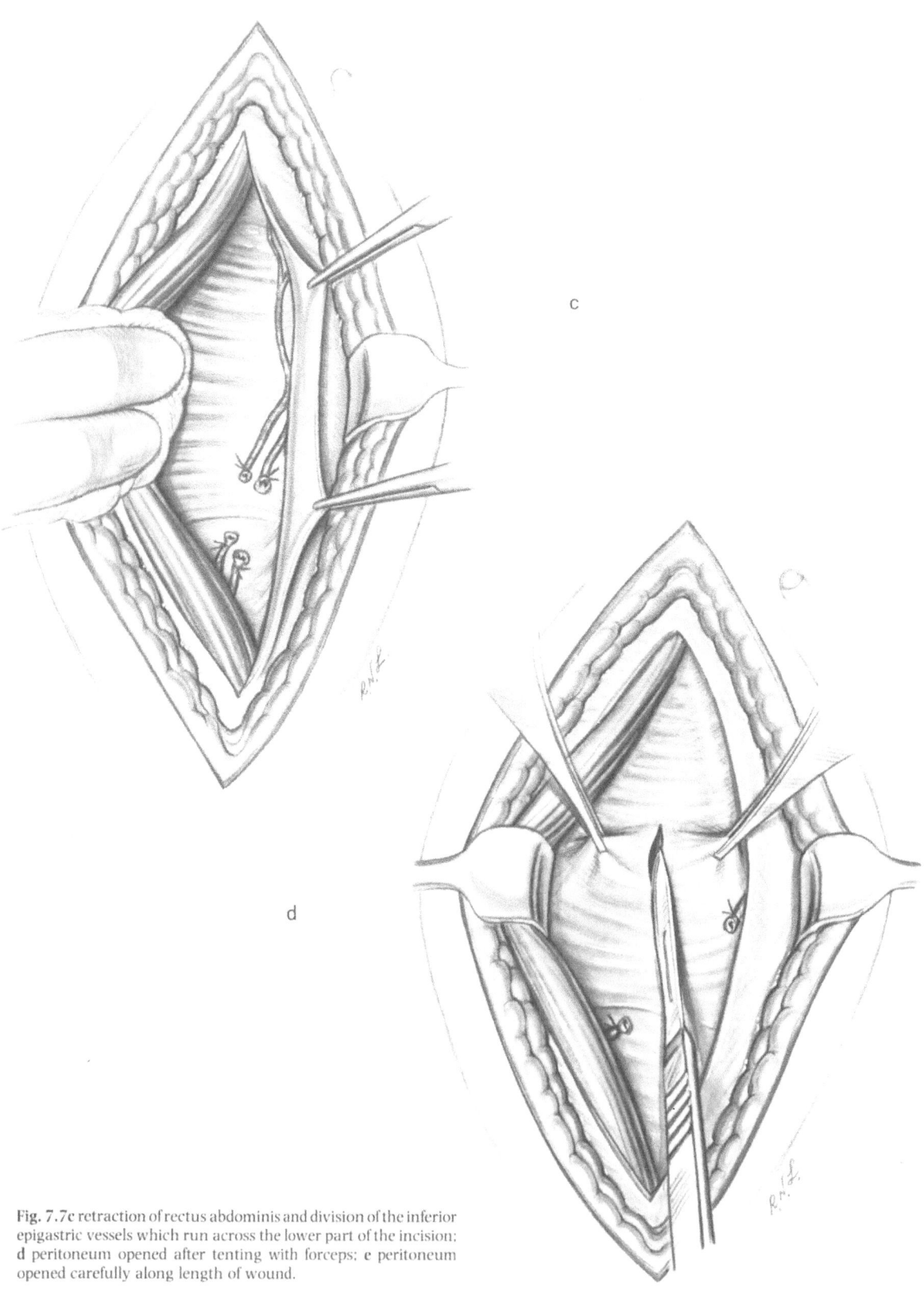

Fig. 7.7c retraction of rectus abdominis and division of the inferior
epigastric vessels which run across the lower part of the incision;
d peritoneum opened after tenting with forceps; **e** peritoneum
opened carefully along length of wound.

Fig. 7.7 (*continued*)

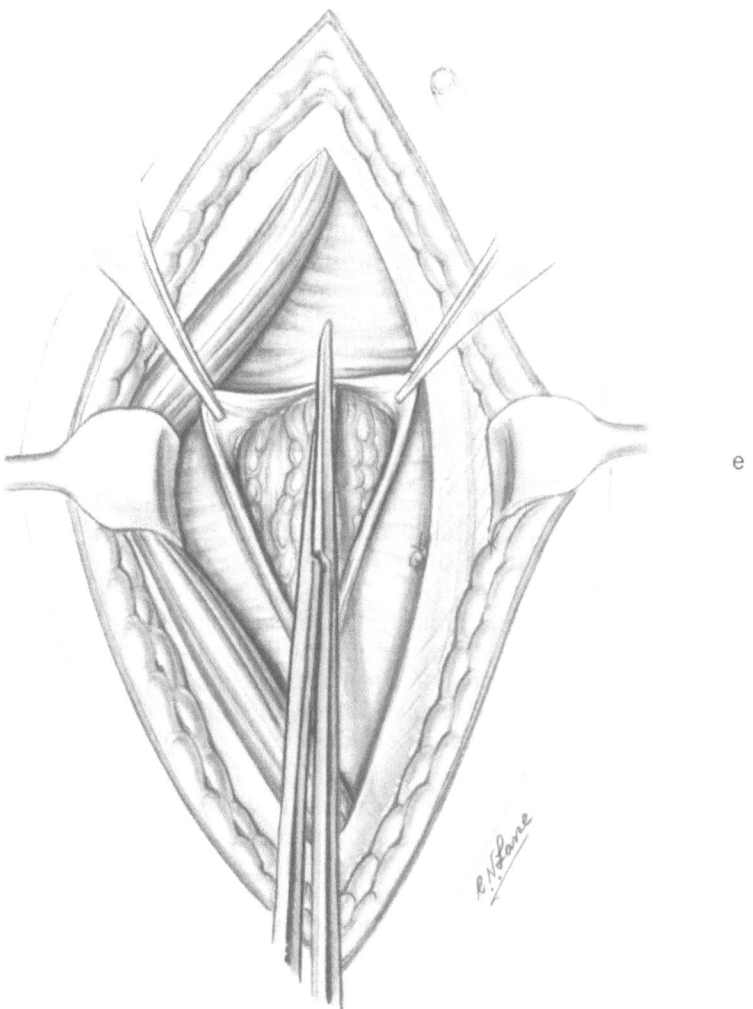

Muscle Split Paramedian

Some surgeons prefer to split the rectus muscle rather than dissecting it free and displacing it laterally. In this technique, the muscle is split longitudinally near its medial border and the peritoneum opened in the same line. The advantage is that the incision can be quickly made and closed and is particularly useful in reopening the scar of a previously performed paramedian incision when it is often very difficult, or sometimes impossible, to dissect the rectus muscle away from the scar tissue of the sheath and only a muscle split is possible under these conditions.

There is the theoretical objection that such an incision may weaken the rectus muscle, but we have failed to find any controlled trial comparing the results of this rectus split incision with the conventional paramedian muscle slide procedure.

Packing

Packing small bowel away into the upper abdomen to give access to the pelvis is useful for most pelvic procedures: ideally, the bowel should be covered with omentum and then packed away, using either wet or dry packs, which for safety are individually tagged with a Spencer Wells forceps. When greater access is required (i.e. during a Wertheim's hysterectomy), small bowel may be packed with a wet swab in an intestinal plastic bag (Foliendeutel–Parke–Davis) and exteriorised for the duration of the operation, without undue desiccation of bowel.

Adhesions

Intra-abdominal fibrous adhesions are a major cause of intestinal obstruction, and by far the most common cause of intra-abdominal adhesions is previous surgical intervention. In addition to obstruction, adhesions may cause visceral dysfunction due to distortion or displacement of an organ within the abdomen or pelvis and persistent pain due to attachment to and traction on the parietes. Although postoperative adhesions can involve any viscus within the abdominal cavity, adhesive obstruction most frequently affects the small intestine.

Since adhesions may have such serious consequences, it is not surprising that a large number of techniques have been devised to prevent their development (Ellis 1971). Only small improvement can be expected unless we look to the underlying pathology. Raftery (1979) has shown that the healing of the peritoneum is a two-stage process. First, there is an initial wave of phagocytic cells responsible for clearing away the traumatic debris in the wound. This is then followed by a wave of subperitoneal perivascular connective tissue cells responsible for healing of the peritoneal defect and formation of the new mesothelium.

It is thought that tissue ischaemia is the initiating stimulus, and adhesions act as vascular grafts to ischaemic tissues. Suturing peritoneal defects under tension and foreign materials contaminating the peritoneal cavity, such as starch glove powder and fragments of gauze, are potent stimuli to adhesion formation. Large peritoneal defects, however, will heal without adhesion formation in the majority of instances, but when attempts are made to oppose wound edges by sutures, adhesions are formed.

Ellis (1962) has shown that injection studies of these adhesions reveal tiny blood vessels running along the adhesion and into the sutured tissue. He concluded that it was not the peritoneal defect that produced adhesions but the presence of devascularised tissue that must unavoidably result from the suturing of the defect.

Damage to the peritoneum, from any cause, results in fibrinous exudate causing adjacent surfaces to stick together forming a fibrinous adhesion. Fibrinolytic activity is absent from the wound during the first 48 h of the healing process. Raftery (1981) further demonstrated that free peritoneal grafting, diathermy of wounds and creation of ischaemic areas of intestine were associated with considerable depression of fibrolytic activity when compared with unsutured peritoneal defects and

also with a significant increase in adhesion formation.

A considerable amount of work, both clinical and experimental, has been published on attempts to prevent adhesions. Ellis (1971) classified the approaches as follows:

1. Prevention of fibrin deposition. This has included the use of a variety of anticoagulants. They have been shown, however, to be of little value and particularly worrying were reports of postoperative haemorrhage and even death in patients who had been given heparin intraperitoneally with a view to preventing adhesion formation.

2. Removal of fibrin. The initial step in formation of adhesions is the adherence of adjacent viscera due to a fibrinous exudate. It is logical, therefore, to try to prevent adhesion formation by the removal of exudate. Lavage, using saline solution and dextrose, has been used but the rapid absorption of these materials makes their efficacy unlikely. Enzymes such as pepsin and trypsin have been used with conflicting reports. The fibrinolytic agents streptokinase and urokinase have reduced the severity but not the complete prevention of adhesions.

3. Mechanical separation of loops of intestine. This particular approach to adhesions has brought about extraordinary surgical ingenuity. Various suggestions have included the distention of the abdominal cavity with oxygen and the stimulation of intestinal peristalsis by prostigmine; one early surgeon gave his patients iron filings mixed with gruel and then passed a magnet over the abdominal wall with the intention of keeping the intestines in constant postoperative motion. Various substances have been introduced into the peritoneal cavity; for example, olive oil, liquid paraffin, amniotic fluid and free grafts of omentum have all been used. There has been initial enthusiasm but most of these methods have exacerbated adhesions rather than reduced them.

4. Inhibition of fibroblastic proliferation. Antihistamines, steroids and cytotoxic agents have been used to inhibit fibroblast proliferation to allow time for reabsorption of fibrin. Large doses of these agents certainly inhibit fibroblast proliferation but they also affect fibroplasia in the wound.

There is little firm evidence that instillation of a substance into the peritoneal cavity is of any clinical value. It may, in fact, cause more problems than it cures.

Although intestinal obstruction from adhesions is a relatively common surgical emergency, the incidence of this complication is not high when compared with the large number of laparotomies which are performed.

Ellis in 1980 showed that we must cease to regard adhesions as evil structures that must be avoided or prevented and must be divided or destroyed whenever they are encountered. Most adhesions are probably completely harmless and may well be beneficial. They undoubtedly act as vascular grafts, thus preventing anastomoses from leaking and devitalised tissue from becoming gangrenous.

To be rational, therefore, we must aim to prevent the development of unnecessary adhesions. We know that adhesions form to areas of peritoneal ischaemia and to sites where foreign bodies are left within the peritoneal cavity. Unnecessary adhesion formation, therefore, may be reduced by meticulous surgical technique including the prevention of granuloma formation from foreign material, for example, glove powder and gauze.

Washing gloves in water does not remove starch completely and may lead to clumping of granules, thus providing a greater stimulus for adhesion formation. It has been suggested that washing in cetrimide and more recently washing in povidone–iodine will remove virtually all of the starch from the surface of the glove. We use the technique described by Fraser (1982): when the gloves are on, 10 ml povidone–iodine surgical scrub is applied. The cleansing process is continued for 1 min during which starch granules on the surface of the gloves are mobilised by the non-ionic surfactant and combine to form blue–black starch iodide. The mixture is then washed off the gloves by pouring 500 ml sterile water from a bottle for at least 30 s. Visual removal of the starch iodide mixture and an aurotactile stick sign confirm a 99·8%–100% removal of starch. A glove (Biogel) has recently been developed (Lennox 1983) that is free of starch, lubrication being achieved by coating only the inner surface with a hydrogel polymer, which is inseparable from the glove rubber. Experiments on rats in our laboratories have shown that this is less likely to produce adhesions than the conventional starch powder glove.

We recommend that peritoneal toilet should be carried out to remove any organic material which may have leaked into the peritoneal cavity. We use a noxytiolin antiseptic mixture. It is preferable that peritoneal defects should be left as raw, oozing surfaces, rather than attempts be made to suture the defect under excessive tension (Raftery 1984). When adhesion formation is considered inevitable because of local tissue ischaemia, the surgeon should attempt to ensure that adhesions develop through structures other than small intestine. An attempt is, therefore, made to draw the omentum over other organs before closing the laparotomy incision.

Ellis and Heddle (1977) showed that closure of the peritoneum in a separate layer plays no significant role in healing the laparotomy wound. In a study using rabbits as experimental animals, they showed there was no significant difference between adhesions to the back of the wound irrespective of whether the peritoneum was sutured or not. Since the strength of healing was not affected, however, there would seem to be nothing to lose by leaving this layer unsutured.

In conclusion, there has been no substitute for meticulous surgical technique with avoidance of contamination of the peritoneal cavity with foreign material and avoidance of suturing peritoneal defects under tension. Most adhesions are harmless and in many instances may be protective. "It is time that the surgeon came to regard adhesions as friends who occasionally misbehave, rather than his enemies" (Ellis 1982).

Wound Closure

The ideal method of closure of the abdominal wound remains to be discovered. It should technically be easy and rapid to perform, entirely free from the complications of dehiscence of the abdominal wound, incisional hernia and persistent sinuses; it should be comfortable and should leave an all but invisible scar.

Closure of the Pfannenstiel incision nearest approaches these ideals. With major laparotomy incisions, work over the past decades has certainly greatly reduced the risk of burst abdomen, but incisional hernia formation and persistent sinuses are still far from uncommon.

Pfannenstiel

Conventionally, the peritoneum is closed with catgut and the rectus sheath with Dexon or nylon. Probably the peritoneal closure can be omitted, and this assertion is based on studies in which the peritoneal layer was left open in a series of midline and paramedian incisions without deleterious effects (Ellis and Heddle 1977). However, we have not seen reports of controlled trials in which this layer has been omitted in the Pfannenstiel incisions.

Midline and Paramedian

There are three technical factors relating to wound failure: tearing of sutures from the tissues, breaking of suture material, and untying of knots. The value of a wide suture bite to prevent the first of these factors is obvious and the first reported laparotomies were closed with that principle. However, under the influence of Halsted in the United States and Moynihan in the United Kingdom the fashion became one of layered closure with exact anatomical apposition of each layer, particularly the peritoneum. It is, however, logical that the surgeon should take wide bites of tissue in closing the abdominal wall, as abdominal wound must be protected against the high intra-abdominal pressures that are known to exist after laparotomy. The integrity of suture technique must be flawless until repair is complete and in the abdominal wound restoration of tensile strength is relatively slowly acquired. The wide bite suture technique (mass closure, Fig. 7.8) has had its advocates since the earliest days of abdominal surgery despite the general trend towards layered closure. There are now many random controlled clinical trials that have suc-

cessfully evaluated the use of mass closure with an acceptably low incidence of burst abdomen or incisional hernia (Goligher et al. 1975; Irvin et al. 1977; Pollock et al. 1979; Bucknall et al. 1982). Mass closure reduced the dehiscence rate in our study from 3·8% to 0·76%.

There are theoretical reasons why the wide bite avoids burst abdomen. Dudley (1970) suggested that the cutting out of sutures relates to the pressure per unit area exerted by them on tissues and the ischaemic necrosis that may follow continual pressure. Jenkins (1976) hypothesised that abdominal wounds lengthen during postoperative abdominal distension and that the tissue bite by a suture in wound closure is related to the length of suture. A suture length: wound length ratio of over 4 : 1 is ideal but anything less than 2·5 : 1 places wounds at risk.

Based on these studies and those I have described in Chap. 10 we therefore advocate the mass closure technique using monofilament nylon.

It is now fully realised, both from clinical studies and from animal experimentation, that healing of the incision takes place by the formation of a dense fibrous scar that unites the apposing faces of the

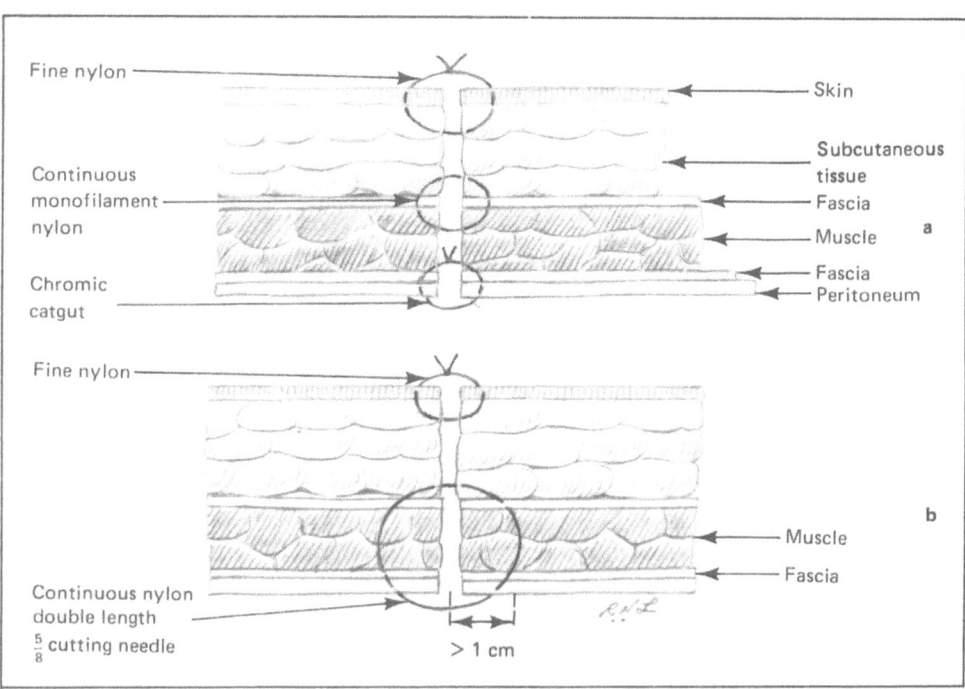

Fig. 7.8a, b. Techniques of abdominal wound closure: **a** layered closure technique; **b** mass closure technique.

laparotomy wound. The purpose of the sutures is to splint the wound edges while this dense fibrous scar deposits and matures. Wide bites must be taken which must be inserted a minimum of 1 cm from the edge of the wound and placed at intervals of less than 1 cm one from the other.

Where possible, omentum is drawn down to cover the abdominal viscera before closure is commenced in order to prevent adhesions between small bowel and the deep layer of the laparotomy incision. We use a hand-held large Moynihan five-eighths needle in order to take wide bites of the full thickness of the abdominal wall and employ number 1 nylon. For the midline incision, all layers of the abdominal wall apart from skin and subcutaneous fat are included in the suture, the skin then being closed (Fig. 7.9a–c). A similar technique is used for the paramedian incision picking up the rectus sheath. The transrectus incision incorporates the medial portion of the rectus muscle in the suture loops. If the peritoneum cannot be included in the suture this is of no consequence.

Some surgeons employ interrupted nylon sutures, either placed simply or by the far and near Smead-Jones technique. To date, there is no available evidence showing whether or not interrupted sutures have any advantage over the continuous technique, which is certainly more rapid.

Drains and ostomy stomas should invariably be brought out through a separate stab wound in order to prevent weakening of the main laparotomy incision.

It should be noted that we have not described the use of tension sutures in closure of the abdominal wall. This is because they are never employed with this technique of primary closure of the abdominal wound. They are painful and give rise to an ugly scar, and there is no evidence in any controlled trial of any value of these sutures in either preventing burst abdomen or incisional hernia if the mass closure technique is employed. The only use for tension sutures is in closure of a burst abdominal incision in those cases where the wound edges are infected and necrotic.

Skin Closure

The factors that need to be considered with skin closure are comfort and cosmesis, ease of postoperative care and avoidance of complications and, of course, speed of closure. Wound disruption resulting from mechanical failure of the closure, haemorrhage and haematoma formation are usually caused by faulty surgical technique rather than the method of closure or the materials used to close

the wound. Fortunately, such complications are uncommon but infection remains a significant complication of wound healing and there is evidence that the choice of suture technique and the materials used in the skin closure may be significant factors in the pathogenesis of this complication (Irvin 1985).

The method of wound closure affects the incidence of infection because all sutures behave as foreign bodies: they generate a variable inflammatory response; they may cause tissue ischaemia; and the interstices of braided sutures may provide a safe refuge for pathogenic bacteria. The adverse effects of wound sutures are particularly apparent in clean-contaminated wounds, and the surgeon should exercise caution in the use of buried suture material in such cases, particularly in the subcutaneous tissues which have little resistance to bacterial proliferation. Fortunately, the prophylactic use of systemic antibiotics provides further protection from wound infection in such cases. Contaminated wounds containing a large bacterial inoculum are likely to become infected almost irrespective of the method of skin closure; some cases are best managed by delayed primary closure of the wound.

If sutures are used the surgeon should use the finest atraumatic sutures compatible with the mechanical requirement of the wound. They should be removed as soon as possible to limit scarring.

Catgut is seldom used as a skin suture but synthetic absorbable sutures are often used as subcuticular sutures.

The non-absorbable sutures include natural materials such as silk and synthetic monofilament and braided (multifilament) materials such as polyesters (Terylene and Dacron), polyamide (Nylon), and polypropylene. Monofilament suture materials are rather less easy to handle than braided sutures but there is little difference in the case of polypropylene, and the monofilament sutures are less likely to predispose to wound infection.

The disadvantages of full-thickness skin sutures are their potential for propagating infection in the subcutaneous tissues, and the undesirable cosmetic sequelae of cross hatching and puncture marks on the skin surface. These disadvantages are countered to some extent by the use of very fine monofilament suture materials, and by early removal of the sutures. Indeed, some surgeons replace the sutures with skin tapes after 3 or 4 days.

Subcuticular sutures placed in the dermal layer of the skin are becoming increasingly popular. A continuous suture technique is usual, and absorbable or non-absorbable materials may be used. Polyglycolic acid and polypropylene are the most

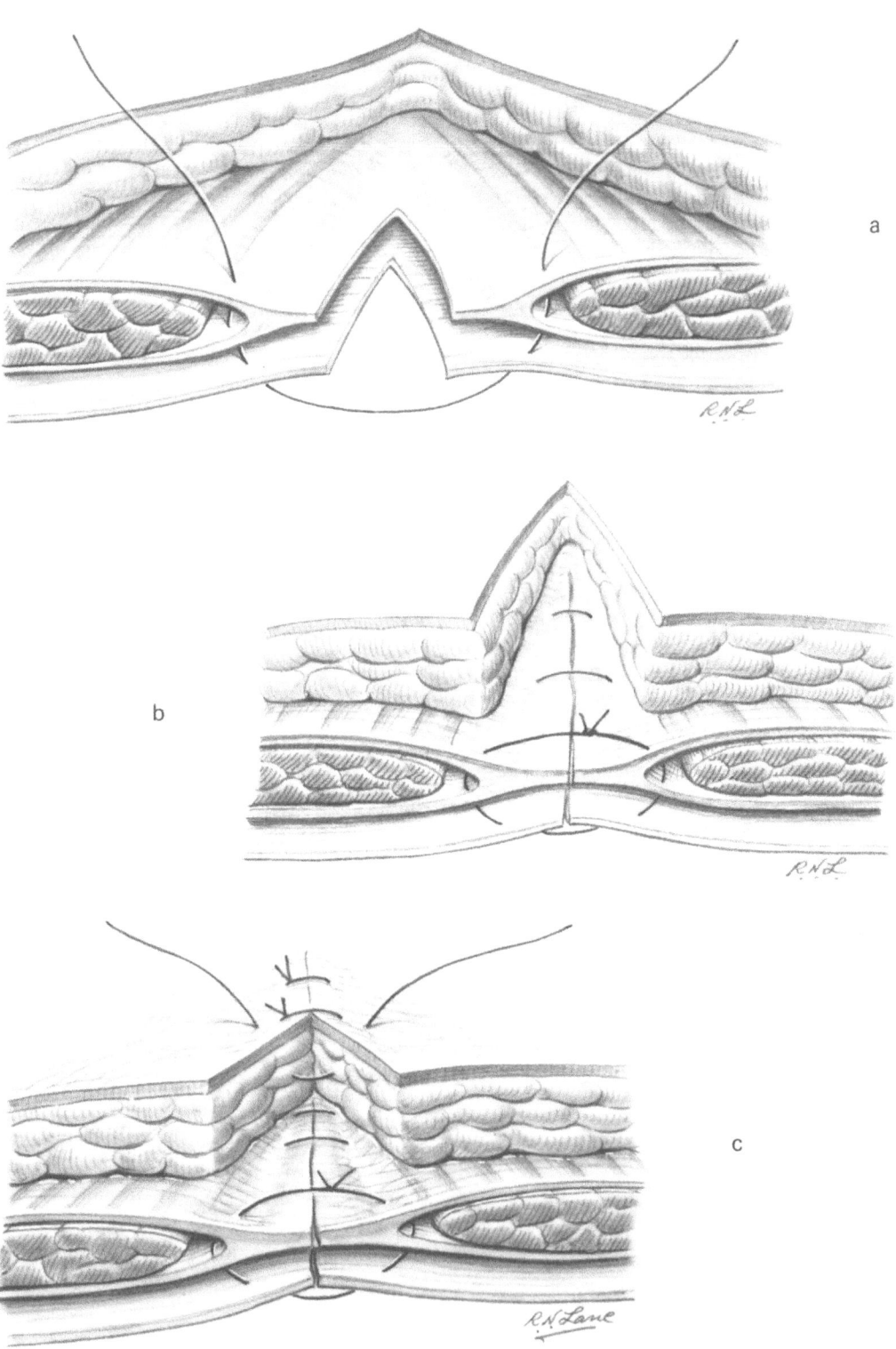

Fig. 7.9. a Midline wound mass closure (see text); **b** midline sheath closure; **c** midline skin closure.

popular. The non-absorbable polypropylene suture is easy to insert since it glides smoothly through the tissues, can be anchored at an appropriate tension with beads and metal collars at each end of the wound, and is easily withdrawn when the wound no longer requires suture support.

The subcuticular technique provides a more comfortable postoperative wound and a superior cosmetic result by comparison with full-thickness skin sutures, although there is probably no significant difference in the incidence of wound sepsis (Bucknall and Ellis 1982). Some surgeons have also adopted a policy of early removal of subcuticular polypropylene sutures in an attempt to avoid suture-related wound infections, using sterile tape to support the wound after a few days. The tape can be applied on completion of the primary wound closure since it is not disrupted by removal of the subcuticular suture.

Steel clips that do not penetrate the full thickness of the skin have been used in wound closure for many years by gynaecologists and occasionally by general surgeons. The use of this type of closure has increased following the introduction of disposable or semidisposable automatic skin staplers. The formation of an incomplete rectangular steel staple secures the edges of the skin wound with little or no invasion of the subcutaneous tissues. Experimental studies have shown that skin stapling causes less tissue damage than skin suturing and is less likely to damage the tissue defences against infection.

In our own studies we found the cosmetic results obtained with staples and clips are similar to those obtained with subcuticular sutures, and they are significantly better than the results of full-thickness skin sutures (Bucknall and Ellis 1982). They are also very quick to insert. Possibly the only real disadvantage of the stapling technique is the substantial cost of the instruments compared with ordinary skin sutures.

Tapes have been used to establish sutureless type of skin closure. The tape that is most commonly used comprises non-woven microporous rayon fibres combined with a polyalkyacrylate adhesive (Steristrip and Reinforced Steristrip, 3M Company). The porous nature of the tape (800 pores/cm^2) prevents accumulation of fluid on the wound surface and discourages secondary bacterial colonisation.

Wounds closed with tape have a greater resistance to infection and usually heal with a better cosmetic result than wounds closed with sutures. Surprisingly, perhaps, tape closures are actually stronger than sutured wounds during the early phase of healing but the taped wounds are rather brittle and these mechanical differences are of little practical significance (Irvin 1985).

Opinions differ with regard to the ease with which accurate and secure apposition of the wound edges may be achieved by tape closure. A perfectly dry skin surface is required, and it is usually advisable to apply an additional adhesive agent to the skin, such as tincture of benzoin. However, problems may arise in achieving accurate apposition of the wound edges in thin subjects or in wounds involving concave surfaces. In such circumstances it may be necessary to supplement the closure with subcutaneous or subcuticular sutures, which reduces the value of the tape closure as a method of avoiding wound infection. Actually, recent experimental evidence suggests that skin staples may be as effective as tape in contaminated wounds and these are our choice for skin closure.

Complications and Their Management

The choice of a particular abdominal incision, the selection of the technique of its closure and the type of suture material to be employed in so doing is to a large extent coloured by the safety of the wound healing which is to be achieved. Failure results at worst in total breakdown of the abdominal incision—"the burst abdomen"—or less dangerous to the patient but still a troublesome complication, initial healing of the wound but subsequent development of an incisional hernia.

Burst Abdomen

Disruption of the abdominal incision may be partial, where either the skin or the peritoneal layer remains intact but where there is rapid development of a massive full-length incisional hernia, or disruption may be complete, where all layers of the abdominal incision tear apart with or without protrusion of the abdominal contents (evisceration).

The published incidence of burst abdomen varies between 0% and 3%. These days, most surgeons would regard the latter figure as extremely high and a fair estimate for all cases would be less than 1%.

The abdominal wound may break down either completely or partially because of one or more of the following reasons:

The Knot May Break or Undo. This is a technical error which is seen from time to time, although it should be avoidable by immaculate technique.

The Suture May Rupture. This occurs either because it is too weak for the tensions placed upon it or because it is rapidly destroyed in the tissues before adequate wound healing has taken place. This factor should be avoidable if the correct size and type of suture material is selected (see Chap. 10).

The Sutures May Cut Through the Tissues. This may occur either because they are placed too close to the wound edge or because excessive weakening of the tissues from such factors as jaundice, uraemia, protein depletion or, undoubtedly the most important, infection.

Wound breakdown will be more likely to occur if the tension placed on the healing wound is increased by abdominal distension or by postoperative coughing or straining.

Although in some instances a single cause can be implicated, more often the cause of wound failure is multifactorial. Indeed, the clinical study of wound healing is complicated by the fact that it is unusual for a single factor to exist in isolation and it may be difficult to determine which of a number of factors has played the important part in wound breakdown. One can visualise the not uncommon situation of a patient undergoing an operation who is suffering from advanced abdominal malignant disease. She may be jaundiced, anaemic and protein depleted. After the operation she may develop an ileus with severe abdominal distension and she may also have a postoperative cough from pulmonary collapse; in addition she may be on cytotoxic treatment. On top of this, we must consider what part the choice of incision, the type of suture material, the technique of closure and the experience of the surgeon may play.

It is an everyday observation that wound healing is rarely a problem in the healthy young patient undergoing routine elective surgery. Problems are likely to be met when the patient is either obese or emaciated, elderly, infected, jaundiced, diabetic, anaemic, alcoholic, protein depleted, vitamin C deficient or suffering from any disease condition being treated with prolonged steroids. Two or more of these factors often coexist.

The number of possible factors affecting healing are legion, both locally at the wound site (blood supply, infection, tension, etc.) and general (vitamin C deficiency, jaundice, uraemia, anaemia, and so on). These are summarised in Table 7.2 (Bucknall 1984).

Table 7.2. Factors affecting healing in surgical practice

Local factors	General factors
Blood supply	Age
Denervation	Anaemia
Haematoma	Anti-inflammatory drugs
Infection—local	Cytotoxic drugs
Irradiation	Diabetes mellitus
Mechanical stress	Hormones
Protection—dressings	Infection—systemic
Surgical technique	Jaundice
Suture material and technique	Malignant disease
Type of tissue	Malnutrition
	Obesity
	Temperature
	Trauma; hypovolaemia and hypoxia
	Uraemia
	Vitamins
	Zinc deficiency

Complete dehiscence of the abdominal wound is associated with a serious mortality rate, as high as 30% in some series, although most reports give an operative mortality in the region of 10%. It is not the wound dehiscence itself which is so lethal but the fact that this complication occurs so often in otherwise generally ill patients. This point was emphasised by Guiney et al. (1966), who noted that, in most cases, the burst abdomen was only one of a number of factors which contributed to the fatal outcome in their study of 232 patients with a 15% mortality.

The best form of treatment is, of course, prevention. A commonsense approach will do much to achieve good and prompt wound healing without complications. In debilitated and aged patients wound healing is retarded, so vitamins, especially vitamin C and a high protein diet, are indicated. Preoperative chest physiotherapy should be instituted in bronchitics and smokers, who must be instructed to stop smoking.

The incision should be no longer than needed. The abdominal fascia must be closed with a nonabsorbable monofilament suture using the mass closure technique. Infection, haematoma and extensive tension should be avoided. Drains should exit through a separate incision or stab incision. A suction tube is placed beneath large skin flaps to prevent fluid collections so that the skin can become adherent to the underlying tissues.

Postoperatively, abdominal distension and pulmonary collapse are avoided as far as possible by nasogastric suction, when the occasion demands, and active physiotherapy.

Disruption of the abdominal laparotomy incision may present in a number of ways. In some cases there is very little warning; the patient's progress appears to be quite satisfactory, but, when the skin sutures are removed 7–10 days postoperatively, the wound disrupts. In other cases, a pink discharge of serosanguineous fluid soaks through the dressings and this is always very suggestive of disruption of the layers of the abdominal wall deep to the skin sutures. This phenomenon represents, in fact, the seepage of blood-stained peritoneal exudate through the skin sutures. The other possibility is that the fluid discharge results from the presence of a large subcutaneous haematoma. One or two of the skin sutures should be removed, preferably in the operating theatre, to investigate this phenomenon. If any separation of the deep layers of the wound has occurred then repair should be carried out at once, but if this is simply a haematoma the fluid is evacuated. In yet other cases, the wound appears to be healing quite normally and then suddenly gives way when the patient is coughing or straining at stool. The phenomenon is surprisingly painless and the patient is amazed to see omentum or a loop of bowel protruding through the wound.

In other cases, there is a stormy postoperative progress with vomiting, distension, respiratory complications and gross suppuration of the wound. An abscess may form and discharge and this is followed by separation of the deep layers of the wound. Inspection may reveal matted omentum or loops of small intestine adherent to the necrotic muscle or fascia in the depths of the wound.

Yet another manifestation is that the patient presents a few days postoperatively with mechanical intestinal obstruction. Exploration reveals that a small part of the abdominal incision has given way and the obstruction has resulted from a knuckle of small bowel trapped within the defect.

Disruption generally occurs between the seventh and tenth postoperative days but may occur as early as the fifth day or be delayed until supporting or stay sutures have been removed. Disruption may occur even later, especially in cases complicated by severe wound infection.

Resuture of the disrupted wound is recommended for the majority of cases, and especially for those in which the edges of the wound are relatively clean, although these may be frayed and torn.

As soon as the condition is recognised, an intramuscular injection of morphine and atropine premedication should be given, and the wound and viscera should be freely bathed with warm normal saline solution and covered with large sterile towels over which a Velcro abdominal support is lightly applied.

When the patient has been moved to the operating room, a nasogastric tube is passed, and the gastric contents are aspirated. The patient is then anaesthetised. The edges of the abdominal wall are then lifted upward, and the prolapsed gut is replaced below the level of the peritoneal edges. Disintegrated fragments of suture material are extracted, and the wound edges are freshened by clipping away necrotic tissue and oedematous skin tags. The sutures will consist of strong monofilament nylon and are inserted 2·5 cm from the margin of the wound and about 2·5 cm apart and are made to transfix all the layers of the abdominal wall on both margins of the wound. The sutures are threaded through 5-cm rubber tubing and firmly tied. For the reapproximation of the skin edges, interrupted nylon sutures are placed between the through-and-through sutures.

The skin sutures are removed on the tenth postoperative day, the through-and-through sutures left in for 3 weeks. Active measures should be taken to combat peritonitis, including gastric suction and decompression, intensive antibiotic therapy and intravenous fluid replacement.

Packing and strapping of the wound only, are indicated: (1) when the patient's condition is such that any secondary operative procedure would be too hazardous, i.e. when the patient is in a critical state and suffering from shock; (2) when the disrupted wound is very foul and freely suppurating; and (3) when there is no gross prolapse of the viscera.

Therefore, in the severely critical case, strapping is to be preferred to resuturing. In the desperate case, the problem is to get the patient safely through the immediate crisis with the least possible interference. As soon as the patient has recovered from the early effects of the wound disruption and the treatment by strapping, and provided there is no evidence of gross infection, secondary suture (when indicated) may then be carried out with much less risk.

It is true that postoperative ventral hernia is an invariable sequel to this method of treatment, but this can be repaired at a later date with comparative safety and success.

Incisional Hernia

Incisional herniae vary from a small insignificant bulge in the wound, only revealed on careful examination when the patient coughs, lifts the legs upwards while in the lying position or sits up, and may not even be noticed by the patient. At the other extreme, the rupture may be very large, unsightly and uncomfortable. If the neck is narrow, there is the risk of strangulation, although this is unusual. Rarely a large thin-walled hernia may be ulcerated, with protrusion of omentum or even the development of an intestinal fistula.

Many surgeons state that incisional herniation is a rarity. In some instances this may be due to excellence of the surgical technique. Goligher et al. (1975) report not a single incisional hernia in 108 laparotomies closed by mass interrupted wire sutures, even though there was one burst abdomen in this group. Donaldson et al. (1982), using the lateral paramedian incision, reported only a single incisional hernia in 231 selected laparotomies. However, we believe that, in the majority of circumstances, the so-called rarity of incisional herniation is due to the fact that patients are not followed up sufficiently and not examined carefully. Our definition of a hernia is any bulge at all in the wound when the patient is examined in the lying position and made to lift the legs upwards, to sit up and to cough. In our study of 1129 major laparotomy wounds followed up for 12 months after operation (Bucknall et al. 1982) we detected a 7·4% incidence of incisional hernias. Others have reported similar findings, for example, Pollock (1981) a 10% herniation rate at 6 months in 961 patients, Johnson et al. (1982) a 13% incidence in 213 laparotomies followed up for 6 months and Irvin et al. (1977) a 4·7% incidence at 6 months in 200 consecutive laparotomies.

Most investigators follow up their patients for 6 or at the most 12 months following laparotomy. Ellis et al. have reported 363 patients whose wounds were soundly healed at 1 year and were reviewed again between $2\frac{1}{2}$ and $5\frac{1}{2}$ years later (Ellis et al. 1983). No less than 21 of these patients (5·8%) were now found to have developed incisional hernias. Six were unaware of the presence of the hernia and none of the patients were inconvenienced by it or requested surgical repair. Interestingly, none of the causal factors which we will discuss later were found to be associated with the development of these late hernias. It is difficult to explain how mature collagen can stretch to form an incisional hernia more than 1 year after sound healing has occurred. However, Harding et al. (1983) from Cardiff, Wales, have also reported late development of incisional hernia in their investigation carried out 3 and 5 years after laparotomy. Akman (1962), in a study of 500 incisional hernias coming to surgery, noted that just over half were present within 6 months of the original operation. Three-quarters had developed within 2 years of surgery and 97% were present within 5 years of the initial laparotomy.

Our study of over 1000 consecutive laparotomies in which there were 19 complete dehiscences and 84 incisional hernias has enabled us to make careful observations on aetiological factors. Herniation was commoner at a statistically significant level in old age, male patients, the obese, patients undergoing large bowel surgery and in incisions greater than 18 cm in length. No significant differences could be found in the type of incision used. Interestingly, there was no difference in incidence between wounds closed by consultants and registrars although the incidence was higher in the hands of senior registrars! The most significant factors were postoperative complications—chest infection, abdominal distension and, most important of all, wound sepsis. Forty-eight per cent of the 179 patients who had developed a wound infection developed an incisional hernia.

Our series included 104 patients whose laparotomies were closed with polyglycolic acid (Dexon) and in this group there were 11·5% wound herniations—significantly higher than in those closed by nylon.

The prospective study by Pollock (1981) of 98 incisional herniae in 961 patients gave similar results to our own—the most important factors being chest complications, male sex, age of 65 and, above all, wound infection. It would certainly seem that the most significant advance in the prevention of herniation in a wound would be the elimination of wound sepsis.

Operations to repair incisional herniae are lesion and beyond the scope of this chapter. In the great majority of cases, a sound repair can, however, be achieved by mass closure with nylon. Only if there has been an extensive loss of tissue from sepsis, trauma or wide surgical excision is there need for mesh implant.

Infection

Infection is the most common complication of wound healing and it is encountered in every surgical speciality. As Lord Moynihan wrote in 1920, "Every operation in surgery is an experiment in bacteriology". Classical wound infection occurring in a wound closed by primary sutures may simply be a source of significant morbidity, but may have disastrous consequences.

It is interesting that, in their early phases, infection and wound healing are remarkably similar processes. Infection leads to a cellular and vascular response to the bacterial injury, and repair then follows the destruction of bacteria and removal of necrotic tissue. Wound healing demonstrates a comparable cellular and vascular response to the mechanical trauma of wounding.

There is now considerable evidence concerning the effect of infection on healing. Delay in healing can be demonstrated experimentally in wounds inoculated with bacteria and there is a decreased tensile strength of contaminated laparotomy wounds from the sixth postoperative day onwards.

The principal biochemical abnormality seems to be a disturbance of collagen metabolism: probably by a depressant effect on fibroblasts. By stimulating fibroblasts and granulation tissue in some way it may, therefore, be possible to encourage healing and there has been some success in increasing capillary growth density by changing the local oxygen concentrations in wounds simply by increasing the inspired oxygen.

The net result of the changes in collagen metabolism is that the collagen content of the wound is reduced. The process is not confined to the wound alone: it extends through the wound edges into unwounded tissues; the wound edges become soft and mechanically weak; and wound sutures will cut out through the softened tissues, resulting in wound disruption.

Infection occurs when the number of organisms exceeds the ability of local tissue defences to handle them and wound infection is defined as the discharge of pus from a surgical incision. The number of organisms that will produce an infection is known and, for most pathogens, is a concentration of 10^6 organisms/g tissue. With smaller numbers, local humoral and cellular defences can dispose of invaders and this is what occurs in contaminated wounds. Contaminated wounds, however, can become infected wounds. This happens when there is a large amount of necrotic tissue present, when certain types of foreign bodies are in the wound or its vicinity, or when something interferes with local tissue defences such as occurs in burns or in patients receiving immunosuppressant drugs. Table 7.3 lists the various factors which contribute to changing a contaminated wound into an infected one.

The best way to deal with infection is to prevent it! Several aspects of prevention are important to the wound healer. To prevent infection we should try to avoid bacterial contamination. If this fails then we must prevent multiplication of any contaminating bacteria.

Any interference with the blood supply will affect the local inflammatory response and favour bacterial growth. This may occur in several ways; in some cases extensive tissue destruction is responsible, particularly in traumatic wounds; in other cases, surgical technique is at fault. The surgeon may unwittingly produce tissue necrosis by rough

Table 7.3. Factors contributing to infection

1. Surgeon	Surgical technique
	Devitalised tissue
	Impaired local circulation
	Haematoma
	Foreign body
2. Organism	Infective nature
	Source: (a) Endogenous, e.g. skin, biliary, colorectal
	(b) Exogenous (cross infection)
3. Patient	Disease, e.g. diabetes, neoplasia, malnutrition, anaemia, chronic granulomatous disease
	Medications, e.g. steroids, cytotoxics, intensive antibiotics, radiotherapy
	Immune response of individual
	Remote active infection

handling of the tissues, by strangulation of tissues during the knotting of ligatures or by the excessive use of surgical diathermy. Gentleness is the key: it will result in less dead tissue, less infection and better healing.

Impaired local blood supply, haematoma and foreign bodies also affect infection and hence healing. The most common foreign bodies are sutures, and certain suture materials are more likely to propagate wound infections. Generally, bulky braided suture materials are more likely to cause trouble than fine monofilament sutures. Wound drains are also foreign bodies and should only be used to remove specific collections or drain dead space. Until recently, it was common practice to drain contaminated wounds as a prophylactic measure against wound infection or abscess formation but there is increasing evidence that drains may be of little value in such circumstances. Wound drainage per se does not therefore appear to reduce infection, but where there is heavy contamination the principle of delayed primary suture is recommended.

Some bacteria are particularly prone to produce infection; these include *Clostridia* species, particularly prevalent after severe soft tissue damage. Radical debridement is the cornerstone of treatment. Actinomycosis and tuberculosis are also associated with extremely poor healing. Most bacteria recovered from surgical wounds however are opportunistic pathogens: they are commensal organisms normally found in the hollow viscera or on the skin surface, and they give rise to wound infections when they are inoculated in the wound in sufficient numbers. We must try hard then to avoid bacterial contamination. Meticulous operative technique is the best method of doing so.

Haematoma

A haematoma is one of the commonest wound-related complications. It is important, not only because of the adverse effects on wound healing, but also because of the nidus it provides for wound infection.

In reconstructive surgery, where haematomas are particularly responsible for skin flap necrosis, the conventional explanation is that haematomas produce internal pressure, which subsequently obstructs the dermal circulation, causing necrosis. Flaps performed experimentally show necrosis only if blood is present beneath; flaps with underlying silicone pillows or serum remain viable. Therefore, haematoma-related necrosis of flaps does not occur solely because of the internal pressure.

A mass of blood, apparently, exerts a toxic effect independent of the level of bacterial contamination. The salvage of flaps overlying haematomas can be improved by evacuation of the underlying blood within 12 h. It should be our aim, however, to try to prevent collections of blood beneath wounds. The importance of surgical technique, with careful attention to haemostasis and gentle handling of tissues, cannot be overemphasised. The recognition of patients at risk is vital. The coagulation mechanism can be disturbed by a number of different factors, including treatment with anticoagulants, haemophilia, thrombocytopenia and fibrinogen deficiency (for example due to liver cirrhosis or disseminated intravascular clotting). Elderly patients are particularly prone because of increased capillary fragility and laxity of tissues.

Where there is a wide area of capillary oozing the use of pressure pads will often be sufficient to secure haemostasis of the smaller vessels and allow minimal use of both ligature and diathermy.

The use of suction drainage or external pressure by dressings on the superficial part of the wound reduces the incidence of haematoma collection, as does the effective closure of dead space, particularly in the obese patient.

If these methods fail it may be advantageous to pack the wound and employ a policy of delayed primary suture after haemostasis some 48 h later.

Topical thrombin has been a recent advance in the prevention of haematoma (Hashemi et al. 1981). In 102 heparinised patients 82·4% of the thrombin-treated group were free of any haematoma while 64·7% of the untreated group developed haematoma. This is especially important as many patients are given low-dose heparin in an attempt to reduce postoperative deep vein thrombosis.

References

Akman PC (1962) A study of 500 incisional hernias. J Int Coll Surg 37:125–142

Bucknall TE, Cox PJ, Ellis H (1982) Burst abdomen and incisional hernia: a prospective study of 1129 major laparotomies. Br Med J 284:931–933

Bucknall TE, Ellis H (1982) Skin closure—a comparison of nylon, polyclycolic acid and staples. Eur Surg Res 14:96–97

Bucknall TE (1984) Factors affecting healing. In: Bucknall TE, Ellis H (eds) Wound healing for surgeons. Bailliere Tindall, London

Donaldson DR, Hegarty JH, Brennan TG, Guillou PJ, Finan PJ, Hall TJ (1982) The lateral paramedian incision—experience with 850 cases. Br J Surg 69:630–632

Dudley HAF (1970) Layered and mass closure of the abdominal wall. Br J Surg 57:664–667

Ellis H (1962) The aetiology of post-operative adhesions—an experimental study. Br J Surg 50:10–16

Ellis H (1971) The cause and prevention of post-operative intra-peritoneal adhesions. Surg Gynecol Obstet 133:497–511

Ellis H, Heddle R (1977) Does the peritoneum need to be closed at laparotomy? Br J Surg 64:733–736

Ellis H (1980) Internal over-healing—the problem of intra-peritoneal adhesions. World J Surg 4:303–306

Ellis H (1982) The causes and prevention of intestinal adhesions. Br J Surg 69:241–243

Ellis H, Gajraj H, George CD (1983) Incisional hernias: when do they occur? Br J Surg 70:290–291

Ellis H, Coleridge-Smith PD, Joyce AD (1984) Abdominal incisions—vertical or transverse?, Postgrad Med J 60:407–410

Ellis H (1984) The abdominal wall. In: Bucknall TE, Ellis H (eds) Wound healing for surgeons. Bailliere Tindall, London

Ellis H, Bucknall TE, Cox PJ (1985) Abdominal incisions and their closure. Current Problems in Surgery, vol. XXII. Year Book Medical Publishers Inc

Fraser I (1982) Simple and effective method of removing starch powder from surgical gloves. Br Med J 284:1835

Goligher JC, Irvin TT, Johnson D, deDombal FT, Hill GL, Horrocks JC (1975) A controlled clinical trial of three methods of closure of laparotomy wounds. Br J Surg 62:823–892

Guiney EJ, Morris PJ, Donaldson GA (1966) Wound dehiscence. A continuing problem in abdominal surgery. Arch Surg 92:47–51

Harding KG, Mudge M, Leinster SJ, Hughes LE (1983) Late development of incisional hernia: an unrecognised problem. Br Med J 286:519–520

Hashemi K, Donaldson LJ, Freeman JW (1981) The use of topical thrombin to reduce wound haematoma in patients receiving low-dose heparin. Curr Med Res Opin 7: 458–462

Irvin TT, Stoddard CJ, Greeny MG, Duthie HL (1977) Abdominal wound healing: a prospective clinical study. Br Med J ii:351–352

Irvin TT (1985) Simple skin closure. Br J Hosp Med 6:325–330

Jenkins TPN (1976) The burst abdominal wound: a mechanical approach. Br J Surg 63:873–876

Johnson CD, Bernhardt LW, Bentley PG (1982) Incisional hernia after mass closure of abdominal incision with Dexon and Prolene. Br J Surg 69:55

Lennox M (1983) Studies on starch-free gloves in adhesions, the problems. In: Lennox M, Ellis H (eds) LRC Products

Pollock AV, Greenall MJ, Evans M (1979) Single layer mass closure of major laparotomies by continuous suturing. J Royal Soc Med 72:889–893

Pollock AV (1981) Laparotomy. J Roy Soc Med 74:480–484

Raftery AT (1979) Regeneration of peritoneum: a fibrinolytic study. J Anat 129:659–664

Raftery AT (1981) Effect of peritoneal trauma on peritoneal fibrinolytic activity and intra-peritoneal adhesion formation. An experimental study in the rat. Eur Surg Res 13:397–401

Raftery AT (1984) Serosae repair. Wound healing for surgeons. Bucknall TE, Ellis H (eds) Bailliere Tindall, London

8 · Scope of Laparotomy

John M. Monaghan

The abdomen should rarely be opened for the purposes of making a diagnosis; in almost all circumstances a firm provisional diagnosis should be made prior to the procedure.

Preoperative Assessment

In order to provide as accurate a diagnosis as possible, the following preoperative assessment techniques should all be considered:

Abdominal and Pelvic Examination

The patient should be fully examined at referral and upon admission to the ward. It is a valuable practice to carry out a pelvic and abdominal examination immediately the patient has been anaesthetised and after the bladder has been catheterised. Not infrequently masses which were thought to be present will be found to have disappeared and vice versa. When the abdominal musculature is relaxed both pelvic and abdominal examinations are greatly facilitated.

Diagnostic Imaging

Contrast radiology of the bowel and urinary tract, ultrasonography, computerised axial tomography (CT scan), and magnetic resonance imaging (MRI) (Chap. 5) are of value in accurately outlining the site and source of intra-abdominal lesions.

However, these investigations are expensive, time consuming and should only be used where appropriate. They also have limitations of resolution which must be appreciated otherwise undue dependence may be placed upon them.

Laboratory Investigations

Laboratory investigations include enzyme studies to determine liver or pancreatic disease and tumour markers where cancers are suspected.

Cytological and Histological Studies

The widespread use of ultrasound has allowed the development of fine needle aspiration techniques which can give the clinician access to remoter parts of the body which often cannot be reached by normal endoscopic methods. The material obtained by fine needle aspiration (FNA), using a Tuohy needle, and other percutaneous biopsy techniques can be processed using standard cytological and histological methods to give an accurate diagnosis of the lesion.

Laparoscopy

Laparoscopy is an accurate and simple way of determining the true nature of abdominal and pelvic pathology without the need for a full laparotomy. Occasionally it is of great value to combine laparoscopy and needle biopsy in order to obtain an accurately directed sample.

Although it is vital to obtain as much prior information as possible about the likely pathology to be found at laparotomy, this requirement should not in any way cause delay in the performance of the procedure. A long, drawn out mechanistic approach to preoperative assessment will not be of value for the majority of patients; for example, the rigid routine of performing a barium enema on all patients with carcinoma of the cervix will rarely yield significant results and will even more rarely alter the management method.

Choice of Incision

The varieties of incision available have been dealt with in detail in Chapter 7; this section will be solely concerned with the reasons for choosing a particular route of entry into the abdomen, their advantages and disadvantages.

Lower Midline Subumbilical Incision (Fig. 8.1a)

Indications

This incision is ideal for access to large pelvic masses, giving excellent access to the whole of the pelvis and to the lower abdomen.

Advantages

Probably the most important advantage of this incision is its simplicity, allowing rapid and easy access to a large part of the lower abdomen and the whole pelvis. It is quickly performed, with minimal bleeding and where necessary can be equally easily extended to allow the surgeon to deliver large tumours from the pelvis or to gain access to upper abdominal lesions.

Disadvantages

The most significant problem associated with this incision is its relative weakness compared with transverse and paramedian incisions. It has a potential for dehiscence and eventual hernia formation. It is also unsightly, causing considerable personal unhappiness.

Low Transverse or Pfannenstiel Incision (Fig. 8.1b)

Indications

This incision should be the method of choice for entering the lower abdomen where the pelvic pathology is known not to be carcinoma or of such a size that the lesion cannot be delivered through the opening. It is also to be recommended for Caesarean sections except where extreme speed is required.

Advantages

The wound is strong and cosmetically satisfying and hernias are extremely rare.

Disadvantages

The major disadvantage is that it cannot be easily extended and gives limited access to the abdomen. It is also a slow method of entering the abdomen and should not be used if the patient is "in extremis". It may also be a bloody procedure with considerable ooze occurring from the rectus muscle and its vessels; drainage of the wound may be necessary.

Interspinous Transverse, Muscle-Cutting Incision (Fig. 8.1c)

Indications

This is a specialised incision used most frequently by the gynaecological oncologist to carry out radical procedures such as Wertheim's hysterectomy and by the author to perform exenterative surgery.

Advantages

The two main advantages are that the incision allows access not only to the pelvis but also to the lower abdomen, giving a clear view of the lower aorta for lymph node dissection, and also facilitates the performance of bypass surgery such as the production of urinary conduits and colostomies.

Disadvantages

The main drawback to the incision is that it cannot be extended easily and because the rectus muscle is cut when the incision is made there is an inherent weakness which may contribute towards dehiscence and hernia development.

Lower Paramedian Incision (Fig. 8.1d)

Indications

This incision continues to be popular with general surgeons; however, it has little place in gynaecological practice except where the operator wishes to leave the contralateral side of the abdomen free for the placing of a stoma.

Advantages

It is said to be stronger than a midline incision with a reduced risk of dehiscence and hernia formation. It is simple to extend the incision into the upper abdomen when more extensive access is required.

Disadvantages

The procedure takes longer to perform than a midline incision, and runs the risk of damaging the blood and nervous supply to the rectus muscle.

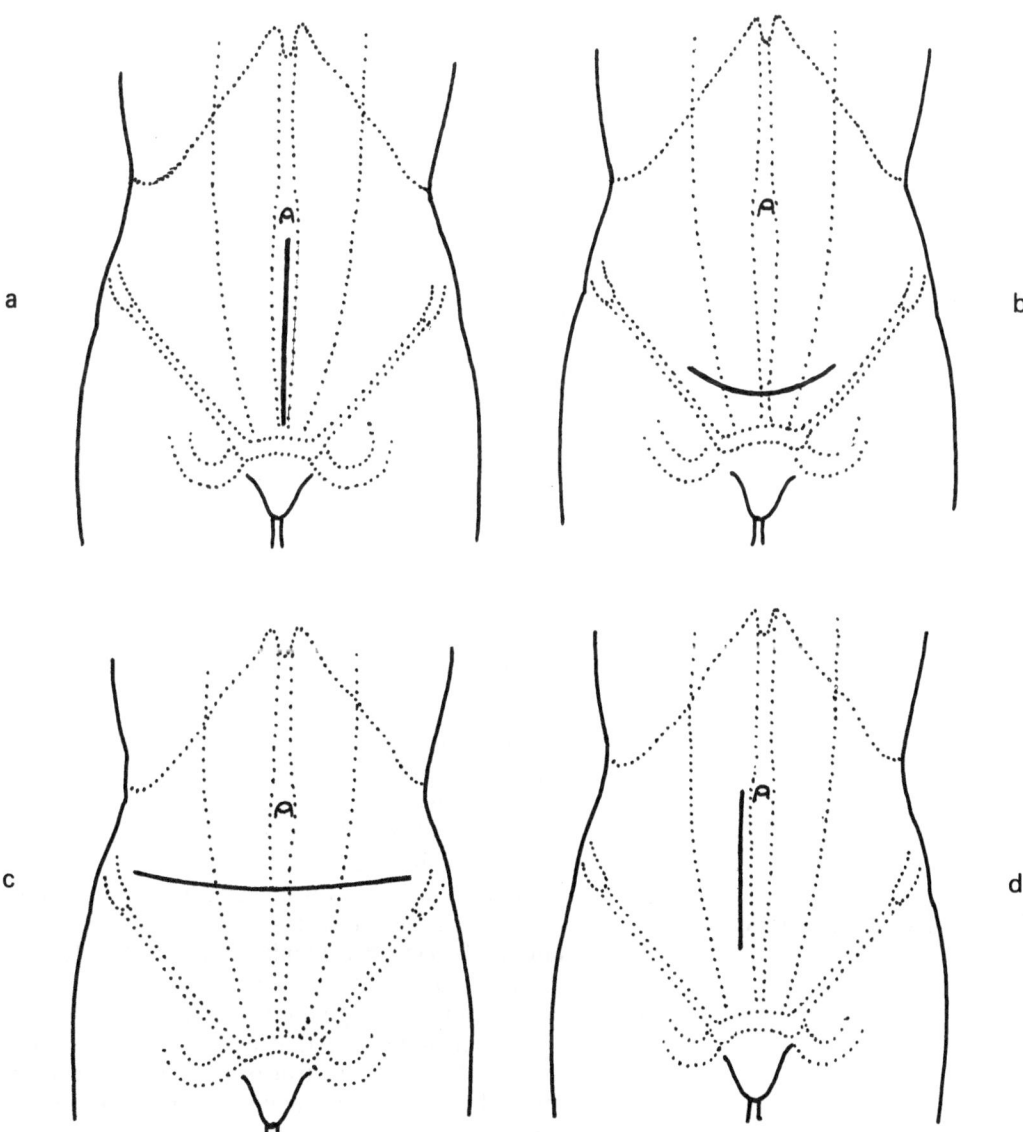

Fig. 8.1.a Lower midline incision; **b** Pfannenstiel incision; **c** interspinous transverse muscle-cutting incision; **d** lower paramedian incision.

Upper Abdominal Incisions

Indications

These incisions will rarely be performed by the gynaecologist and are in the province of the general surgeon.

Changing the Incision

All surgeons will at some time find that they have entered the abdomen using an incision which is inappropriate for the required procedure. It will then be necessary for the operator to make an alteration to his initial incision; the choices available will include:

1. Direct extension of the initial incision is clearly the easiest and most convenient choice. Unfortunately this can only be performed if the original incision was a midline or paramedian. It is therefore clear that if there is the slightest possibility of the need to extend that the primary choice of incision should be one of these two.

2. Secondary incision at an angle to the original may be performed but is very unsatisfactory, with a significant risk of devitalisation at the junction of the two wounds, frequently resulting in difficulties with wound healing.

3. Closure of the original wound and performing a new and more appropriate incision is often the best course of action. This course of action often provokes the comment from senior colleagues that "the green was only reached in two". The patient will often benefit from this approach as the procedure of choice will be facilitated by the use of the correct incision.

Procedure of Laparotomy

Technique

Palpation

The gynaecologist must develop the habit of accurately palpating the pelvic and abdominal organs in a methodical and meticulous manner, similar attention being paid to the pelvic side wall, the posterior abdominal wall, the dome of the diaphragm and the posterior surface of the anterior abdominal wall. The surgeon should assiduously practice gentle palpation of all intra-abdominal structures so that he builds up in his mind a tactile picture of every organ. This includes the kidneys, spleen, pancreas, liver, gall-bladder and small and large bowel. Only in this way will he develop the necessary skills instantly to recognise normal from abnormal by touch alone.

Inspection

Visual inspection of the pelvic organs is routinely performed by gynaecologists; however, many are remiss in not performing a visual inspection of abdominal structures. The author recommends using palpation as a preliminary screening device and then careful visual inspection of any areas which appear to be abnormal. This is of particular importance in cases of carcinoma especially of the ovary where accurate assessment and documentation of the full extent of the intra-abdominal disease is mandatory.

Access to the upper abdomen may be obtained by either extending the incision or by elevating the anterior abdominal wall by traction so that the liver, dome of diaphragm and both the infracolic and gastric omentum can be directly visualised.

Sampling

It is important that prior to contaminating the abdomen with blood from the wound edge the surgeon should carefully collect samples of any fluid or pus that may be present within the abdominal and pelvic cavity. A sterile universal container is used to collect ascitic fluid and a bacteriology swab is used to sample pus or other evidence of infection.

If there is intraperitoneal spread of a carcinoma with multiple small metastases present on the peritoneal surfaces, it is often tempting to remove the most accessible and be satisfied that an adequate biopsy has been taken. This is a practice to be eschewed if possible; the metastasis often represents the most aggressive part of a carcinoma and consequently is often poorly differentiated, thus leaving the pathologist with an extremely difficult task in determining the origin of the carcinoma.

It is recommended that a considerable effort is made to determine the true origin of any carcinoma and a biopsy of the original tumour mass made. This biopsy should be of an adequate size so that a number of studies can be performed upon it, e.g. mucin stains to differentiate between carcinomata of the bowel and the ovaries.

Recording Information

Operation records all too frequently leave a lot to be desired in accuracy and content. It is not of great value to write long procedure notes detailing every minor move in what is a standard procedure, but it is vital to record findings fully. This is best done by using either a standard proforma or tick list which is filled in at the time of surgery by an assistant or immediately afterwards by the surgeon himself. This approach is particularly important when dealing with cancer patients where a knowledge of the exact stage of the disease will have a major influence on the type of future management the patient may require.

If the surgeon has plans to analyse his data on a future occasion he should carefully prepare the proformata so that they can be used to collect information in a manner which will allow direct transfer to a microcomputer. There are a number of simple inexpensive data management software packages available which are invaluable to the clinician who wishes to regularly update, evaluate and analyse his records.

Operative Findings

The gynaecologist must make a careful assessment of the abdomen every time he carries out a procedure:

1. Definition
2. Diagnosis
3. Management
   a) Operate
   b) Do nothing
   c) Call for another opinion
   d) Close the abdomen and refer
   e) Drain

Unexpected Findings

Extravasations

Pus

1. Always take a specimen in a bacteriological container for culture and sensitivity testing.
2. Identify the source of the infection.
3. Remove the source of the infection.
4. Drain the area affected.
5. Local cleansing with antiseptics such as Noxyflex and intraoperative intravenous antibiotics.

6. Close the abdomen and treat the patient with systemic antibiotics.

Blood

1. Identify the source of the bleeding.
2. Control the haemorrhage by the most appropriate method.
3. Actively replace blood lost with appropriate materials.

Ascites

1. Collect a specimen of fluid in a clean universal container.
2. Send for cytological assessment for the presence of malignant cells.
3. Send for bacteriological studies, taking care not to forget the possibility of infections such as tuberculosis.
4. Make a careful inspection of the upper abdomen particularly the liver for evidence of cirrhosis; *do not biopsy the liver.*

Bowel Contents

1. Take a specimen and send for bacteriological assessment, culture and sensitivity.
2. Identify the source of the leakage, and be sure to determine whether there is one leak or a number.
3. Remove as much of the leaked material as possible and carry out meticulous peritoneal lavage.
4. Begin broad-spectrum antibiotics intravenously immediately. Sensitivities obtained later may modify the choice of drugs used.
5. If it is a simple task to close the bowel defect do so; if bowel resection is necessary and specialist help is required, call for a general surgical colleague.

Bile

Leakage of bile into the abdominal cavity is extremely rare without prior surgical interference but may occur from an empyema. Bile is extremely irritating to the peritoneum, producing an intense peritonitis with extreme pain.

MANAGEMENT

1. A specimen should be taken for culture and sensitivity of any bacterial content.
2. The patient is started on a broad spectrum antibiotic.
3. Drainage of the site of leakage instituted.
4. As leakage is so often associated with infection surgical procedures are often not possible or prudent, therefore drainage and conservative

measures allowing the infection to settle are the optimal first steps. Surgical management can be carried out as an interval procedure.

Pancreatic Fluid

Pancreatic fluid is made up of proteolytic enzymes so it has an extremely corrosive effect upon intra-abdominal structures. The body's natural response is to localise the leaking fluid with the formation of a pancreatic pseudocyst, often developing within the lesser omentum. It is rare to find leakage of pancreatic fluid occurring spontaneously, except in association with acute pancreatitis. Leakage most frequently follows surgery to the stomach or gall bladder or following abdominal trauma.

There is usually a large mass lying between the stomach and the transverse colon; occasionally the mass may be between liver and stomach or behind or below the transverse colon.

MANAGEMENT
1. If the problem is found at laparotomy, expert surgical advice should be sought.
2. The treatment of choice is to make a communication between the encysted fluid and the stomach, a cystogastrostomy.
3. Where a pancreatic fistula has developed there is considerable danger to the patient because of the excessive loss of fluid and electrolytes which occurs.
4. The fistulous opening also undergoes proteolysis and requires careful protection with acidic barrier creams.
5. Dependent drainage is the treatment of choice.

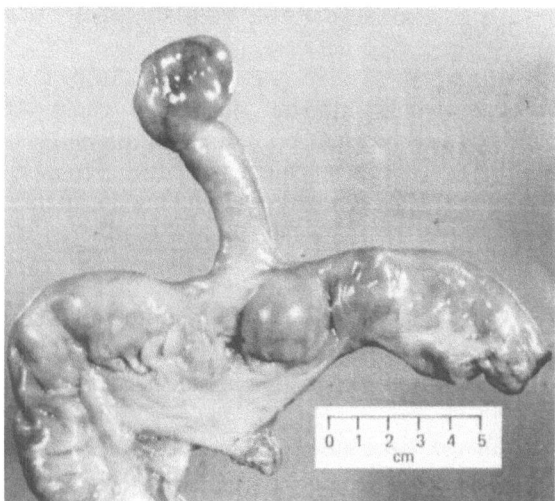

Fig. 8.2. Meckel's diverticulum.

Bowel

Meckel's Diverticulum

Meckel's diverticulum is a developmental residuum of the vitellointestinal duct, connecting the distal part of the ileum to the umbilicus. The abnormality may be patent producing a fistulous communication with the umbilicus, or more frequently it is present as a small outpouching of the small intestine, usually 3–5 cm long, linked to the posterior part of the umbilicus by a band or short duct (Fig. 8.2).

The most common problem that may arise is that of inflammation, which may be intermittent, mimicking appendicitis. Occasionally the band may provoke adhesions or obstructive symptoms due to torsion.

DIAGNOSIS. This is best made by carefully inspecting the terminal few feet of the small intestine when the adherent band is readily apparent.

MANAGEMENT. If the structure is present as a band all that is required is for it to be resected between ligatures; if the diverticulum is of any size it is better to resect it in similar manner to that required for the appendix, taking care not to narrow the ileum.

Carcinoma

Small bowel carcinoma is relatively rare but that of the large bowel is not, particularly of the ascending and descending colon. Ascending colon cancer is second most common and tends to occur predominantly in older women. This is the group of patients which the gynaecologist will frequently find give him a surprise at laparotomy. Either of these cancer sites can be mistaken for ovarian masses; they commonly collect a covering of omentum, can be misdiagnosed on ultrasound as multicystic tumours and may appear on clinical examination to arise from the pelvis. Contrast radiology of the large bowel is the most accurate diagnostic tool but is not always performed by the gynaecologist.

DIAGNOSIS. The gynaecologist will pick up the thickened mass of the carcinoma during his general inspection of the abdominal viscera at the onset of the laparotomy. The site of the cancer should be accurately defined, the mesentery inspected for evidence of nodal spread and the liver examined for metastases.

MANAGEMENT. The gynaecologist should call upon a surgical colleague to assist him in the assessment; if the lesion is thought to be resectable it can be

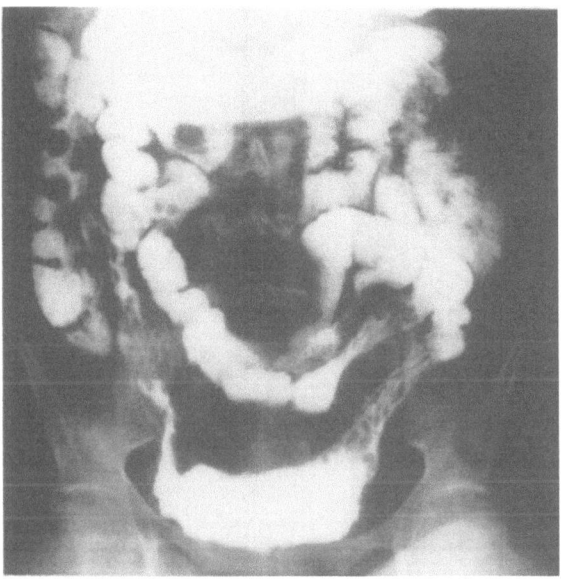

Fig. 8.3. Radiographic appearance of Crohn's disease.

carried out immediately with intravenous antibiotic cover. A resection with primary anastomosis is usually possible, a procedure which is often more easily performed using stapling devices.

Regional Ileitis *(Crohn's Disease)*

This granulomatous inflammation of the bowel, commonly developing in young adults, may affect any part of the tract from mouth to anus but is most frequently seen in the terminal ileum. Preoperative

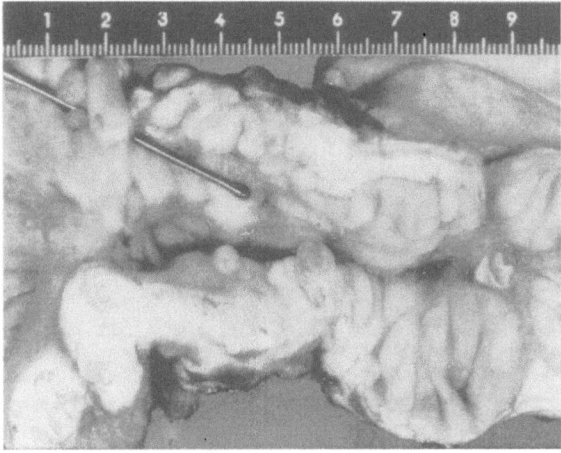

Fig. 8.4. Fistula developed in small bowel affected by Crohn's disease.

diagnosis is best made using barium studies of the bowel (Fig. 8.3).

DIAGNOSIS. The disease is characterised by diarrhoea, weight loss and intermittent abdominal pain. It is not unusual for the abdomen to be opened because of abdominal pain misdiagnosed as of tubal or ovarian origin; the bowel will be found to be enlarged over a short segment or segments, as "skip" lesions frequently occur. The bowel is thickened "brawny", weeping, covered with a dull greyish exudate and may have the mesenteric fat extending over the bowel surface. Occasionally the bowel is adherent to surrounding structures, a frequent precursor of fistula formation (Fig. 8.4).

MANAGEMENT. The most important function that the gynaecologist can serve is fully to document the extent of the disease and to call for assistance from a surgical colleague. If assistance is not readily available the wisest course of action is to close the abdomen following the accurate recording of the findings. **A biopsy of the bowel should *not* be taken** as this only increases the risk of fistula formation.

Ulcerative Colitis

This inflammatory condition of the bowel is frequently found to occur in young women and is not an uncommon finding at laparotomy. The disease is characterised by debilitating diarrhoea and abdominal pain with weight loss and a high risk of malignant change in the affected bowel. The ulceration usually begins in the distal large bowel and progresses proximally; if the ileocaecal valve is incompetent the terminal ileum may also be involved though this is unusual (Figs. 8.5, 8.6).

DIAGNOSIS. It is uncommon to find this condition as an incidental finding as the symptoms are so characteristic; however, if affected bowel is found it is important not to carry out primary surgical procedures or biopsies.

MANAGEMENT. Conservative medical treatment is the first line of management. Surgery is reserved for those cases where life is threatened, or where there are complications or a risk of neoplastic change.

Diverticulitis and Diverticulosis of the Colon

This usually occurs in an older group of patients; consequently it is not often mistaken for salpingitis, ectopic pregnancy or other conditions related to the menstrual years. Occasionally a perforated diverticulum may present to the gynaecologist, who mistakenly diagnoses an ovarian or tubovarian abscess.

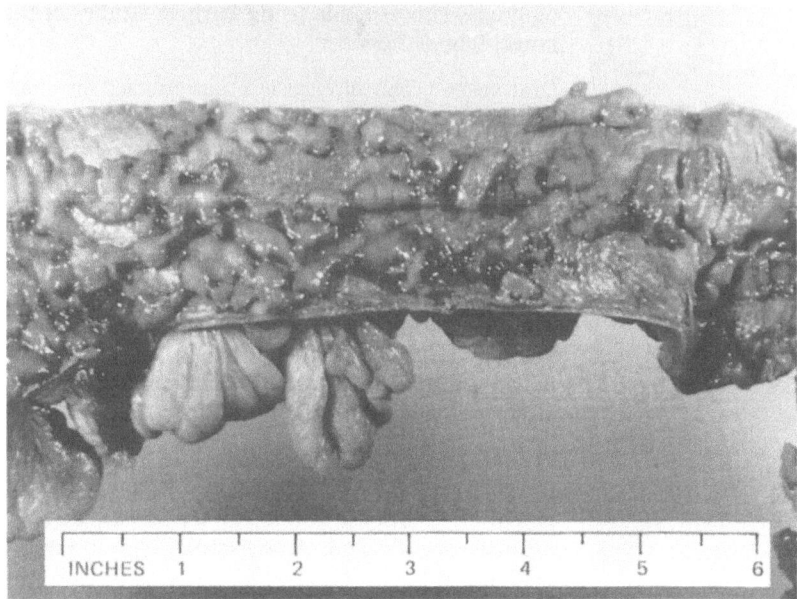

Fig. 8.5. Ulcerative colitis.

DIAGNOSIS. Upon entering the abdomen the descending colon or sigmoid loop will be found to have a perforation releasing faeces and/or pus into the peritoneal cavity; frequently the mass which has been inadvertently diagnosed as an ovarian lesion will be seen to be an abscess localising the perforation, sealing off the leaking bowel contents.

MANAGEMENT. If the bowel contents have leaked into the abdominal cavity the entire area should be carefully cleansed and lavage of the cavity per-

formed with antiseptic solutions. The area of perforation should be drained and a defunctioning colostomy performed proximal to the perforation. Where a diverticular abscess has formed the site should be drained, ideally retroperitoneally, and a proximal defunctioning colostomy performed.

If the site of perforation is localised and identifiable the segment of bowel may be isolated and resected or exteriorised. Immediate antibiotic treatment is begun in theatre using an intravenous broad-spectrum Gram-negative and bacteroides-

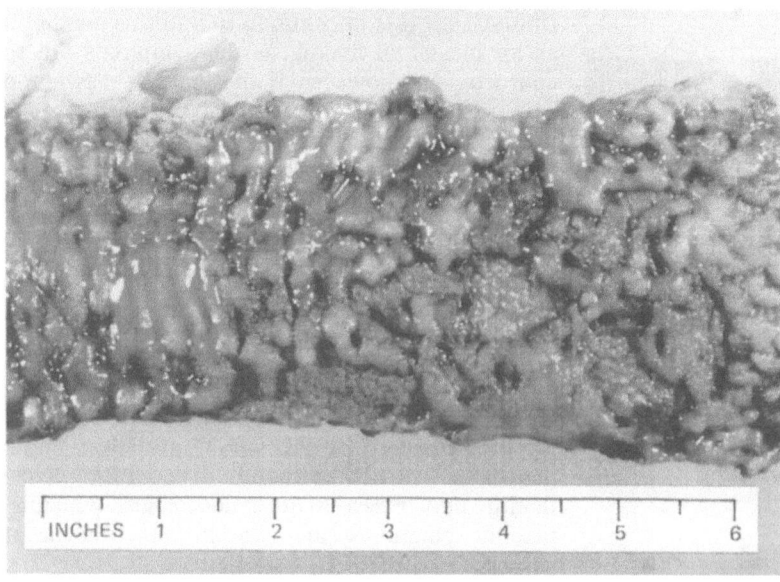

Fig. 8.6. Ulcerative colitis (close up).

specific combination. The patient is in great danger of developing septic shock, which must be pre-empted.

A perforated colon diverticulum is a life-threatening condition.

Acute Appendicitis

This condition, which spans all age groups but is particularly common in the young, is not uncommonly found at laparotomy by gynaecologists.

DIAGNOSIS. As the abdomen is opened pus may be visible within the abdominal cavity; this should be swabbed and the swab sent for culture and sensitivity. If the appendicitis has been contained by omentum there may be a large mass in the right iliac fossa containing the organ. All too frequently the appendix is simply inflamed and engorged often with faecoliths contained within the appendiceal lumen. In gynaecological practice appendicitis can mimic pelvic pathology when it lies close to or over the brim of the pelvis.

MANAGEMENT. The appendix should be removed, a procedure well within the surgical compass of the gynaecologist, and often simple to perform because of the relatively large incisions used by the gynaecologist. It is important to put the patient on an antibiotic and carefully to invaginate the stump of the appendix using a purse string technique.

Appendix Abscess

Unfortunately the gynaecologist may be called to see patients who have mistakenly been diagnosed as having pelvic inflammatory disease whereas when the abdomen is opened it is found that the seat of infection is the appendix. This error is most commonly seen when the appendix is extending into the pelvis or lying close to the right ovary.

DIAGNOSIS. This is not always easy especially when the pelvic organs and small bowel are involved in the infected mass. It may be possible to identify the base of the appendix close to the mass.

MANAGEMENT. This will depend on the extent of the infection and the involvement of other organs. In general the inexperienced gynaecologist should simply swab the pus from the abdomen, send a sample for culture, clean the area and drain any obvious abscess cavity. An interval appendicectomy can be performed after the infection has been controlled with antibiotics.

Great care should be exercised in placing the drain so that fistula formation can be avoided. Similarly the habit of separating adhesions with a swab on the finger must be eschewed or fistulae will result.

Mesenteric Adenitis

This is a diagnosis which is often difficult to substantiate; it most commonly occurs in children and lasts for a brief period followed by full recovery. It is not uncommon for the child to be subjected to appendicectomy which does appear to remove the chance of future episodes.

DIAGNOSIS. This is not easily made at laparotomy and is usually a diagnosis of exclusion. Mesenteric nodes may be palpable but it is difficult to be certain that they are pathological.

MANAGEMENT. A conservative approach is recommended but where there is the slightest possibility of appendicitis the appendix should be removed.

Tuberculosis

Tuberculosis of the bowel is a relatively uncommon finding at laparotomy; it can mimic regional ileitis in its hypertrophic form or ulcerative colitis in its ulcerative form. When the condition affects the peritoneum small vesicles are found which can give the appearance of deciduosis peritonei. Ascitic fluid may also be present which should be sent for culture and protein assessment.

DIAGNOSIS. This is best made by culture of fluid within the peritoneal cavity and the use of contrast radiology of the bowel.

MANAGEMENT. Surgery is rarely required except where perforation has occurred. The abdomen should be closed without drainage and chemotherapy instituted.

Endometriosis Affecting the Bowel

This common condition will only rarely directly involve the bowel and produce complications. Although it is common to see extensive involvement of the pouch of Douglas, the rectum and sigmoid colon will usually function normally. Occasionally the condition will deeply invade the wall of the large bowel and produce obstruction mimicking carcinoma because of the constriction of the lumen consequent upon the scarring process.

DIAGNOSIS. Unfortunately the diagnosis is not made until the bowel has been resected and the pathologist has inspected the specimen histologically.

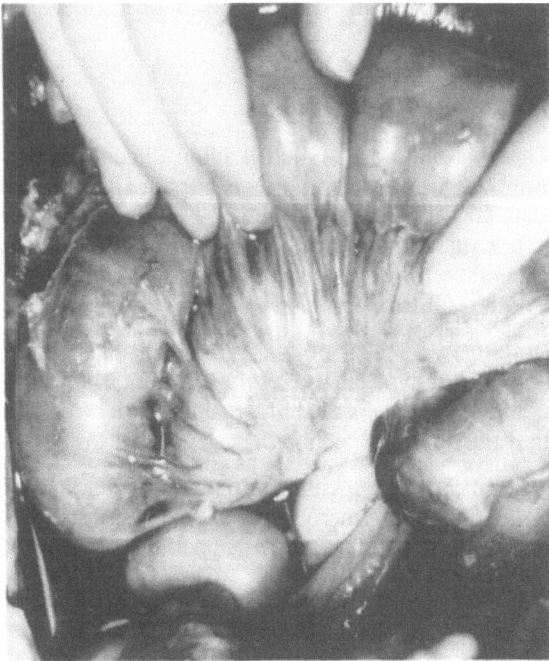

Fig. 8.7. Torsion of the small bowel.

MANAGEMENT.   If there is other evidence of endometriosis in the pelvis the best management is conservative, using Danazol over at least 6 months. This can be followed by inspection of the pelvis with the laparoscope.

Mechanical Disturbances

Torsion (Fig. 8.7), herniation and intussusception (Figs. 8.8, 8.9) all have characteristic appearances

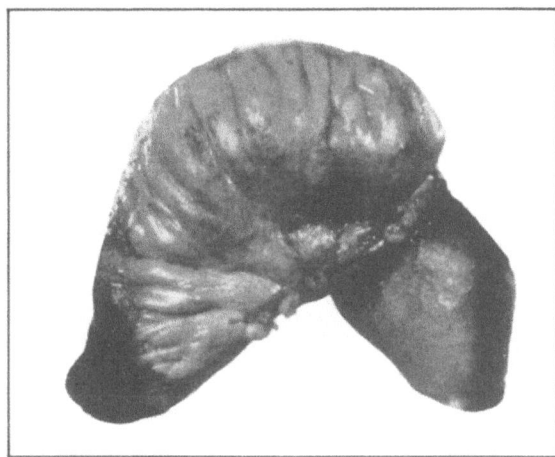

Fig. 8.8. Intussusception of the small bowel, external appearance.

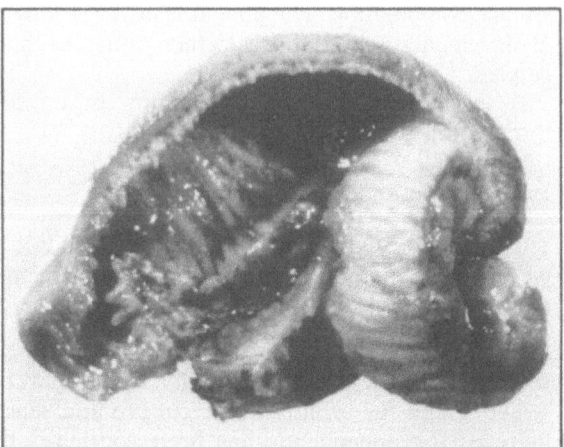

Fig. 8.9. Intussusception of the small bowel, internal appearance.

which should be dealt with by a skilled general surgeon. It is the duty of the gynaecologist to call for assistance from the surgeon rather than attempt to treat these problems with the possible exception of uncomplicated torsion.

Prolonged mechanical disturbance may lead to infarction; this dangerous condition which predominantly affects the small bowel requires rapid and skilful management. The gynaecologist is again recommended to call for surgical assistance.

Radiotherapy damage

This is not infrequently found at laparotomy.

DIAGNOSIS.   The bowel is characteristically pale and immobile with a thickened dead-looking wall; the damage is frequently in segments and particularly affects the terminal ileum after pelvic irradiation (Fig. 8.10).

MANAGEMENT.   Radiotherapy damage calls for delicate handling, taking great care not to put tension on the bowel or its mesentery and not to manipulate the bowel with either swabs or instruments more than is absolutely necessary. Too much handling can result in the development of fistulae or at least provoke severe haemorrhages in the wall of the bowel which may later break down. Unless an oncologist or general surgeon is available who is used to handling irradiated tissue the abdomen should be closed and the patient referred.

Liver

Congenital Abnormalities

The liver is rarely the site of significant congenital anomalies, the most common and important being

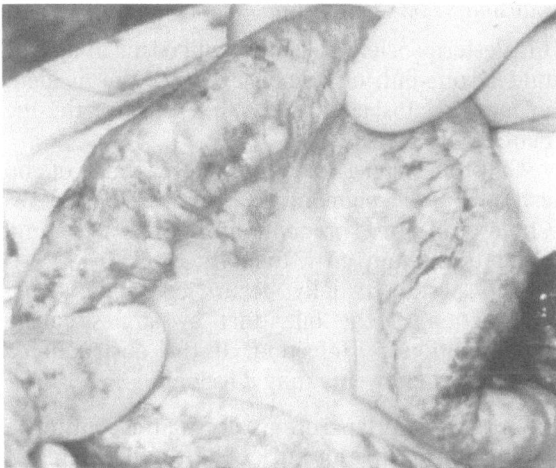

Fig. 8.10. Radiotherapy damage to small bowel.

polycystic disease and cavernous haemangiomas.

DIAGNOSIS. The liver is usually enlarged by soft bulbous protrusions (Fig. 8.11), polycystic disease being not uncommonly associated with a similar condition of the kidneys.

MANAGEMENT. It is best to simply record the findings and not to carry out any operative procedure.

Carcinoma

In Western medical practice the vast majority of carcinomas of the liver are secondary. The commonest sites for the primary tumours are those of the gastrointestinal tract, the breast, melanomas and, in later stages, tumours of the genital organs. In Africa and the Far East malignant hepatoma

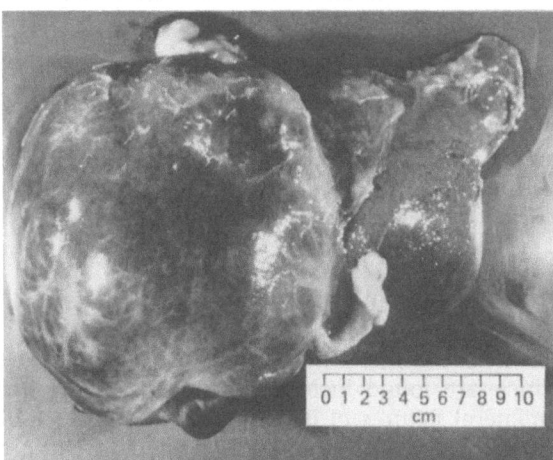

Fig. 8.11. Polycystic disease of the liver.

is common, most probably due to environmental factors. The most likely carcinogen is aflatoxin derived from the fungus *Aspergillus flavus*, which is frequently found on nuts and maize.

DIAGNOSIS. Unfortunately the diagnosis is usually made at a late stage and occasionally at laparotomy which has been carried out for intra-abdominal pain usually produced by haemorrhage from the cancer. Ascites may be present.

At laparotomy the liver is found to be irregularly enlarged; sometimes only one lobe or part of a lobe is affected and treatment may be possible.

MANAGEMENT. A surgical opinion must be sought and an assessment of operability made. It may be possible to resect a lobe or segment of the liver if the tumour is small; however, the long-term survivals are extremely poor. Surgery is the best method of management, chemotherapy only having a temporary palliative effect.

Infection, Hepatitis, Amoebiasis, Hydatid Cyst

Infections and infestations of the liver are rarely met with in surgical practice.

DIAGNOSIS. When hepatitis is present the liver will appear engorged, enlarged and hot.

Amoebic abscesses are usually single and situated in the right lobe; the abscess is large and thin walled and contains a liquid which is characteristically described as looking like "anchovy sauce". The abscess may rupture into the abdominal cavity, producing the symptoms of an acute abdomen.

Hydatid cysts are formed by infestation of the liver with the embryos of the tapeworm of the dog; they are most commonly found in sheep-rearing areas where man, dog and sheep live in close proximity. The cyst commonly calcify producing classical X-ray pictures.

MANAGEMENT. Hepatitis should be allowed to work out its course with general supportive therapy. Amoebiasis is best treated by the use of metronidazole, with the addition of aspiration of the abscess if the response is not rapid. Hydatid cyst should be resected with a margin of normal liver tissue around, clearly a task for the experienced surgeon, to whom referral should be made.

Cirrhosis

In Western society the commonest cause of cirrhosis of the liver is excessive alcohol intake. In Africa, China and the Middle East, schistosomiasis is a common causative agent. Cirrhosis consequent upon chronic hepatitis is relatively rare. Portal hypertension develops and the characteristic portasystemic shunting occurs usually at the junction of the oesophagus, the fundus of the stomach, around the umbilicus and at the anus. Ascites is a common development but its cause may be misdiagnosed and culminate in a laparotomy. Usually these manifestations are clear before the abdomen is opened.

DIAGNOSIS. If cirrhosis has not been suspected prior to laparotomy, palpation and inspection of the liver makes the diagnosis obvious. The liver is shrunken, often of a yellow hue and nodular. This nodularity may be of a micronodular or macronodular type, the former developing nodules a few millimetres in diameter and the latter more irregular large protruberances which can be mistaken for tumour involvement.

MANAGEMENT. Sampling of the ascitic fluid and accurate recording of findings is the most important management to be carried out by the gynaecologist. He should remember that this condition is often associated with bleeding disorders; therefore he should take exceptional care not to traumatise tissues and should inaugurate haematological studies including: thrombin time, kaolin cephalin clotting time, prothrombin time and platelet count.

Vitamin K, fresh frozen plasma, factor concentrates and platelet transfusions may all be required to manage the bleeding problems.

It is therefore clear that referral and transfer to a unit skilled in managing these complex problems is mandatory.

Gall Bladder

Congenital Abnormalities

These are extremely common, most of which are minor variations and aberrations of the blood supply and its relationship to the cystic and bile ducts. Cystic change of the bile duct occasionally occurs (choledochal cyst).

DIAGNOSIS. A gynaecologist simply inspecting the gall bladder will not usually notice the congenital variations of the vasculature, but would be expected to recognise a choledochal cyst if of significant size.

MANAGEMENT. A surgical opinion should be called or the abdomen closed and the patient referred to a surgeon. Ultrasound can be used to confirm the diagnosis. The preferred course of action is to resect the cystic part of the duct and perform a choledochojejunostomy (Roux-en-Y). Malignant change can occur in long-standing untreated cysts.

Gallstones and Cholecystitis

In Western society gallstones will occur in approximately one-fifth of women aged 40; the incidence in men is considerably less (one-third of the incidence in women).

Gallstones consist of either aggregations of cholesterol or bile pigments or mixtures of the two. Cholesterol stones predominantly occur in younger patients and may grow to a large size.

Cholecystitis usually occurs consequent upon obstruction of the bile duct by stones causing inflammation or infection. If the obstruction is chronic an empyema may develop.

DIAGNOSIS. At laparotomy during the routine palpation of the inferior surface of the liver enlargements of the gall bladder can be readily felt and stones can be palpated through the thin wall of the gall bladder.

MANAGEMENT. The finding should be documented and the patient referred to a surgical opinion after recovery from the laparotomy.

Carcinoma of the gall bladder is extremely rare and invariably fatal.

Urinary Tract

Abnormalities of the urinary tract rarely impinge upon the abdominal cavity; however, this does not excuse the gynaecologist from examining the tract. He should particularly look for:

Hydronephrosis and Hydroureter

These are caused by obstruction due to intrinsic pressure from carcinoma or stones, or extrinsic pressure, from carcinoma, scarring and radiotherapy changes.

The bladder should also be carefully inspected to exclude carcinoma.

MANAGEMENT. The findings should be carefully documented and if an expert general surgical or urological opinion is not immediately available the patient should be referred as soon as possible in the postoperative period.

Pelvic Organs

The most common deformities of the pelvic organs which are found incidentally at laparotomy are unilateral failures of development and failures of fusion of the Mullerian ducts producing varying degrees of double uterus. All manner of variation will be seen from true double uterus (uterus didelphus) to a small dimple in the fundus which may be associated with a small intrauterine septum.

The problems are not infrequently associated with non-development of parts of the renal tract.

MANAGEMENT. The findings should be recorded and no surgical action taken. If there is associated infertility this problem can be investigated and a planned surgical approach made at a later date.

Haematocolpos

This should not be found as a surprise finding at a laparotomy if a proper pelvic examination has been performed. The imperforate vagina is obvious and the diagnosis easy to make. The uterus should not be touched abdominally; the vagina is opened and free drainage instituted.

Fibroids

These common benign tumours of the uterine wall are probably the most commonly found incidental finding at laparotomy.

DIAGNOSIS. The appearances of the tumours are very characteristic enlarging the uterus with smooth firm nodules of varying sizes. They may be solitary or multiple, reaching enormous size and, depending upon their position, present interesting surgical exercises during their removal.

MANAGEMENT. If the patient has already consented to a procedure involving removal of the uterus, the presence of fibroids does not produce a problem. They should be removed together with the uterus.

In younger patients who may wish to have further pregnancies myomectomy may be necessary; however, the trainee gynaecologist should be very careful not to embark on this procedure without either the consent of the patient or a considerable degree of experience.

Pregnancy presents some difficult management problems for the gynaecologist. It is not uncommon for fibroids to undergo a process of "red degeneration" during pregnancy. This problem may present as abdominal pain which is localised to the pregnant uterus or alongside it. If the abdomen has been opened and a degenerating fibroid is found it should be treated conservatively. The abdomen is closed and the patient treated with analgesics until the degeneration settles down. *Under no circumstances should the gynaecologist resect the fibroid.* The risks of haemorrhage are enormous, and the records of patients who have eventually lost the pregnancy and the uterus as the result of this manoeuvre are legion.

Pyometra and serometra

These two conditions are associated with carcinoma of the cervix and its radiotherapeutic treatment. Pyometra will develop when either the carcinoma of the cervix or the radiation treatment has totally obstructed the cervical canal and the fluid which has built up in the uterus has become infected. A serometra usually occurs after radiation treatment; the fluid which builds up remains sterile. The diagnosis should not be made at laparotomy if adequate vaginal assessment has been made and proper attention paid to the patient's history.

MANAGEMENT. The problem should be treated entirely from the vaginal aspect as disastrous consequences may ensue if a pyometra is opened into the abdomen. Drainage must be adequate to prevent a recurrence.

Endometriosis

This enigmatic disease, still without an adequate explanation of its origin, can manifest itself in many different ways. It is therefore not surprising that this is a diagnosis often made at laparotomy.

DIAGNOSIS. The disease is relatively simple to recognise, with its small, fresh, red, papular appearance or the "burnt matchhead" pattern surrounded by small patches of scar. In extreme cases the ovaries are cystic, developing the classical "chocolate cysts" full of dark-brown altered blood. These cyst are difficult to resect because of their lack of a capsule and usually rupture, releasing the irritant contents into the abdominal cavity.

When the process has been going on for a long time, the uterus may be fixed in retroversion, with dense adhesions to surrounding structures, particularly the rectum and sigmoid colon loop. Occasionally the condition may present because of the tendency to affect other organs in the pelvis, including obstruction of the bowel imitating cancer formation.

MANAGEMENT. If there is only a small amount of endometriosis and the patient is young and wishes to have further pregnancies, the abdomen should be closed and medical treatment initiated with Danazol.

If there is evidence of chocolate cysts or more extensive disease and reproductive function is still required, then the cyst should be resected, preserving any small amounts of normal ovarian tissue which may be present. The abdomen is then closed and medical treatment with Danazol begun.

If the patient has no further desire for pregnancies then the surgical treatment can be more radical, removing all visible evidence of endometriosis.

However, it should be remembered that surgical treatment without ovarian removal or their subsequent functional control with Danazol is not certain to cause cessation of the continuing development of the disease. The vogue for hysterectomy alone has little scientific evidence to support it as a treatment for endometriosis.

Malignant Conditions of the Uterus, Including Carcinoma of the Corpus, Cervix and Carcinomatous Change in Fibroids

DIAGNOSIS. It is unusual for these problems to be undiagnosed at the time of laparotomy; however, if the circumstance arises it is most important not to perform any procedure which may jeopardise later definitive treatment. For example, removal of the uterus by simple hysterectomy will make subsequent successful treatment of a carcinoma of the cervix extremely difficult. Disease limited to the uterus is difficult to diagnose without histological confirmation; if necessary this can be obtained with frozen section biopsy at the time of laparotomy.

MANAGEMENT. If there is evidence of spread from the uterus to the pelvic side wall or beyond, the most important step is to comprehensively document the findings, sampling lymph nodes where appropriate and marking the site of tumour metastases with metal marker clips.

Fallopian Tube and Ovarian Carcinoma

These two conditions may be first diagnosed at laparotomy; often unfortunately when they are not expected.

DIAGNOSIS. The typical findings are of a carcinomatous mass arising from the ovaries or tubes, commonly bilateral, and with evidence of widespread intraperitoneal spread particularly to the omentum and diaphragm.

MANAGEMENT. Each of these carcinomas should be managed in the same way.

Ascitic fluid should be sampled and sent for cytology. Specimens should be taken from the pelvis and the paracolic gutters. The whole abdomen must be carefully explored and the findings recorded.

The carcinoma should be removed completely, together with the uterus, the omentum and any deposits on the bowel or the peritoneum. The aim should be to achieve complete surgical removal, or if this is impossible, "debulking" to a point at which no tumour mass greater than 2 cm in diameter remains. If the carcinoma is invading the peritoneum it is often possible to clear the tumour by carrying out a retroperitoneal dissection removing the tumour and peritoneum together. This technique is particularly valuable in the pelvis.

Posterior Abdominal Wall

Neurofibromata, Congenital Cysts, Anterior Myelomeningocoele and Associated Congenital Abnormalities of the Sacrum and Pelvis

All these conditions have been reported to occur but are very rare. The most frequently found is the neurofibroma which appears as a soft fibrous fleshy mass commonly lying alongside the rectum and displacing it sideways. The masses tend to grow to a large size, frequently developing a false capsule in the manner of uterine fibroids. The gynaecologist must take great care to identify structures such as the ureters before any attempts at removal are made. The surgery is usually simple but can lead the gynaecologist into territory with which he is unfamiliar.

Second-Look Laparotomy

Principle

The term second-look laparotomy has been coined to describe a secondary laparotomy performed on patients with ovarian cancer to assess the status of intra-abdominal disease after a course of treatment.

This course of treatment usually consists of a primary laparotomy at which the patient's disease is staged, and optimal resection of the cancer is performed, ideally to a point at which only microscopic disease remains. The patient is then treated with a series of courses of chemotherapy with a view to clearing any residual microscopic disease.

Indications

The second-look laparotomy is therefore performed on patients who are clinically free of tumour after a course of chemotherapy, and should be differentiated from what the author descibes as second-chance laparotomy. Those patients with the best chance of having a negative second-look procedure are those who had the following factors:

1. Less than 0·5 cm of residual disease at first operation
2. The use of *cis*-platinum as a chemotherapeutic agent
3. Patient less than or equal to 50 years

These factors increase the likelihood of cytologically and histologically negative second-look procedure.

Procedure

The operation consists of a thorough examination of the entire abdomen and pelvis carried out through a long midline incision.

Any free peritoneal fluid is taken for cytological examination and washings of the pelvis and paracolic regions are carried out by instilling between 200 and 400 ml of normal saline into the abdominal cavity, taking care to allow the fluid to travel around the peritoneal surfaces. Some surgeons enthusiastically "shake" the patient but this is not necessary. The fluid is then withdrawn from each area in turn and collected in universal containers. The specimens are immediately sent for cytological examination, which is best performed on the concentrated material produced after light centrifugation of the fluid.

Any evidence of "burnt out" tumour is removed and sent for histopathological examination. The sites of major tumour masses are either removed or sampled and carefully measured and documented. The diaphragm is inspected and sampled cytologically.

Pelvic and para-aortic lymph nodes should also be carefully inspected and sampled. The entire length of the bowel is examined and any remnants of omentum which remain are removed and sent for analysis.

If any single specimen shows cytological or histological evidence of malignant cells the second-look laparotomy is considered POSITIVE.

Comment

Some authorities criticise the use of second-look laparotomy on the grounds that even if positive little can be done as a second-line treatment. This is thought to be particularly so if cis-platinum has been used as the first-line drug. The author feels that even when this is the case the second-look procedure should be performed if only for the acquisition of information about the state of the abdominal contents. These data are invaluable when decisions are made as to the timing of cessation of treatment. At the present time non-invasive techniques of assessing the internal state of the abdomen, including ultrasound and CAT scan, are not as accurate as the open laparotomy.

A negative second-look laparotomy is a good indicator of tumour clearance although there is evidence that up to 25% of patients with negative second-look procedures may subsequently relapse.

Second-Chance Laparotomy

The author has used this term to allude to the circumstance where a second laparotomy is performed with a view to achieving optimal removal of tumour prior to giving a full course of chemotherapy. The surgery may be carried out a short period after the inadequate primary laparotomy, or it may follow a short series of pulses of chemotherapy. The aim of the procedure is to reduce the tumour burden so as to make the chemotherapy more effective.

Indications

The author feels that this can be an invaluable procedure, especially in the circumstances where inadequate primary surgery has been performed. There are considerable doubts about its value after a series of courses of chemotherapy.

Acknowledgements

The author is indebted to Dr. J. Sunter, Consulting Pathologist, of the Queen Elizabeth Hospital, Gateshead, for Figs. 8.2, 8.5, 8.6, 8.7, 8.8, 8.9, and to Mr. I. Miller, Consultant Surgeon of the Queen Elizabeth Hospital, Gateshead, for Figs. 8.3 and 8.4.

Suggested Reading

Bailey H., Love M. (1984) Short practice of surgery. In: Rains A, Ritchie H (eds) 19th edn. HK Lewis, London

Bonney's Gynaecological Surgery (1986) Monaghan JM (ed) 9th edn. Bailliere Tindall, London

Bucknall T, Ellis H (1984) Wound healing for surgeons. Bailliere Tindall, London

9 · Instruments Old and New

Stuart L. Stanton

Introduction

Instruments are probably the most neglected part of our surgical training: a senior house officer uses the instruments the registrar uses, who in turn usually takes whatever is in the hospital pack. The days have long departed when the newly appointed consultant was invited to submit his list of instrument requirements. Thus, nowadays, there is frequently little opportunity to question or consider the type of instrument we use.

Very few of us watch our gynaecological or surgical colleagues operate and miss the opportunity of seeing changes in techniques or use of innovative practice.

This chapter critically reviews the choice of instruments and is a personal account of instruments which some gynaecologists and myself have found useful in our surgical practice.

Care and Choice of Instruments

The care and choice of instrument is frequently delegated to the nursing staff with little medical input: unless we indicate our preference, we are hardly justified in complaining if instruments are imperfect or unsatisfactory.

The surface of the instrument is important. To avoid reflection of operating lights which dazzle the surgeon, many instruments are now satin-finished or black, instead of being chromium plated. About 75% of instruments are made of stainless steel, which resists rust, takes a fine point and retains a clean cutting edge. The instrument is protected against corrosion by a process known as "passivation", which involves exposing the metal to the atmosphere and certain oxidising agents. A thin protective film of chromic oxide is laid down. Repeated use and exposure to the atmosphere actually increases this passivation process.

However, instruments can still discolour, due to water spot, staining or corrosion. Water spotting is due to the deposition of sodium, calcium or magnesium contained in the local water, which precipitates onto the instrument due to faulty autoclaving and inadequate exhaustion of steam.

Stains have three main causes:

1. Rust-coloured film is due to deposition of foreign particles left inside newly installed steam pipes. This is usually a temporary phenomenon. In some areas, it may result from a higher concentration of iron compound in the water.

2. Bluish-grey stain is caused by some cold sterilising solutions, which produce this discoloration.

3. Brown stain, which is due to the hospital water containing polyphosphates, which have a copper-solubilising action on the steriliser, causing a layer of copper to be deposited by electrolytic action on the instrument.

Corrosion is due to:

1. Inadequate cleaning and drying immediately after use
2. Contact with corrosive sterilising solutions (e.g. Lysol) or too long exposure to sterilising solutions, especially cold soap solutions
3. Exposure to tap rather than distilled or demin-eralised water
4. Detergent agents
5. Faulty autoclaving

Blood and saline are two common causes of cor-rosion: instruments should be thoroughly cleaned, particularly around serrations, ratchets and box hinges. After surgery, ALL instruments on the trolley (not just those used) should be cleaned and dismantled where appropriate and dried. Ultrasonic cleaning is an ideal method of removing debris from difficult joints; however, chromium-plated instru-ments should NOT be ultrasonically cleaned, as flaking of chromium plating can occur.

Proper care and usage of instruments is import-ant if they are to remain effective and retain the precision action for which they are designed. All too often, one can see misuse of instruments by nursing and medical staff.

1. Arterial clamps or haemostats are designed to clamp blood vessels and should not be used as towel clips, suction tube clamps or pliers. Abnor-mal straining will lead to misalignment of the jaws or fracture of the jaws and hinge.
2. Needle holders are designed for different sizes of needles and use of too large a needle will lead to misalignment of the jaws and damage to the serrated edge, with weakening of the holding power.

3. Scissors should be used to cut the tissue for which they are intended. Inappropriate use (i.e. suture cutting by fine dissection scissors) will blunt the cutting edge.

Choice of Instruments

The instrument should be comfortable to hold and use and do the job you want it for. The handles, length and axis are all important. The Turner-Warwick needle holder is an example of a purpose-built and elegantly fashioned instrument: it is well balanced and very functional (Fig. 9.1) (Down's Instruments).

When choosing clamps, it is important to ensure that on light clamping the jaws do not overlap: if they are serrated, the teeth must mesh properly. The box hinge can be checked by grasping the handles in either hand and juggling it. If it is too loose, misalignment of the jaw will occur on closing, or it may spring open during use. That will also occur if the ratchet is worn and this can be checked by engaging the instrument on the first tooth, holding it at the joint and tapping the ratchet portion against a firm object; if the instrument opens, it is faulty.

The best dissection scissors have a tungsten carbide insert along the cutting edge and should *never* be used for cutting sutures. Scissors are best tested by their cutting aptitude at the tip of the blades and should be able to cut four layers of gauze at the tips. When closed, the shanks should be in good approximation.

A needle holder should be tested by placing the correct size needle in the instrument and locking the instrument on the second ratchet. It should be difficult for the needle to be rotated by hand; if not, the instrument needs repair. The best needle holders

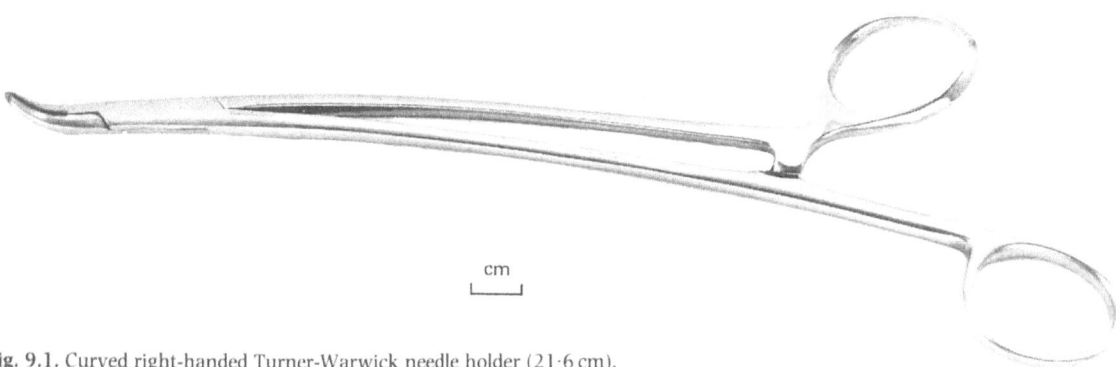

cm

Fig. 9.1. Curved right-handed Turner-Warwick needle holder (21·6 cm).

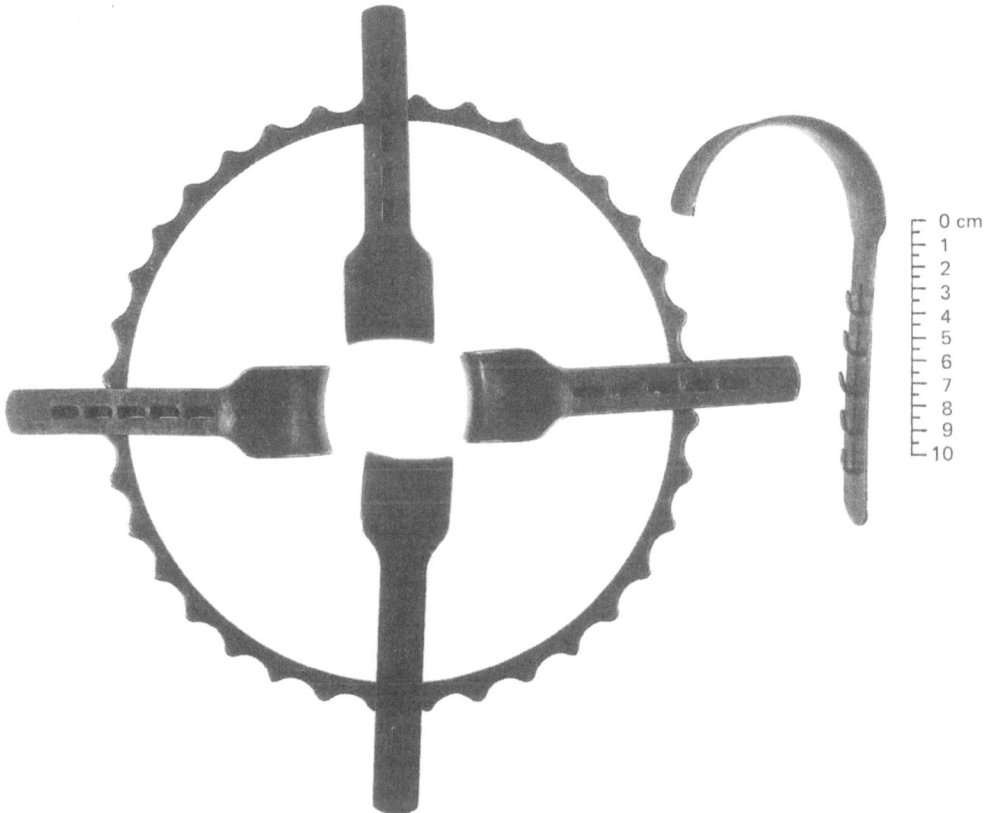

Fig. 9.2. Denis Browne matt black ring retractor (30 cm) with four shallow blades and one deep blade.

have serrated tungsten carbide inserts, which should be replaced once the serrations begin to wear down.

What's New and Old

This list is by no means complete. It contains those instruments which have been found to be particularly useful.

Retractors

Efficient retraction makes pelvic surgery easier, frees the assistant to assist and provides a better field of view for the surgical team and onlookers.

A retractor ought to be adjustable, easy to use and free of small detachable parts, which could get lost in the depths of the pelvis or on the theatre floor. The ring type of retractor meets many of these criteria. Many versions exist, e.g. Kirschner, Buchwalter, Denis Browne. I prefer the latter, which is circular and is available in three different internal diameters (23, 30 and 37 cm) (Fig. 9.2). The blades, usually four in number, are available in wide, narrow, shallow or deep size and are clawed or smooth at the extremity (Genito-Urinary Instruments, London).

Clamps and Forceps

There is a wide range of clamps, reflecting different surgical needs and personal preferences. The ideal clamp should be easy to apply and retain the tissues securely; theoretically, serrations should be parallel, rather than at right angles to the jaws (Fig. 9.3). There seems little point in having the large jaws with which most gynaecological clamps are provided: this only serves to encourage the inclusion of an unnecessarily large pedicle. It is preferable to dissect away superfluous tissue and leave a smaller pedicle with less risk of slipping.

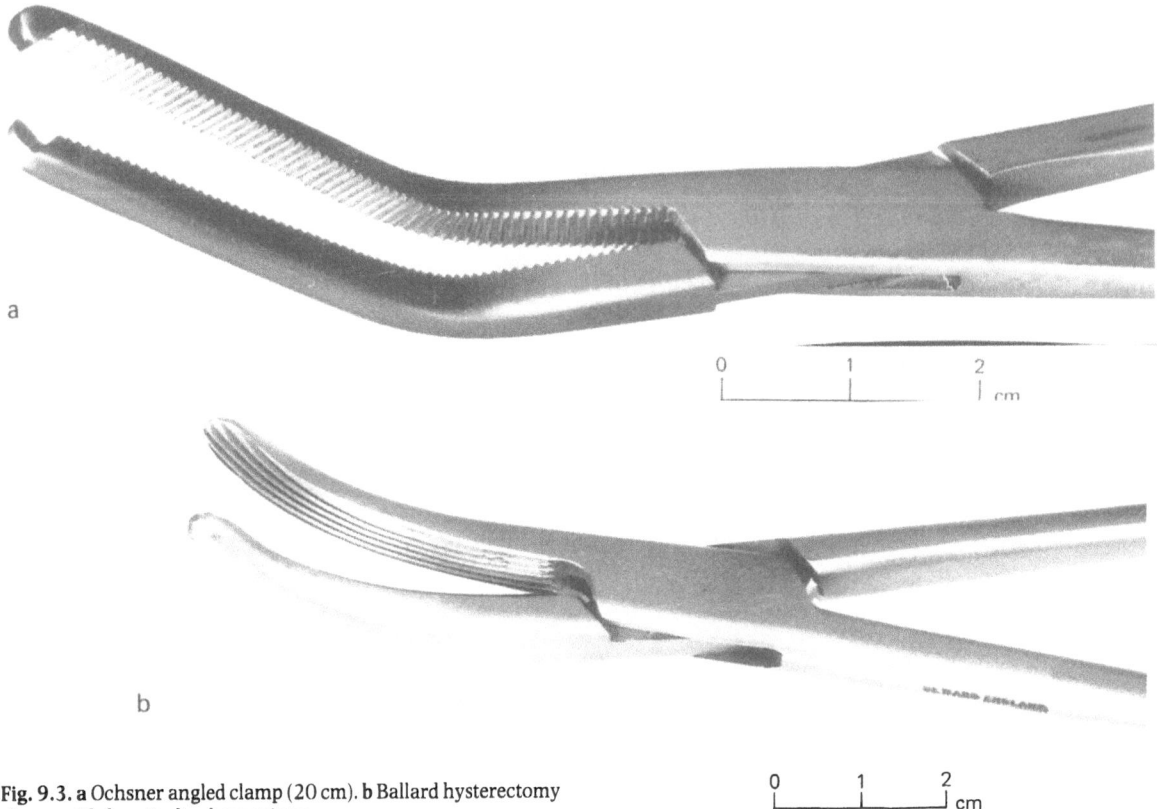

a

b

Fig. 9.3. a Ochsner angled clamp (20 cm). **b** Ballard hysterectomy clamp with longitudinal serrations.

For abdominal and vaginal hysterectomy, I prefer the straight and curved 8″ Rogers clamp (Codman) (Fig. 9.4). The clamp is light and well balanced, with fine longitudinal vascular toothing which give more secure retention of pedicles than the conventional uninterrupted serrations. Similar clamps, with a greater variety of jaw curvature, are found in designs by Martin and Zeppelin: the latter has a slightly different style of serration (Fig. 9.5). Both are more expensive than the Rogers. I do not like the conventional heavy hysterectomy clamp with its terminal claw (to prevent the pedicle slipping), which is traumatic and sometimes makes it difficult to free the clamp (Fig. 9.6).

John Monaghan (1986, personal communication) likes the Navratil (or Meig's) clamp (Fig. 9.7) for ligating vessels deep within the pelvis: the right angle of the small head of the instrument allows a tie to be accurately positioned. The tie is placed around either the head or points of the instrument and when the assistant moves the forceps backwards or forwards, the opposite end automatically comes within the loop, allowing the surgeon to confidently tie the vessel.

For clamping discrete pedicles, Chris Hudson (1986, personal communication) and Monaghan prefer the Zeppelin curved tissue forceps.

Needle Holders

My standard needle holder is the straight Mayo-Hegar (20·3 cm), which is light but strong and well balanced (Fig. 9.8). The Turner-Warwick curved needle holder (21·6 cm), available for the right or left hand, is admirable for vaginal repair of inaccessible fistulae high in the vault or deep in the pelvis (John Lawson 1986, personal communication) (Fig. 9.1).

For the colposuspension and sling procedure and more difficult inaccessible suturing within the pelvis, I prefer the angled jaw Finochietto needle holder (21·6 cm) (Fig. 9.9).

Scissors

Scissors are a personal preference: Monaghan prefers the angled Mayo (or Bonney) for accurate dissection (Fig. 9.10). They are sturdy and with relatively blunt ends and do little damage when separating tissues, whereas the blades are powerful enough with the strong leverage of the long handles to cut the tough scar tissue which follows irradiation.

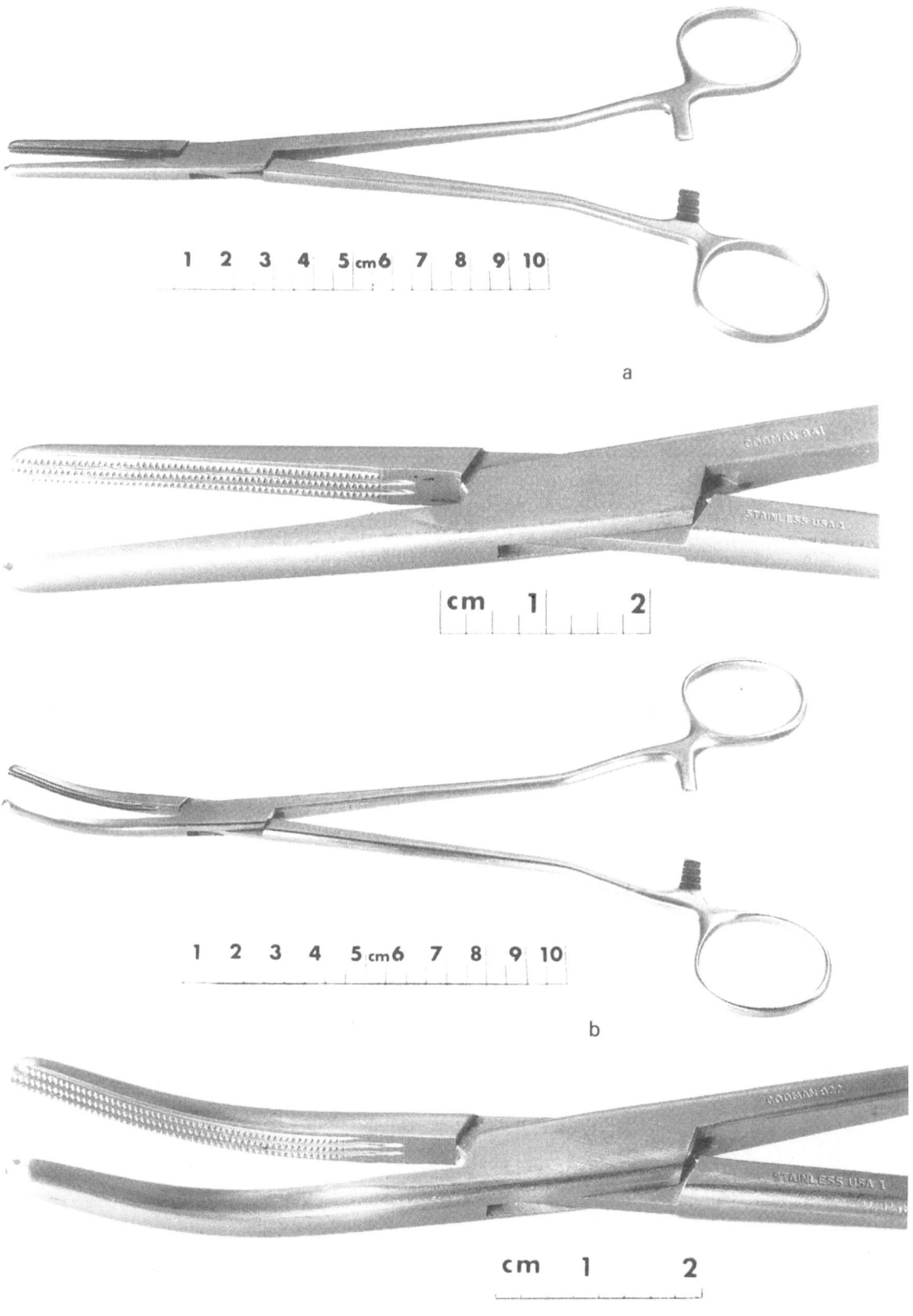

Fig. 9.4. a Straight Roger's clamp (21·6 cm) with close-up. **b** Curved Roger's clamp (21·6 cm) with close-up.

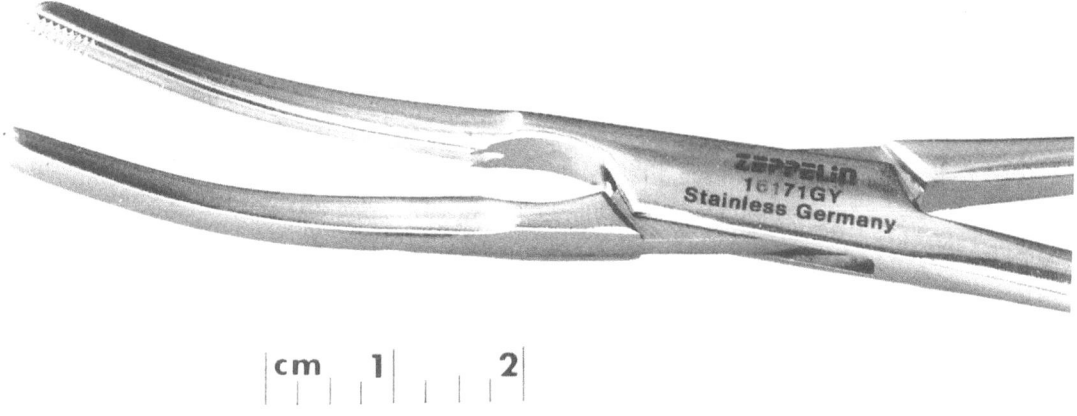

Fig. 9.5. Zeppelin adnexal forceps (16171 G) (19·0 cm).

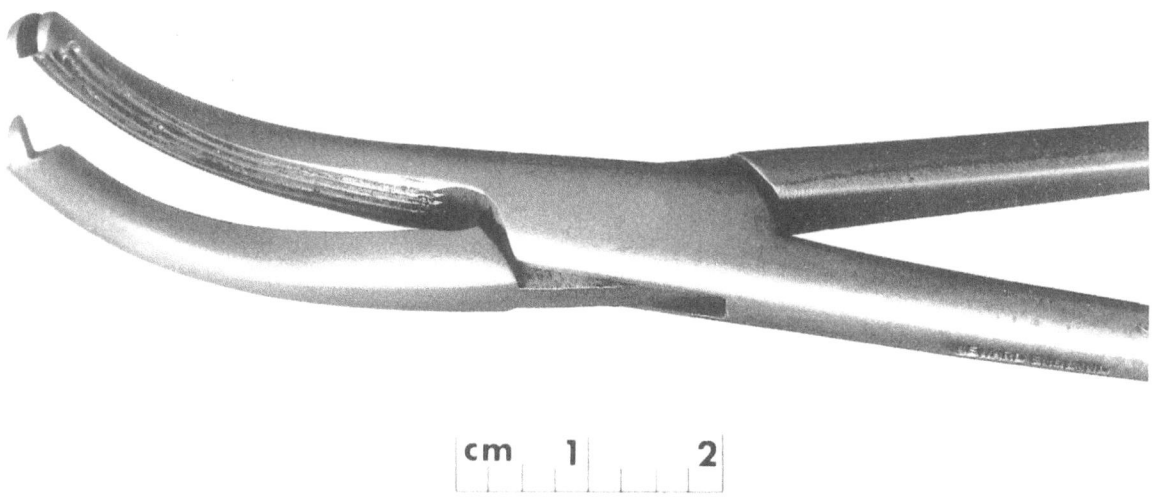

Fig. 9.6. McCullogh's hysterectomy clamp (22·9 cm).

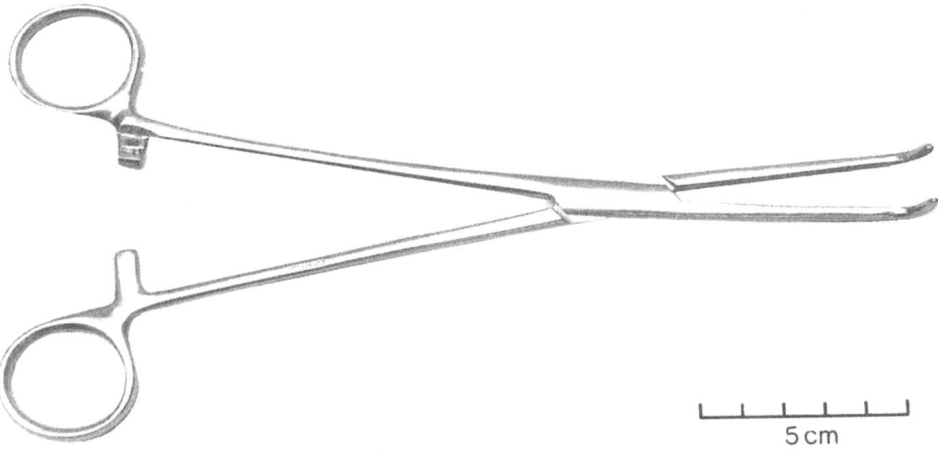

Fig. 9.7. Navratil curved forceps (23·5 cm).

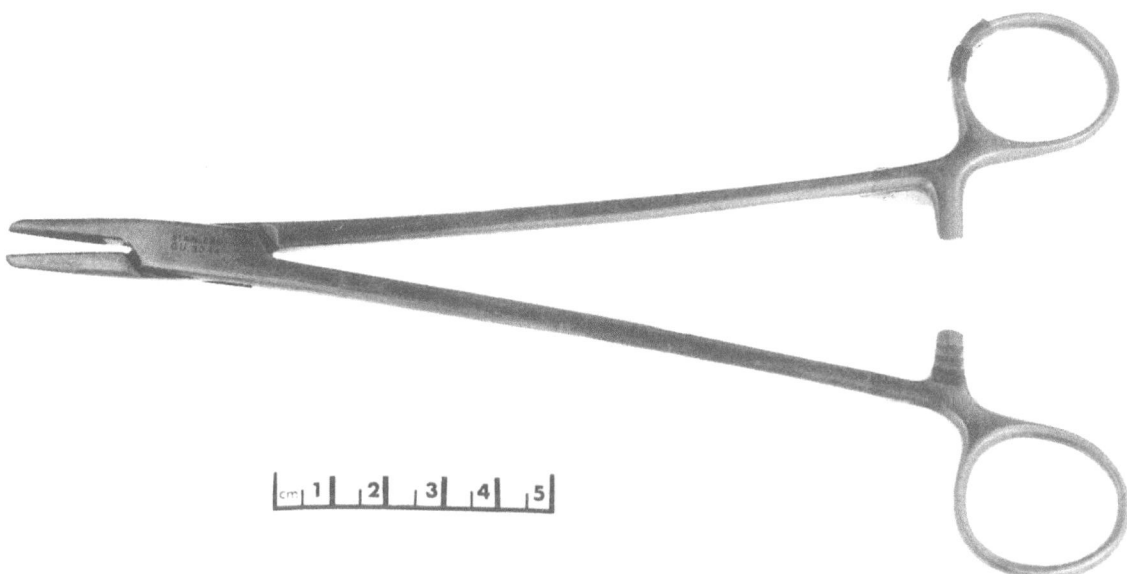

Fig. 9.8. Mayo-Hegar straight needle holder (19 cm).

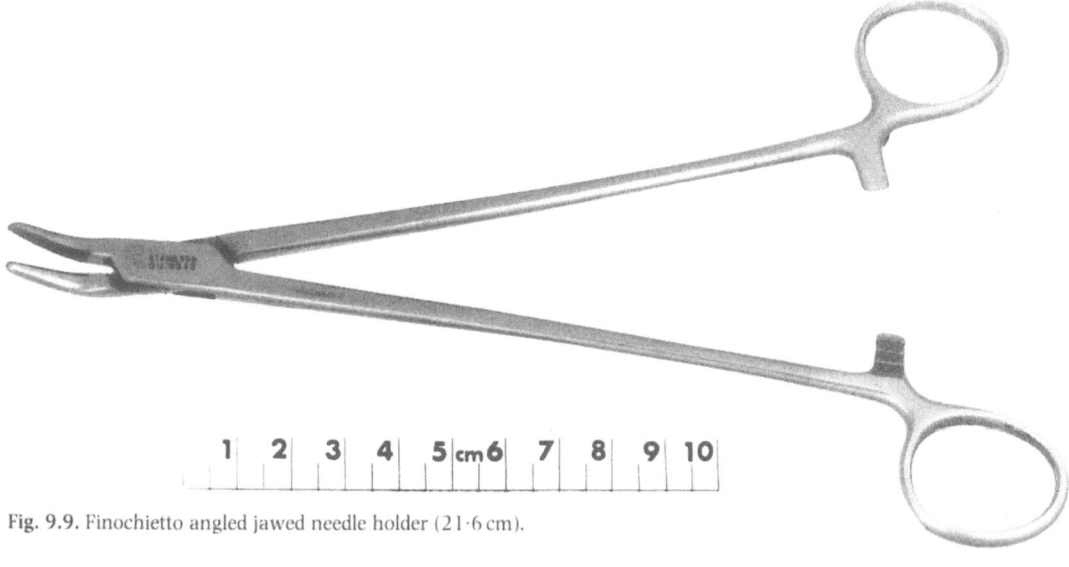

Fig. 9.9. Finochietto angled jawed needle holder (21·6 cm).

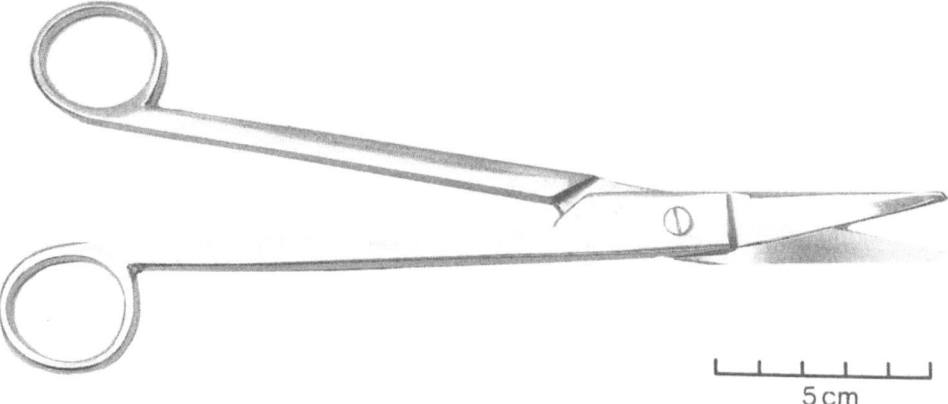

Fig. 9.10. Angled Mayo scissors (21·6 cm).

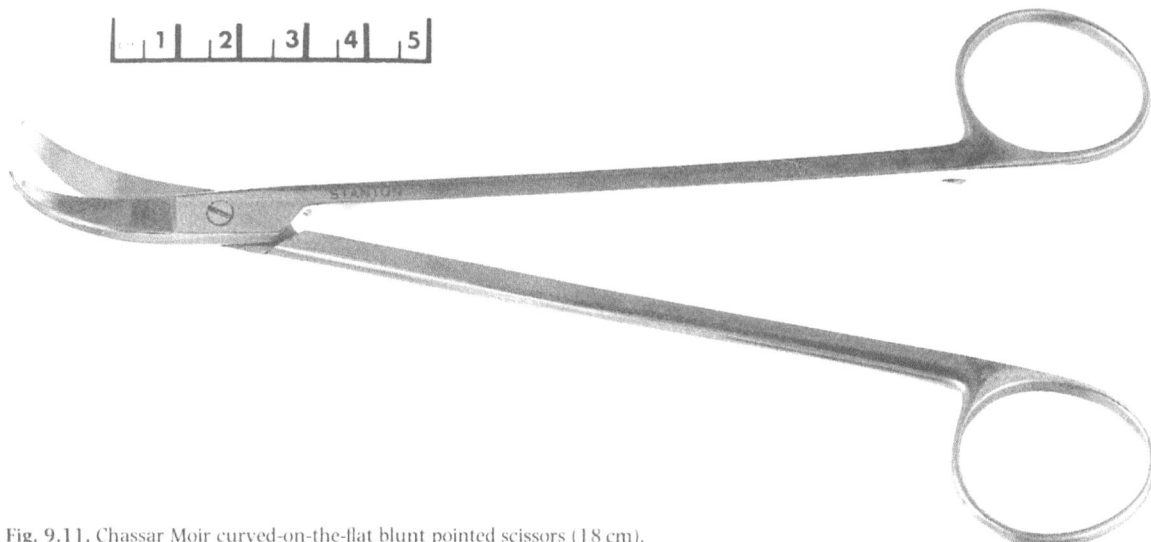

Fig. 9.11. Chassar Moir curved-on-the-flat blunt pointed scissors (18 cm).

For repair of fistulae, both Lawson and Hudson (1986) prefer the curved or flat angled Chassar Moir scissors (Fig. 9.11). For routine dissection, I prefer the curved Mayo (18 cm) with fairly blunted ends and for retropubic and deep pelvic dissection, I like the Metzenbaum scissors (23 cm) (Fig. 9.12).

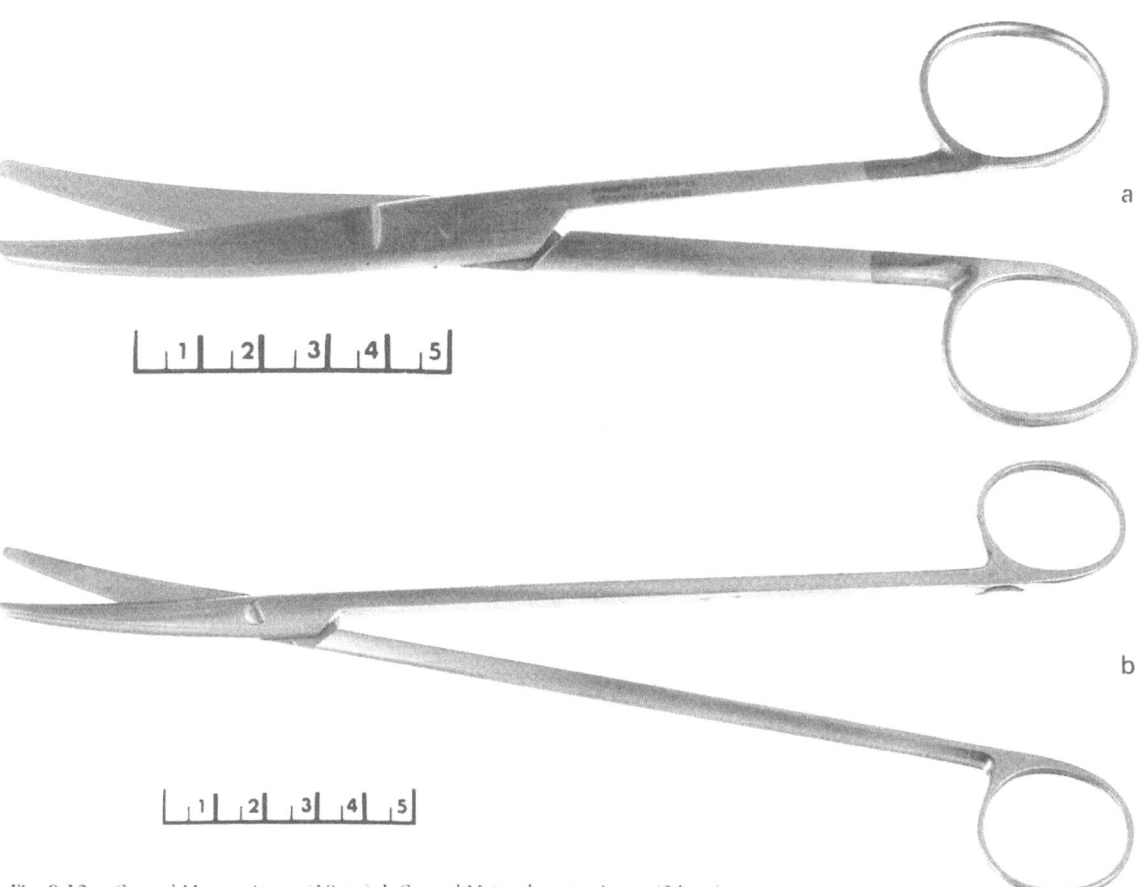

Fig. 9.12. a Curved Mayo scissors (18 cm). b Curved Metzenbaum scissors (24 cm).

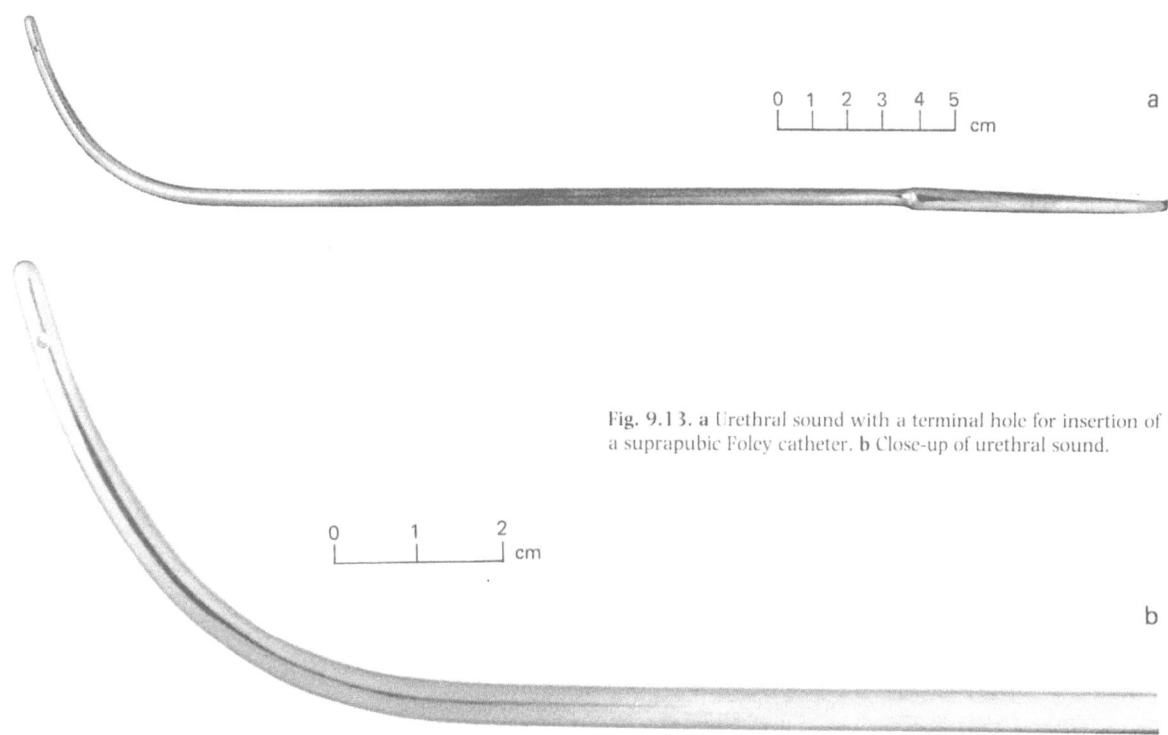

Fig. 9.13. a Urethral sound with a terminal hole for insertion of a suprapubic Foley catheter. b Close-up of urethral sound.

Suprapubic Catheter Introducers

There are many suprapubic catheters of varying size, complexity and retaining ability (Schmidt 1986). The Foley urethral catheter is in many ways ideal for suprapubic use—it is cheap and available in many sizes and the balloon allows good retention. It is simple to insert and use. There are two main methods of insertion. A urethral sound, with a hole drilled just distal to the tip (Fig. 9.13), is inserted via the urethra into a partially filled bladder. Under either local or general anaesthesia, the instrument is pushed through the anterior bladder wall and then through a small incision in the anterior abdominal wall, where it is tied to the end of a Foley catheter, using the distal hole. This is pulled into the bladder and out through the urethra and the sound detached. The catheter is drawn back into the bladder and the balloon inflated.

Alternatively, an Ansari suprapubic cystostomy needle may be used (Fig. 9.14) (Ansari and Rutenbergs 1970). This consists of three parts—the stylet or obturator and inner and outer sheaths. The inner and outer sheaths have fenestrations along their entire lengths. When assembled, the fenestrations are 180° away from each other.

A 180° rotation of the inner sheath in either direction will then align both fenestrations and allow lateral withdrawal of the catheter from the introducer. The bladder is filled, a small incision made about one to two finger breadths above the pubis and the cystostomy needle inserted into the bladder. The obturator is removed, a Foley catheter introduced and the balloon inflated. The needle is withdrawn by rotating the inner and outer sheaths to align both fenestrated portions.

Stapling Devices

Mechanical stapling of tissues originated with the work of Hulti and Fischer in Budapest, when they demonstrated a stapling device for gastrectomy in 1908, in which fine wire staples were placed in double staggered rows (Steichen and Ravitch 1984). Their device was superseded after some 20 years by the now better known Von Petz stapler, which laid a single Indian file of staples, later modified to a double row. Since then, however, stapling devices have reverted to double staggered rows (where possible), using fine wire staples. Stapling was introduced into the United States in the 1920s,

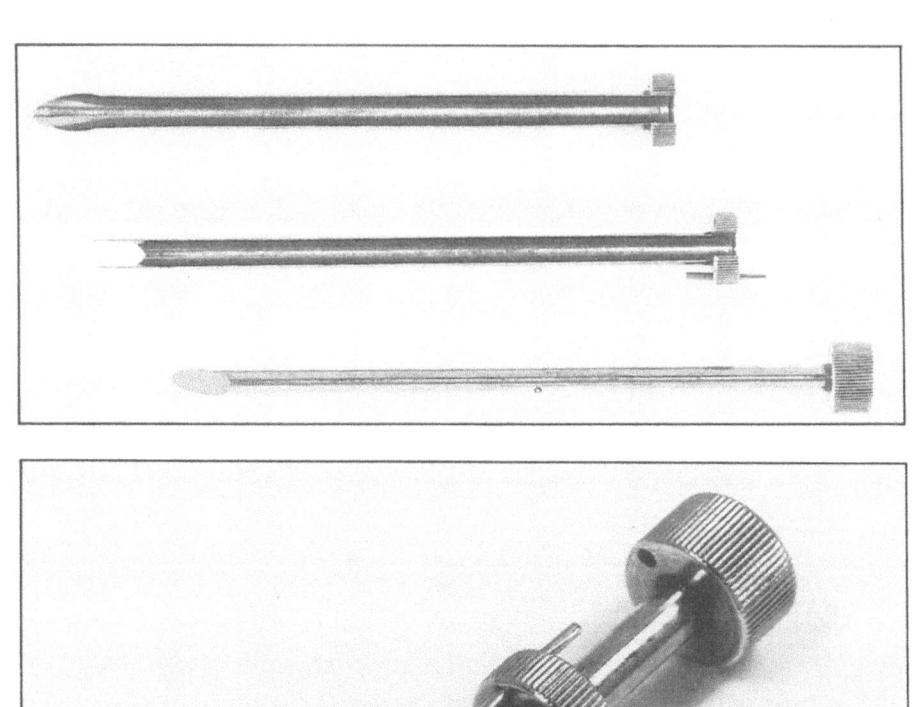

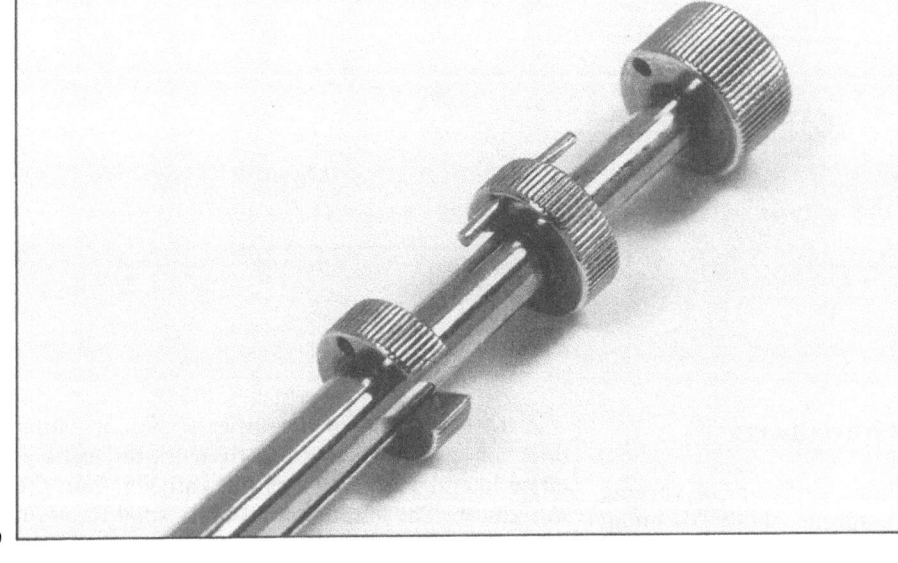

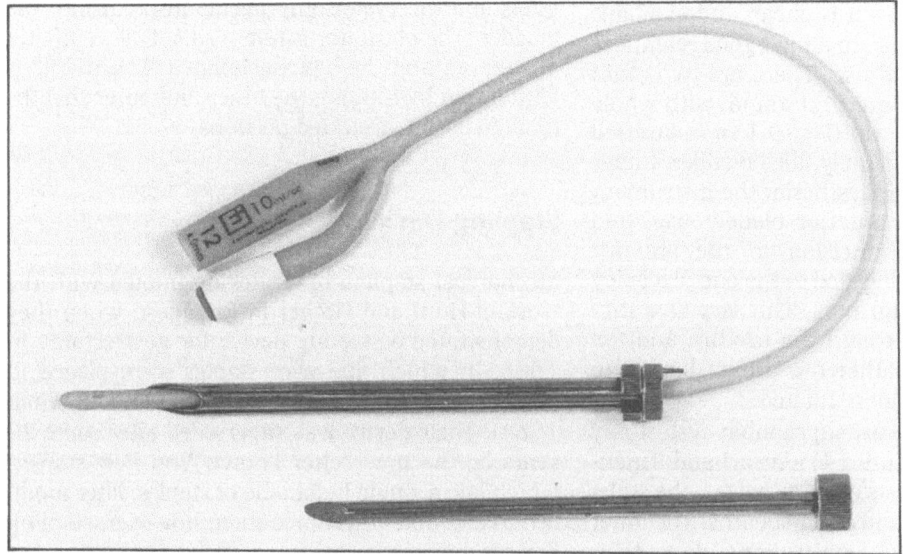

Fig. 9.14a-c. Ansari suprapubic cystostomy needle for insertion of a suprapubic Foley catheter. **a** Obturator, inner and outer sheaths; **b** needle assembled; **c** sheaths assembled and catheter in place and obturator withdrawn.

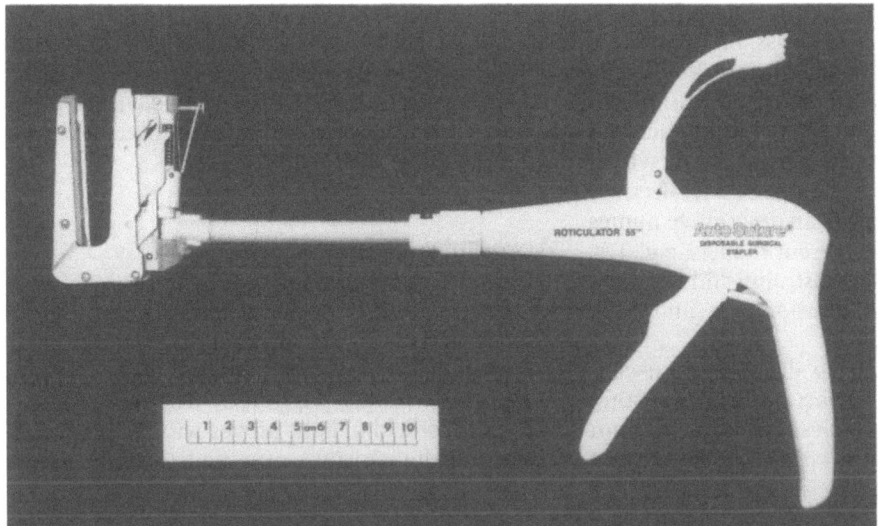

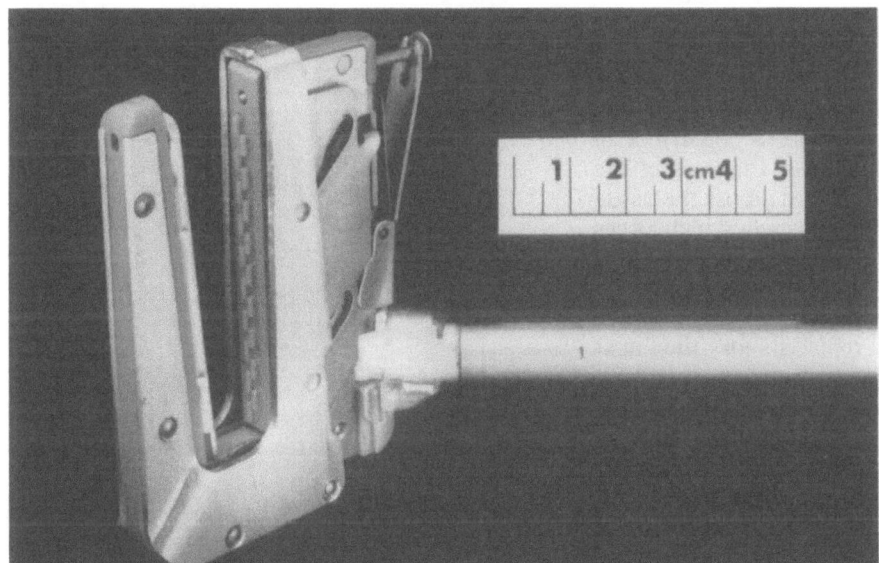

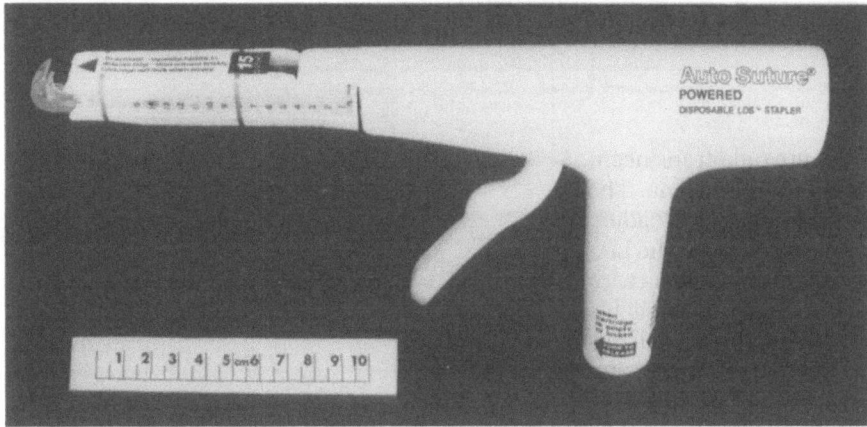

Fig. 9.15. a Autosuture suture disposable Roticulator 55; **b** close-up of head, angled and rotated; **c** autosuture ligating and dividing powered stapler.

but the major developments continued in Europe
and in the 1950s; it was the Russians who were
foremost in stapling for bowel closure and anastomoses. The first generation of American instruments appeared in the late 1960s, manufactured
by the United States Surgical Corporation, which
remains the principal manufacturer today. Because
of patent law, initials rather than descriptive names
are used to designate the different models; e.g. TA,
Thoracoabdominal; GIA, Gastrointestinal anastomosis; EEA, End-to-end anastomosis; and LDS,
Ligating and dividing stapler.

For the gynaecologist, two devices are useful.
First is the TA 55[1], which places a linear everting
double line of staggered staples, 30, 55 or 90 mm
long and with staple lengths either 3·5 or 4·8 mm,
depending on tissue thickness. The most recent
development has been the production of a flexible
head instrument, the Roticulator 55[1] (Fig. 9.15),
which rotates through 320° and articulates
through 120° and uses either stainless steel or absorbable staples (the latter is awaiting a product
licence here and is available only in the United
States at present: the staples are a copolymer of
lactic and glycolic acids). To use, the jaws of the
stapling device are opened, placed across the tissue
to be stapled and the handle squeezed, which forces
staples through the tissues and against the firm
anvil. All staples are fired simultaneously and each
is transformed into the shape of a capital "B". Once
used, the cartridge is replaced for the next
manœuvre. The TA 55 can be used to clamp
adnexal tissue at either abdominal or vaginal hysterectomy and closure of the vaginal vault at
abdominal hysterectomy (Beresford 1984). The
Roticulator 55 is designed to overcome difficult
access to the adnexae or vault. The advantages of
both models are:

1. Closer resection of the vagina
2. Less granulation tissue
3. Speed

In addition, absorbable staples are radiotranslucent
and will not be extruded through the vagina. The
disadvantages are cost (Premium TA 55 loading
unit = £43.34 + VAT). The second device is the LDS
instrument[1], which clips vessels, ligates them twice
and divides tissue between the clips. It is available
as a disposable power device, driven by a small gas
cylinder contained in the handle. Again, speed and
ease of surgery are the main advantages, with cost

1 Obtainable through Autosuture UK Ltd (a subsidiary of United
  States Surgical Corporation), 2 King's Ride Park, King's Ride,
  Ascot, Berks SL5 8BP.

remaining the main disadvantage (£54.84 + VAT).
Its main application is in the division of gastric,
mesenteric and omental vessels.

Skin closure using staples is well known and
advocates will support the ability to achieve good
wound closure with a neat scar.

Accessory Lights

Fibre optic headlights are a valuable ancillary to
difficult deep pelvic or vaginal surgery, providing
an intensive, adjustable light, exactly where the
surgeon is working (Fig. 9.16). The disadvantages
are that the field of light moves with the operator's
head and the assistant may find the field of view

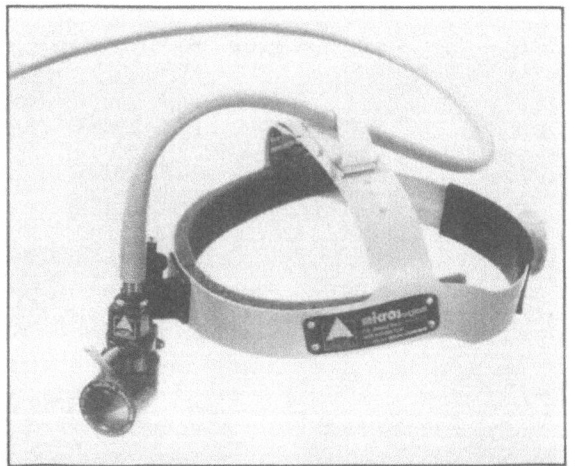

a

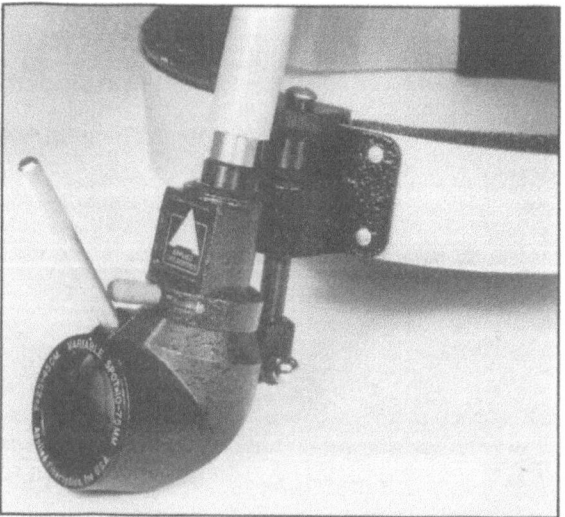

b

Fig. 9.16. a Fibre optic headlight. b Close-up showing coaxial
rotary headlight with variable spot (spot range, 2–8 cm, and focal
distance, 46 cm).

has a changing light distribution, which may be uncomfortable over a long period. He too may need a personal headlight!

There are also fibre optic light attachments for suckers, retractors and speculae (Codman Ltd).

Acknowledgements. I acknowledge with thanks the help and advice provided by Sir Rustam Feroze, Professor Chris Hudson, Mr. John Lawson, Mr. John Monaghan and Dr. Julian Ward. Mr. H. Broadbridge and Mr. N. Watkin of Codman Ltd and Mr. J. Farrell of Auto Suture UK Ltd have provided invaluable technical advice. Much useful information has been obtained from the booklet *The care and handling of surgical instruments,* published by Codman Ltd. TA (Thoracoabdominal), GIA (Gastrointestinal anastomosis), EEA (End-to-end anastomosis) and LDS (Ligating and dividing stapler) are all trademarks of United States Surgical Corporation.

References

Ansari A, Rutenbergs B (1970) Needle suprapubic cystostomy: a new and simple technique. Obstet Gynec 35:814–819

Beresford J (1984) Anastomotic stapling techniques in abdominal hysterectomy. Surgical Clinics of North America, vol 64. Ravitch M, Steichen F (eds) Saunders, Philadelphia, pp 609–618

Schmidt R (1986) Post-operative catheter drainage. In: Stanton, Tanagho (eds) Surgery of female incontinence, 2nd edn. Springer, Berlin Heidelberg New York, pp 267–273

Steichen F, Ravitch M (1984) Stapling in surgery. Year Book Medical Publishers Inc, Chicago, pp 3–77

10 · Recent Advances in Suture Material

Timothy E. Bucknall

Pathophysiology

Stages in Wound Healing

When the surgeon brings wound edges together he is trying to create a favourable situation for the patient's body to repair the wound. However, many other significant factors influence normal healing. The patient is more likely to heal normally if in good health without chronic illness such as diabetes or cancer. Adequate nutrition is an important requirement particularly protein, essential amino acids and vitamins, especially vitamin C. Respiratory dysfunction, which results in poor oxygen delivery to injured tissues, makes the wound more vulnerable to infection and slowed healing. An obese patient because of a thick layer of subcutaneous fat leading to haematoma and infection, a patient on high doses of steroids depressing the initial inflammatory response and reducing collagen synthesis, a jaundiced or uraemic patient with depressed fibroblast activity—all require extra care to ensure sound healing. Yet even the young, fit, well-nourished patient may not escape postoperative infection, haemorrhage or wound disruption if the surgery is not of the highest standard and aseptic technique is not followed.

The healing process is initiated at the moment of wounding, whether this is following trauma or scalpel. There is an initial brief period of vasoconstriction followed by vasodilatation and an increase in blood flow. The blood clots and a local inflammatory response is activated.

As a large number of platelets come into contact with the wound they disintegrate and release thromboplastin which changes prothrombin to thrombin in the presence of calcium. Thrombin reacts with fibrinogen to form threads of fibrin which create a network, trapping erythrocytes pulling them by contraction into a mass called a clot.

Platelets, because of their adhesive character, seal vessels mechanically as well as stimulate blood vessel contraction. As the fibrin contracts blood vessels are pulled together beneath the clots. Phagocytes clear away debris and fibroblasts begin their process of repair.

Three stages of wound healing are now recognised. There is a brief inflammatory (lag or substrate) phase followed by a proliferative and then remodelling phase.

Inflammatory Phase

This phase usually lasts about 4 days after wounding; but the duration is directly related to the extent and nature of the wounding agent. The vascular response includes dilatation of blood vessels with exudation of plasma protein, increased permeability of cells and their transport into the wounded area. Lymphatic flow is accelerated. Blood loss is controlled by platelet plugs and the fibrin network starts to fill with blood cells (Fig. 10.1a). After about 12 h the cellular response starts. Polymorphs arrive and enzymatic debridement begins. This may also stimulate subsequent fibroplasia. Later in this phase

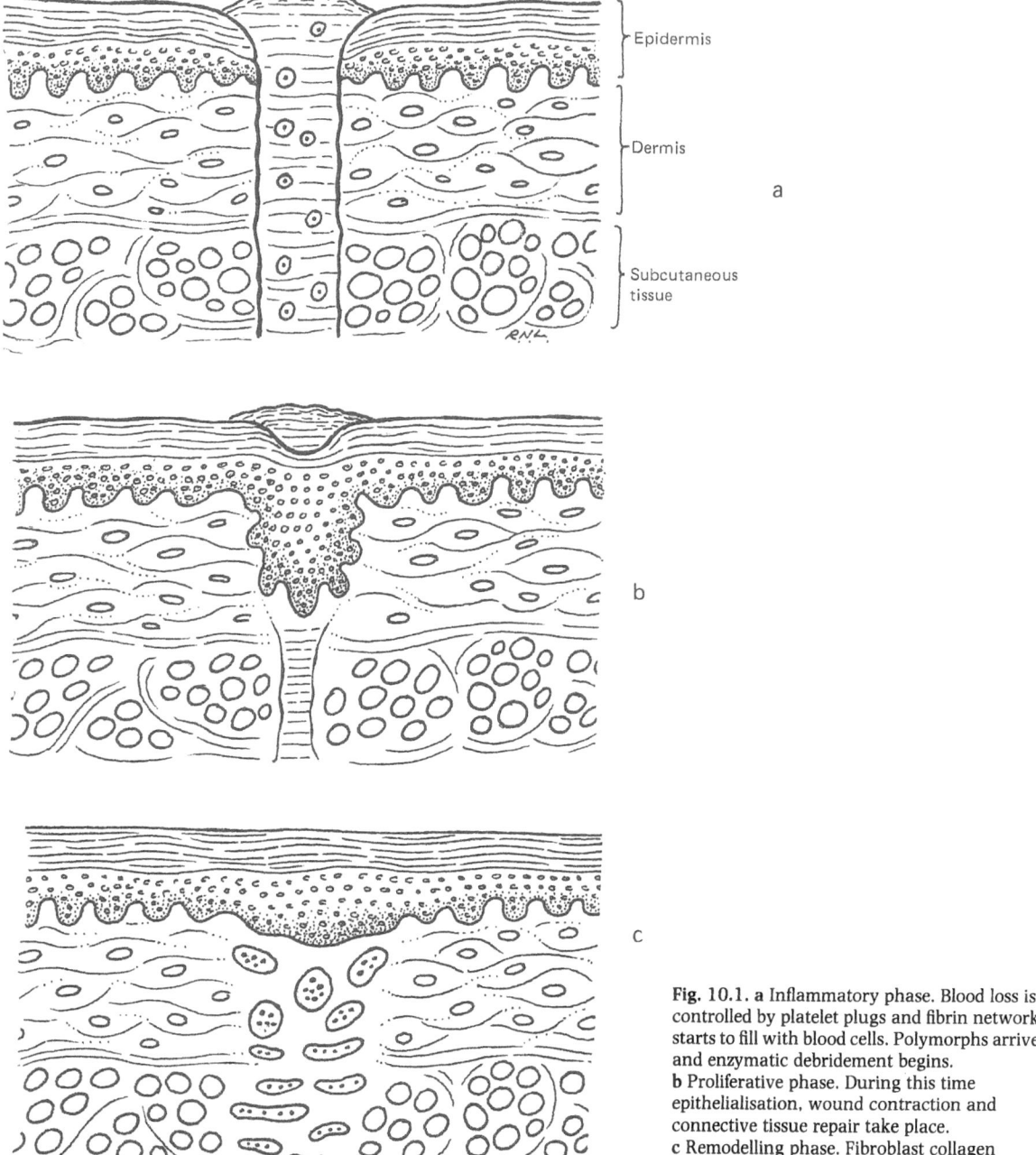

Fig. 10.1. a Inflammatory phase. Blood loss is controlled by platelet plugs and fibrin network starts to fill with blood cells. Polymorphs arrive and enzymatic debridement begins.
b Proliferative phase. During this time epithelialisation, wound contraction and connective tissue repair take place.
c Remodelling phase. Fibroblast collagen undergoes orientation and polymerisation which may take many months.

lymphocytes, macrophages, round cells, mast cells and monocytes arrive and release enzymes and polysaccharides which participate in the break-down and absorption of debris and in resorption of collagen. This phase therefore prepares the wound for healing without any gain in strength. *It is essential that sutures are responsible for the total strength at this stage.*

Proliferation Phase

This phase extends from the 5th to approximately the 20th postoperative day although this may be delayed in the presence of infection or other factor. During this time epithelialisation, wound contraction and connective tissue repair take place (Fig. 10.1b).

Epithelialisation is a combination of cell movement and new cell formation, with surface coverage of the open wound its primary purpose. Epithelialisation also provides some tensile strength. In the clean surgical wound, the epidermis migrates along the cut edge into the dermis. It does not bridge the gap directly across the wound surface. Rather, there is downward growth of epithelium from both sides, meeting at the depths of the dermis. Very small wounds may close entirely by epithelial repair.

Wound contraction is a remarkable phenomenon by which large, open, soft tissue wounds in some body areas close without scarring or cicatrisation. During wound contraction, the surrounding skin is stretched towards the centre of the wound. The nature of wound contraction is intimately related to the function of fibroblasts; these cells have unique metabolic capabilities. Fibroblasts appear to originate locally in the wound as part of the body's complex response to injury and are responsible for laying down collagen, on which the surgeon depends.

During this phase the wound is rapidly gaining strength but does not attain its final strength until the wound has remodelled.

Remodelling Phase

The activities of the fibroblast are crucial in the synthesis of collagen which provides the strength of the healed wound. The fibroblast secretes a precursor of collagen into the wound. These new fibrils aggregate or join pre-existing fibrils to form the collagen fibre. It then differentiates into mature collagen and disappears as a cell. Collagen orientation and polymerisation continue slowly adding to the strength of the wound (Fig. 10.1c). The remodelling phase (a resorptive or differentiating phase) begins in the 3rd week after wounding and may continue for many months. Even 100 days postoperatively, a wound will not have regained the original tensile strength of the tissues.

During the immediate postoperative period, rest and relative immobility of the patient are important to successful early healing. During the remodelling phase, however, appropriate patient activity with concomitant stress and strain on the repaired wound is essential for gain in tensile strength to be substantial thereafter. The migration, realignment and remodelling activities of the fibroblast are stimulated by stress and strain.

Theory and Role of Suture Material

Sutures provide the total strength of a wound for the first few postoperative days. Within 14 days 25%–30% of the original strength has been restored. The more significant gain in wound tensile strength begins with the work of the fibroblast and continues for many weeks and months. No suture will increase the rate of normal wound healing but if sutures are not used correctly the individual characteristic of various materials and the site of their placement can interfere with normal healing. For example, subcutaneous fat does not tolerate any suture material particularly well. But when silk is placed in fat, vulnerability of that layer to infection is greatly increased. Silk is a foreign protein which can act as a nidus for infection.

The absorption of surgical gut creates a relatively high level of inflammatory reaction in tissues. In critical repair situations such as nerve, tendon and blood vessel, minimal tissue reaction to suture material is highly desirable. The use of surgical gut would therefore be contraindicated in those cases.

Synthetic non-absorbable sutures (polyester, polyamide, polypropylene) are stronger than natural fibres (silk and cotton). The synthetics provoke relatively little tissue reaction. They can be used in the presence of infection, but are a bit more difficult to handle and tie securely than are the natural fibres.

Stainless steel wire is the strongest of all suture materials, the least reactive in the presence of infection, and can be tied in secure knots. However, it is more difficult to handle and place in tissues than other non-absorbable materials.

Synthetic absorbable sutures (polyglycolic acid, polyglactin, polydioxanone) provoke much less tissue reaction than does surgical gut. Their tensile strengths in vivo are longer lasting than surgical gut. In comparable sizes, polyglycolic acid suture is stronger than gut. Body tissues slowly hydrolyse this suture while surgical gut is absorbed by phagocytosis. These are becoming increasingly popular and used extensively by gynaecologists with good results. They should not however, be used where prolonged strength is required.

Adverse Influences

There are several adverse influences of sutures materials because they are essentially foreign bodies and are therefore likely to cause infection (Table 10.1). They are also prone to cause other reactions because of the body's response to them. The individual effects are dealt with in the next section.

Table 10.1. The possible causes of tissue changes associated with sutures. (Williams 1971)

1. Infection
2. Secondary neoplasm
3. Postoperative fibrosis
4. Physical effect of the suture as a static foreign body
5. Physical trauma resulting from movement of suture
6. Failure of suture to perform satisfactorily
7. Response to the material or its degradation products

Infection is the most significant problem but recently a good deal of interest has centred on secondary neoplasm in association with sutures. O'Dwyer et al. (1985) have tested commonly used surgical sutures and their abilities to adhere tumour cells. Most of the sutures tested adhered significant tumour cells, the least adherent being the monofilament synthetic non-absorbables, for example, prolene; thus providing further evidence, if we needed it, that suturing is not a simple procedure.

Classification of Suture Materials

The choice of suture material is frequently motivated by an emotional rather than a scientific thought process (Capperauld 1975). This is due mainly to a lack of knowledge by the surgeon of the physical and biological properties inherent to individual suture materials and the relevance of these properties to the clinical situation, where rates of healing and tissue response vary considerably. Surgical technique is more important than the suture material used in any given clinical situation. However, a detailed knowledge of the material selected will lead to a more scientific approach to the problem of wound closure and, hopefully, to consistent and reproducible results regardless of the clinical situation. The surgeon should be aware of the normal strength of the tissues to be sutured, and the time required for the wound to regain its strength. Other essential considerations are suture tensile strength, the rate at which the material loses its strength in vivo, and the interaction expected between suture and tissue. Weighing all these factors enables a well-informed choice of suture.

Suture materials are either absorbable or non-absorbable. The absorbable materials lose tensile strength over a given period and progressively undergo absorption, with a corresponding loss of mass or volume. The time taken for a material to absorb is always in excess of that for total tensile strength loss to occur. Non-absorbable sutures, by definition, do not absorb, but some, especially those

of biological origin, lose strength without any change in the mass of the suture material. In other non-absorbables, especially those of synthetic or polymeric origin, there is never any loss of tensile strength or change in mass following implantation.

A further classification of suture material is based on the origin of the raw material either from a biological source (animal or plant) or from man-made fibres. Classification can be broadened by reference to the structure of the suture materials—some are monofilament and others are multifilament, where the multifilament is either braided or twisted to form a suture. Suture materials can also be classified as dyed or undyed, where visibility is improved by the inclusion of an approved non-toxic dye.

Table 10.2. Classification of sutures

Absorbable	
Catgut	Biological origin from sheep or ox; twisted, "monofilament"; undyed and uncoated
Collagen	Biological origin from ox; rolled "monofilament"; undyed and uncoated
Glycolide	Man-made homopolymer; braided multifilament; dyed or undyed; coated or uncoated. Trade name Dexon (PGA, polyglycolic acid)
Glycolide and lactide	Man-made copolymer; braided multifilament; dyed or undyed; coated or uncoated. Trade name Vicryl. Ratio of glycolide to lactide is 90/10 (polyglactin 910)
Polydioxanone	Man-made copolymer; monofilament; dyed or undyed. Trade name PDS (polydioxanone suture)
Non-absorbable	
Silk	Biological origin from silkworm; braided multifilament; dyed or undyed; coated or uncoated. Trade name Mersilk.
Linen	Biological origin from flax plant; twisted multifilament; dyed or undyed
Cotton	Biological origin from cotton seed plant; twisted multifilament; dyed or undyed
Polyester	Man-made; multifilament; dyed or undyed; coated or uncoated. Trade name Mersilene or Ethibond (polybutylate coat)
Polyamide	Man-made; monofilament or multifilament; dyed or undyed; generic name Nylon 6 or Nylon 66. Trade names Ethilon (monofilament) and Nurolon (multifilament)
Polypropylene	Man-made; monofilament; dyed or undyed. Trade name Prolene
Steel	Man-made; monofilament or multifilament

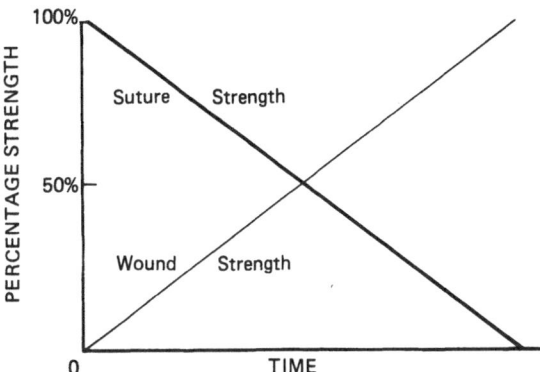

Fig. 10.2. Ideal absorbable suture performance.

Finally, the surface characteristics can be altered by application of coatings, some of which will reduce the capillarity of the material and others will alter its coefficient of friction by reducing the drag factor and hence ease the passage of the suture through tissues and facilitate knotting. Table 10.2 classifies the different sutures available.

Suture Selection

The purpose of a suture is to hold the wound in apposition until such time as the healing process is sufficiently advanced to make its continued presence in the tissues unnecessary. The ideal suture, that is, one which could be used on all occasions, the surgeon merely having to select the size of suture and needle, does not exist. Indeed it is highly unlikely that one single material which will perform in every clinical situation will ever be invented. The surgeon will always be faced with a large selection of suture materials and have to make a decision on which is the best for a particular surgical procedure.

The holding of a wound together in the initial postoperative period is entirely dependent on the suture. However, as healing progresses, the contribution made by the suture gradually decreases until finally it is redundant, since the support function has been taken over by the healed wound (Fig. 10.2). The remaining tensile strength of the healing tissues gives the true tensile strength of the wound at any given point. However, as shown in Fig. 10.3 the rate of repair of tensile strength in individual tissues varies. The suture chosen should lose strength and absorb at the same time as the tissue gains strength and heals, thus avoiding complications caused by the continued presence of a foreign body. Non-absorbable material in the biliary tree or urinary tract, for example, may lead to stone formation, and anastomotic ulcers may arise in the gastrointestinal tract in relation to retained suture material.

As seen in Fig. 10.3 an absorbable suture which retains up to 50% of its tensile strength for at least 14 days would suffice for bladder, colon and stomach, but skin has only 10% or 11% of its original tensile strength at 14 days. Paradoxically, skin sutures are removed at 7–10 days, when the tensile strength of the wound is very weak. However, Forrester (1972) claims that the skin wound does not break down because of the protective action of the elastin. Fascial tissue can take as long as 9 months to regain 75% of its original tensile strength (Douglas 1952). A non-absorbable or absorbable material with prolonged tensile strength retention would be preferable for tissues taking a long time to regain their original tensile strength.

It is advisable to keep the volume of the suture to a minimum, as all suture materials are foreign bodies. The smallest size of suture material which will hold the tissues in apposition without breaking should be used and the correct knot should be tied to maintain security. The ideal knot for synthetic materials is a double throw followed by a single throw followed by a third double throw. Howes and Harvey in 1929 calculated the limits of strength of particular tissues by calculating the "pull out value" of a loop of suture from these tissues. If the breaking strength of the suture material is matched to the pull out value of the tissue, the appropriate size can be selected (Table 10.3).

Surgeons often use sutures two or even three sizes larger than is really necessary to hold the wound together. There is no merit in having a suture very much stronger than the pull out value

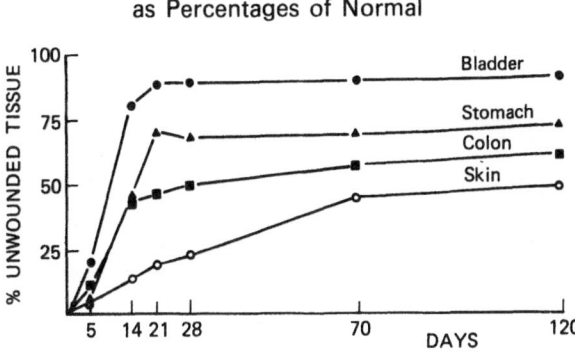

Fig. 10.3. Wound breaking strengths as percentages of normal.

Table 10.3. Choosing the size of suture

Tissue	Suture pull-out value (kg)	Breaking strength in kilograms and size of catgut	Breaking strength in kilograms and size of silk
Fat	0·2	0·31 6/0	0·20 7/0
Peritoneum	0·86	1·50 5/0	0·82 5/0
Muscle	1·27	1·70 4/0	1·70 4/0
Fascia	3·77	3·70 2/0	3·70 2/0

of the tissue, since this merely increases the foreign body volume. Additional throws on the knot compound this situation, since many extrusions and suture sinuses occur as a result of a large knot.

There is often confusion over suture material sizing and at present two systems are used in Europe. The metric system is expressed as a metric number representing the diameter of the suture in tenths of a millimetre. A comparison of the metric number and the former empirical gauge system is shown in Table 10.4.

Table 10.4. Metric gauging of suture material

Metric number	Former gauge	
	Catgut/collagen	Non-absorbables Synthetic absorbables
0·1	–	–
0·2	–	10/0
0·3	–	9/0
0·3	–	8/0
0·4	–	8/0 Virgin silk
0·5	8/0	7/0
0·7	7/0	6/0
1	6/0	5/0
1·5	5/0	4/0
2	4/0	3/0
3	3/0	2/0
3·5	2/0	0
4	0	1
5	1	2
6	2	3 and 4
7	3	5
8	4	6

The metric gauging system of suture materials indicates the actual diameter of materials. It has been adopted by both the European and the United States Pharmacopoeia. The metric number represents the diameter of the suture in tenths of a millimetre.

Tissue reaction is an important aspect of suture selection, and it can be demonstrated either by tissue culture or by animal implantation. The reaction which occurs in the first few days around a suture material is mainly due to the trauma of implantation and, therefore, tissue culture is the better method of assessing early reaction. The reaction to trauma settles after 7 days and a more reliable implantation technique can be used. The material absorbs, then a reaction must occur, especially of the absorption process is one of proteolysis. Certain materials may show a secondary reaction after 3 or 6 months due to the breaking of polymeric bonds and biodegradation without loss in mass or volume.

It should also be remembered that all suture materials show a difference between the knot pull strength and the straight pull strength. When a knot is placed on a suture material, the strength at the knot can be 10%–40% weaker, depending on the material. When a suture fails it always breaks at the knot, unless some damage has been inflicted on the material. The commonest cause of damage is iatrogenic, due to rough handling, defective surgical instruments or inadvertent crushing (Fig. 10.4), monofilament polypropylene being specially prone to instrument damage.

Sterilisation of suture materials also alters their characteristics. Most suture materials are sterilised by gamma irradiation from a cobalt-60 source or

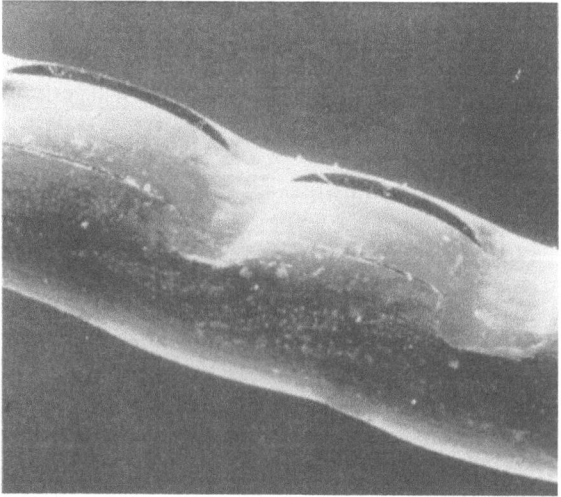

Fig. 10.4. This is a scanning electron micrograph of a piece of 3/0 polypropylene (Prolene) which has been damaged using a crushing clamp. This suture may break in situ following this damage.

by ethylene oxide gas. Sterilisation will reduce the tensile strength by approximately 10%. Repeated sterilisation can lead to sutures which have a low tensile strength and subsequent failure in use.

Another important physical characteristic of a suture material is its extensibility. This is the amount of "give" or stretch in a material, or elongation, before the break point occurs. Many materials will return to their original strength following extension short of breaking, while others will remain elongated. Some materials can elongate as much as 30% before breaking and hence are useful where postoperative oedema is expected to occur and the "give" in the suture prevents cross hatching on the underlying tissue.

Absorbable Sutures

These fall into two categories, namely catgut and collagen of biological origin, and the synthetic absorbables made from polyglycolide, polyglactide or polydioxanone.

Catgut and Collagen. Both are produced in the plain and chromic form. Modern catgut with improved processing is almost 100% pure collagen. The tensile strength loss and absorption profile can be altered by treatment with chromic sulphate to produce chromic catgut; the untreated material produces plain catgut. Many references in the past to catgut being allergenic are probably false. The allergy described was due to dichromate, which was used when catgut was sterilised with iodine. The allergies were, therefore, due either to the iodine or to the dichromate.

Chromic catgut retains its tensile strength for 30 days and is totally absorbed by 90 days. Plain catgut retains its tensile strength for 15 days and is totally absorbed by 60 days. Both forms produce a greater tissue reaction than do the synthetic absorbable materials. Chromic catgut produces a polymorphonuclear reaction while plain catgut tends to elicit a small lymphocytic-type reaction. Both materials are absorbed by proteolytic enzymes, released from the lysosomes within the polymorphonuclear cell. After total absorption only a small scar is left.

Plain and chromic collagen behave similarly to plain and chromic catgut. The collagen is derived from ox Achilles tendon and is extruded as a flat strip then rolled up like a Swiss roll to form a monofilament type suture. The absorption and tensile strength loss profiles are similar to catgut, but the collagen suture tends to be less reactive. Both collagen and catgut handle well and have been

traditionally accepted. Indeed, today, 120 years after Lister, catgut is still the most popular absorbable suture.

Synthetic Absorbable Sutures. At present three synthetic absorbable sutures are available, Dexon, Vicryl and PDS. Dexon, which is the homopolymer of glycolide, was introduced in 1970. Vicryl, which is the copolymer of glycolide and lactide (in the ratio of 90% glycolide to 10% lactide), followed a few years later. These materials are similar in many respects; both are braided and both are polyester. Dexon can be self-coloured or dyed green and can be uncoated or coated with a lubricant to reduce its coefficient of friction. Vicryl can be self-coloured or dyed violet and can also be coated with a lubricant. The coating on Vicryl consists of calcium stearate, lactide and glycolide. Both sutures elicit a minimal tissue reaction but the tensile strength loss and absorption pattern varies slightly. Dexon has lost all tensile strength in 30 days and absorbs in 90 days. Vicryl loses all tensile strength in 32 days and absorbs in 70 days. Absorption in both cases is by hydrolysis and a minimal scar remains. Both sutures produce a giant cell tissue reaction (Capperauld 1971) but the significance of this is unknown. A comparison of the tensile loss profiles is shown in Fig. 10.5.

The latest synthetic absorbable suture is made from the homopolymer of polydioxanone and is called PDS. It differs significantly from the other two absorbables as it is monofilament. The tensile strength loss and absorption profile differ also. PDS takes 56 days to lose its tensile strength and 108 days to absorb. This material also elicits a minimal tissue reaction and is absorbed by hydrolysis. It is produced in a translucent and violet dyed form. PDS represents a significant step forward from the early days of synthetic absorbables, since its tensile

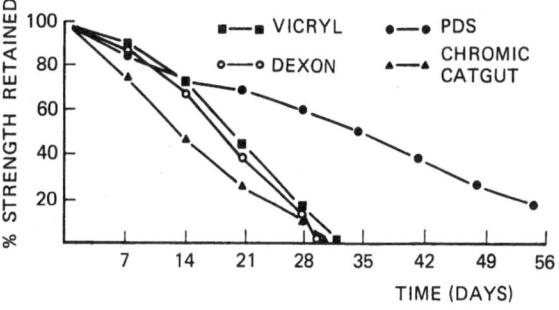

Fig. 10.5. In vivo breaking strength of absorbable sutures.

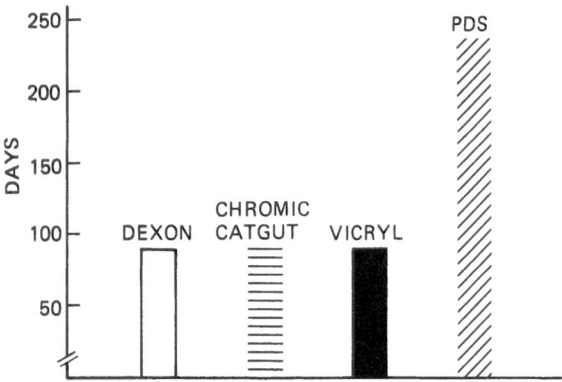

Fig. 10.6. Absorption time of absorbable sutures.

strength retention profile allows it to be used safely in some of the slower healing tissues where previously a non-absorbable was indicated. A comparison of the absorption profile of all the absorbable sutures is shown in Fig. 10.6.

All the synthetic absorbable materials are sterilised by ethylene oxide, since exposure to gamma irradiation causes premature in vivo tensile strength loss. They should not be resterilised by autoclaving as this leads to premature hydrolysis and a radical change in physical characteristics, especially loss of tensile strength.

Non-absorbable Sutures

Silk. Silk is derived from the cocoon of the silkworm and is one of the commonest suture materials used today, mainly because of its excellent handling and knotting properties. It is a braided material and is conventionally dyed black either with a log wood dye or with material such as thional black or sulphosol G. It is normally sterilised by gamma irradiation. Silk can be coated with silicone to reduce its coefficient of friction. Traditionally, it is coated with varying amounts of wax to reduce capillarity and increase stiffness.

Cotton. Cotton is derived from the cotton seed and is traditionally produced as a twisted suture. It is extremely popular as a suture material in the United States. Tissue reaction of cotton is similar to that of silk and linen. All three have a brisker tissue reaction than any of the synthetic non-absorbable sutures. Cotton is sterilised by ethylene oxide.

Linen. Linen is derived from the flax plant and is produced as a twisted material. As described above,

it tends to have a fairly brisk tissue reaction. Sterilisation is by ethylene oxide. It is the only suture material that tends to gain tensile strength when wet.

Synthetic Non-absorbable Sutures

Polyesters. Polyesters were introduced in the 1950s and are probably better known as terelene or Dacron. They are extruded from a homopolymer and braided. They have extremely high tensile strength and relatively low tissue reactions. Coating agents such as PTFE and polybutalate have been used to reduce the coefficient of friction. Tensile strength loss is minimal, making these sutures valuable for support work.

Polyamide. Polyamide, better known as nylon, is manufactured as a monofilament or braided suture. Tensile strength loss is approximately 25% after 2 years. The fibre in the monofilament form tends to be stiff, but certain manufacturers overcome this by adding a pliabilising fluid to the material in the foil pack. Nylon has a "memory" (tending to return to its original state) and hence tends to have a lower knot security index than does polyester. It is very non-reactive in tissues.

Polypropylene. Prolene is produced as a monofilament and the dye is added in the melt prior to extrusion. It has an extremely high initial tensile strength, which it retains apparently indefinitely when implanted in vivo. It has an extension to break of 30%. It is known to be the least thrombogenic of all suture materials and hence is ideal for vascular anastomoses or repair. Although it has a low coefficient of friction and hence passes through the tissues readily, it has a high knot security index. This is because the material deforms when knotted on itself and so maintains the stability of the knot. Polypropylene should be handled with care as it is very liable to surface damage. It is sterilised by ethylene oxide, since gamma irradiation destroys its high tensile strength.

Steel. This is produced both as monifilament and a braid. Steel is inherently a difficult material to handle and if kinked will fracture. Its use has therefore declined.

Suture Technique

The techniques of suture use depend to a large extent on the particular tissues or wounds. Abdominal wounds should be closed en mass, bowel anastomoses with inverting sutures and so on.

General aspects of technique include careful apposition of wound edges, avoidance of strangulation and secure knotting (Irvin 1981). Sutures should be inserted away from the immediate wound edge as the edges themselves are weakened by collagenolysis for several days following wound closure and sutures may cut out if they are too close.

Minimising trauma is of fundamental importance for uncomplicated wound healing. This requires that the tissue is treated meticulously during suturing. The tissue should not be constricted by a suture and ligatures comprising a large amount of tissue outside a vessel are avoided. Dead space, and accordingly the risk of haematoma or seroma, should be avoided by correct application of sutures. Wound edges are joined loosely since there is always some postoperative swelling.

The selection of suture technique is a matter of the surgeon's expertise so long as the fundamental principles are respected. It must be pointed out that continuous sutures have certain disadvantages, since wound dehiscence may occur if the suture material breaks or if the knot fails. Interrupted sutures are safer in this case and moreover may result in less disturbance of the circulation.

Taylor (1938) described the surgeon's knot and this should be used. Monofilament materials generally have poor knotting characteristics and special care must be exercised.

Recommended Sutures for Particular Functions

Moynihan in 1920 laid down the requirements for an ideal suture. It should be free from infection, be non-irritant to tissue, achieve its purpose and, if appropriate, disappear when its work is finished. As we have seen, this ideal does not exist and we must, therefore, choose the best material available for a given task. As an example we have chosen abdominal wall closure.

Wound dehiscence, herniation and sinus formation have been shown to be closely related to sutures and infection in abdominal surgery (Bucknall 1981). Catgut, for example, has been rejected as the suture of choice following alarmingly high burst abdomen rates (Goligher et al. 1975). Keill et al. (1973) reported a 72·3% wound infection rate prior to bursting, as compared with 3·4% for normal wounds.

To find the ideal suture available for a potentially infected abdominal closure we performed a series of experiments (Bucknall et al. 1983). These experiments included tensiometry and electron microscope investigation.

Sutures were implanted into the back of rats, previously infected by local injection of *Staphylococcus aureus*. Sutures were removed at 10-, 30- and 70-day intervals and their strengths measured. Sutures were also examined by electron microscopy. Nylon, in both monofilament and braided forms, retained its strength during the entire test period. Silk sutures, normally regarded as being non-absorbable, in fact lost up to 83% of their original strength after 70 days. Polyglycolic acid rapidly lost strength after implantation and by 30 days only 4% of the original strength remained. It is interesting to note that infection slowed absorption. However, as it takes up to 70 days for abdominal wall to heal, the results for the polyglycolic acid sutures were disturbing.

Electron microscopy was used to test the hypothesis that bacteria could become entrapped within the braid of multifilamentous material. Bacteria were found lodging in the interstices of all infected multifilamentous material, particularly silk and nylon (Figs. 10.7, 10.8) where a vigorous polymorphonuclear cell reaction between the strands continued to 70 days. In the non-infected sutures, fibroblasts and giant cells appeared earlier (Fig. 10.9) probably because there were no polymorphs preventing their ingress. Suture strands remained tightly bound in the non-infected state (Fig. 10.10) in contrast to the infected sutures, where pus cells were seen between the strands (Fig. 10.11). Polyglycolic acid showed little cellular reaction in the non-infected state (Fig. 10.12) until giant cells invaded and quickly absorbed the suture (Fig. 10.13). The giant cell invasion was slowed by infection (Fig. 10.14) and consequently strands of polyglycolic acid remained at 70 days (Fig. 10.15). These strands were therefore acting as foreign bodies without any strength.

The reaction around monofilament nylon was minimal and a fibrous capsule appeared at 10 days (Fig. 10.16), even in the presence of infection. There was, therefore, nowhere for the bacteria to lodge within the monofilament suture unless, of course, the suture was knotted. The knots provided space in which bacteria could become enmeshed. This can lead to wound sinus formation in clinical practice (Fig. 10.17) and a method of sealing knots would be a real advance.

The closest to the ideal suture for abdominal wound closure is, therefore, a monofilament, non-absorbable suture—in this case, nylon. There were

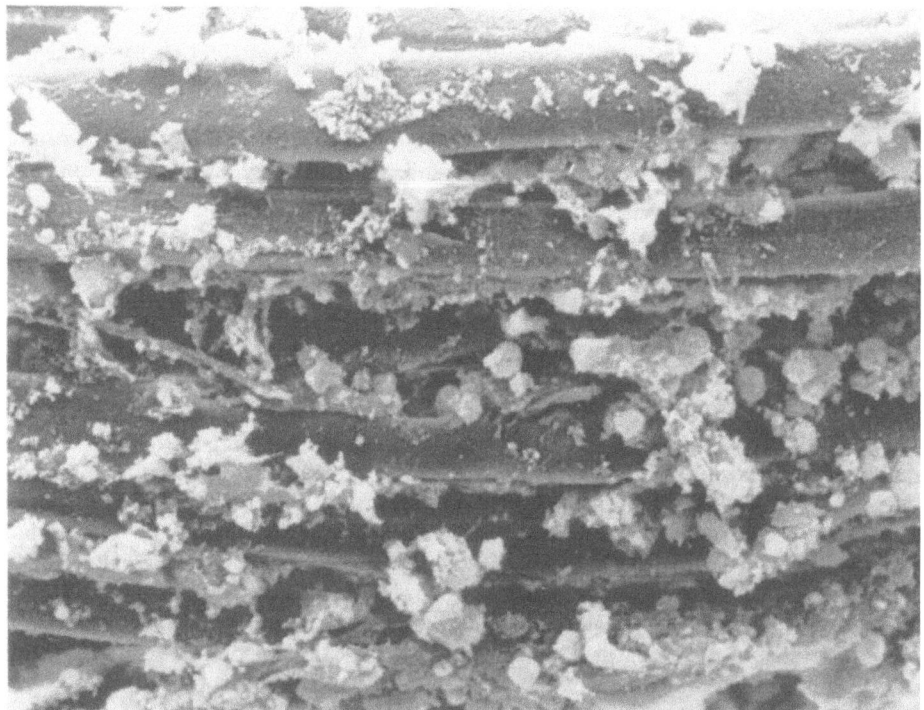

Fig. 10.7. Electron micrograph of infected silk at 70 days. There was marked polymorph reaction.

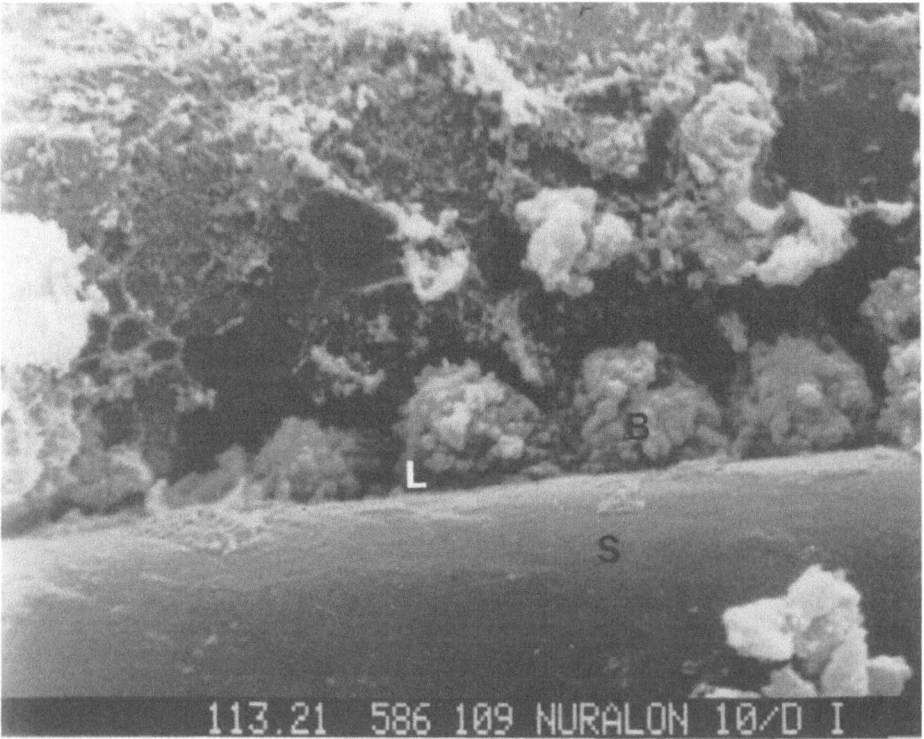

Fig. 10.8. Electron micrograph of infected multifilament nylon at 10 days showing white cells (L) surrounded with bacteria (B) between the suture strands (S).

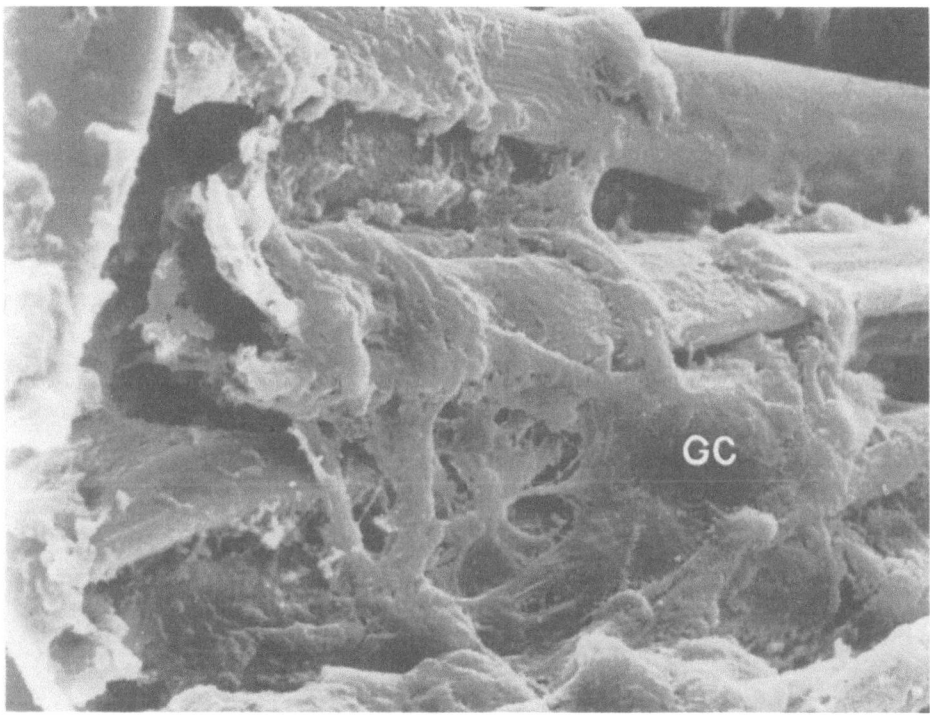

Fig. 10.9. Non-infected silk at 70 days. Strands have been almost completely engulfed by giant cells (*GC*).

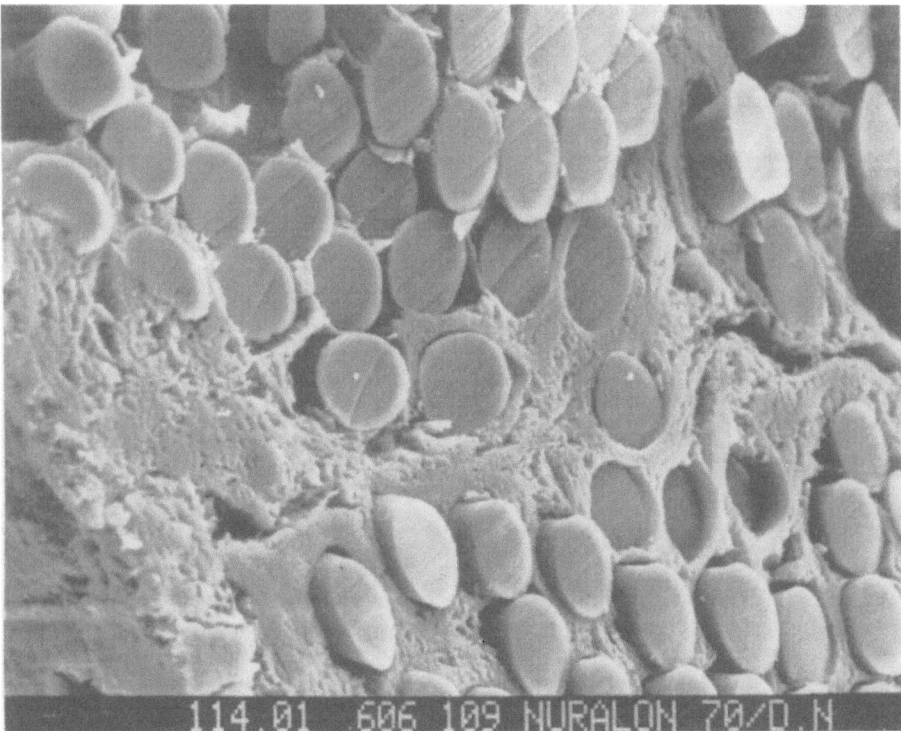

Fig. 10.10. Non-infected multifilament nylon at 70 days. Fibrous tissue ingrowth is seen around the suture strands. A well-defined fibrous capsule surrounds the whole structure.

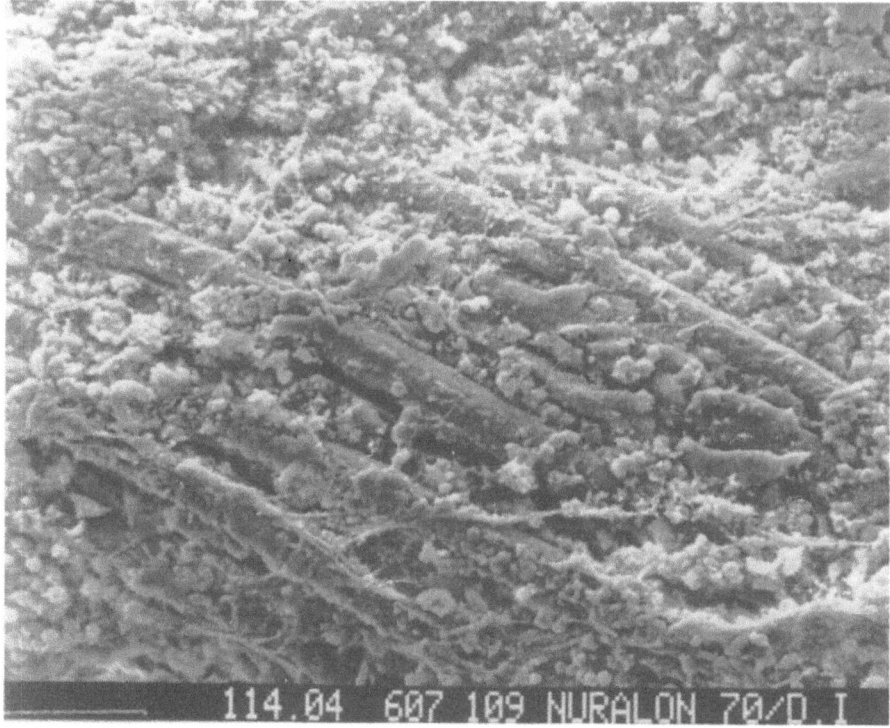

Fig. 10.11. Infected multifilament nylon at 70 days. Pus remains between the strands.

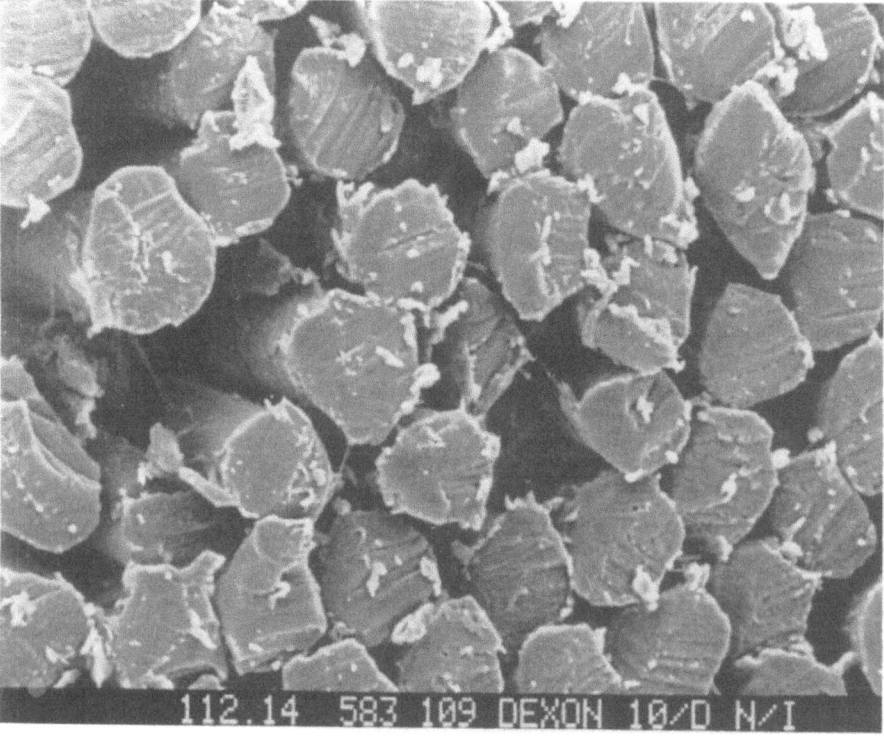

Fig. 10.12. Non-infected Dexon at 10 days. There is no absorption at this time. Strands are still tightly packed, with very little cellular reaction.

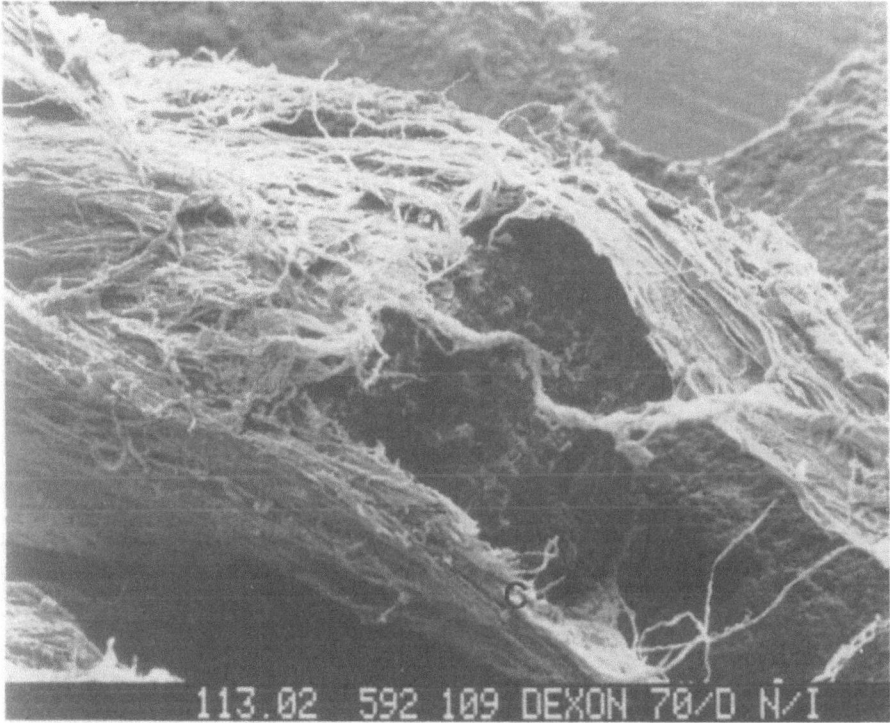

Fig. 10.13. Non-infected Dexon at 70 days. There is 80% absorption with a hollow appearance of the capsule (*C*).

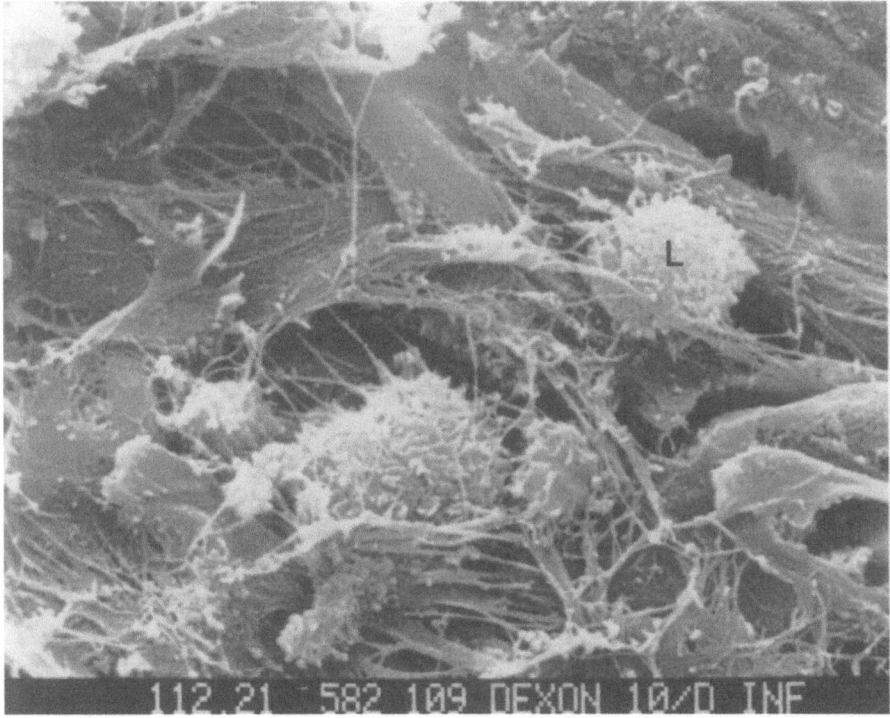

Fig. 10.14. Infected Dexon at 10 days. There is a marked cellular infiltration of the strands. Polymorphonuclear cells (*L*) are seen with attached strands of fibrin and bacteria.

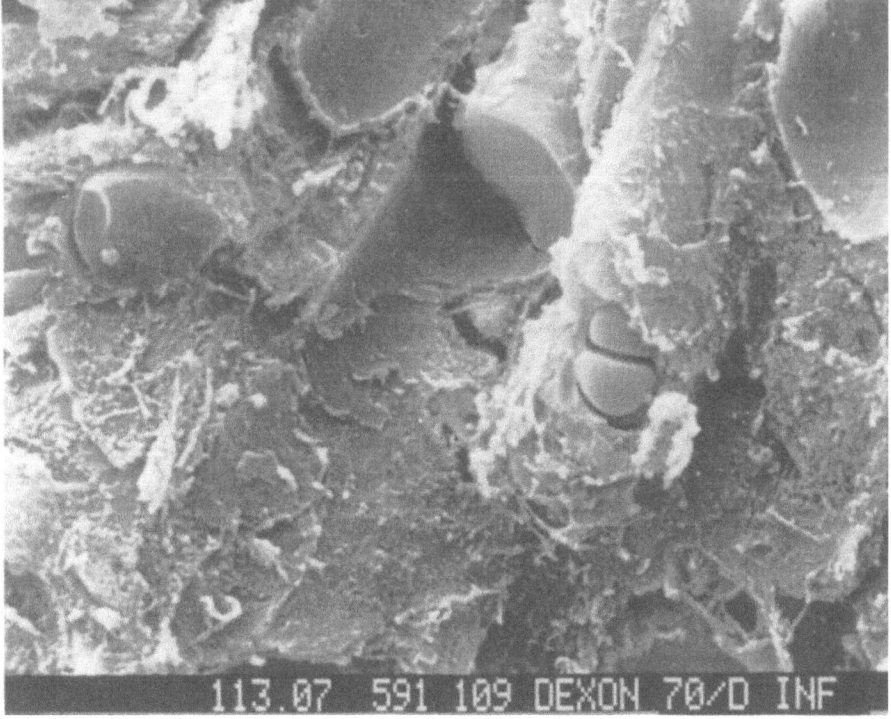

Fig. 10.15. Infected Dexon at 70 days. Only 50% of the suture is absorbed. The cellular component is greater than in the non-infected Dexon.

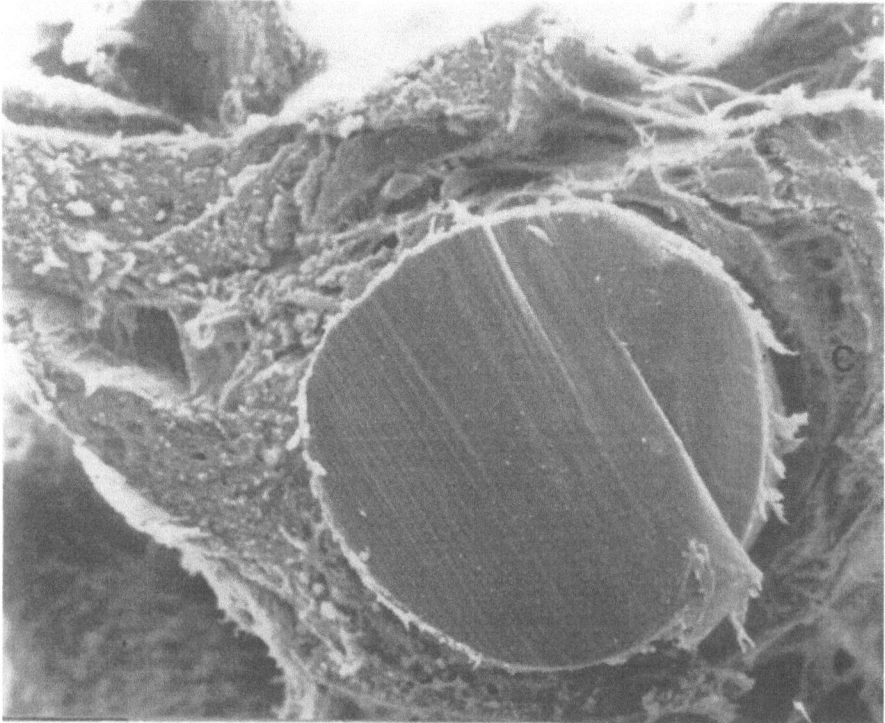

Fig. 10.16. Infected monofilament nylon at 10 days. Slightly increased cellular components when compared with the non-infected suture, but still only a very small reaction zone. A fibrous capsule has developed (C).

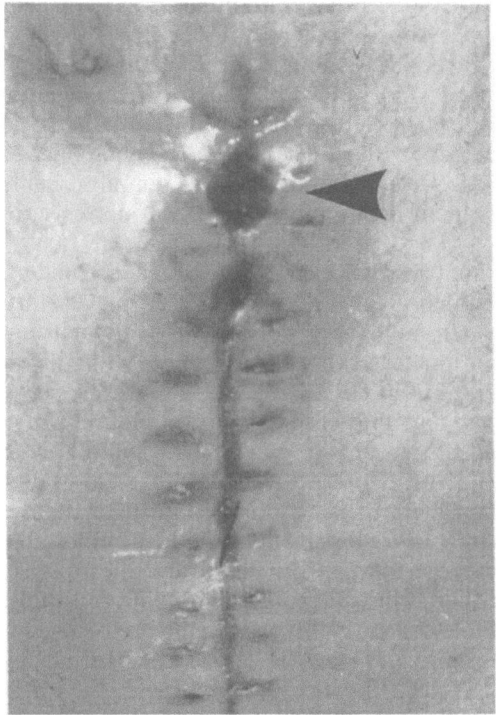
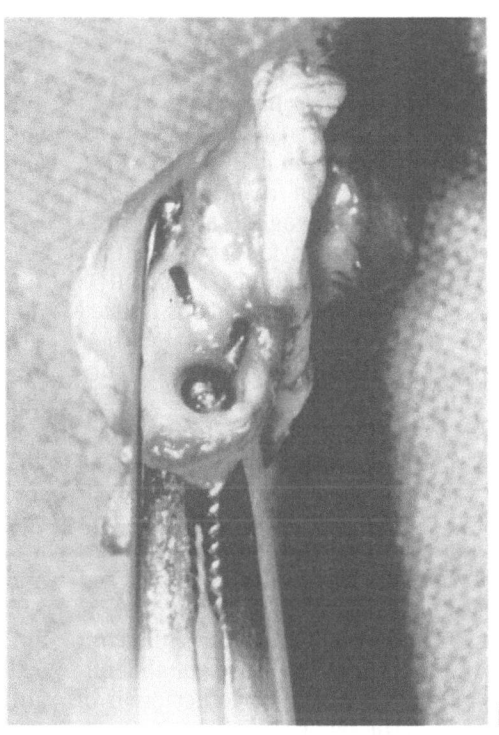

Fig. 10.17. a Abdominal wound sinus caused by a knotted suture (*arrowed*). b Excised suture knot with pus.

no places for bacteria to "hide" and, as well as this being desirable in not potentiating wound infection, it is also important in reducing sinus formation. The strength of the sutures should be sufficient to hold abdominal fascia together even if healing were delayed by infection. This was confirmed in a clinical trial in which we compared monofilament nylon with polyglycolic acid in the mass closure of abdominal wounds (Bucknall and Ellis 1981). There was significantly higher wound failure rate with polyglycolic acid. Also the expected advantage of the absorbable polyglycolic acid suture, in terms of zero sinus formation rate, was not seen (11·5% with polyglycolic acid, 9·5% with nylon), presumably due to infection delaying the complete absorption of the suture, allowing it to act as a foreign body.

We have there illustrated that the choice of suture material has a significant bearing on the success of subsequent wound repair. There is no question that if one selects a large enough suture, even though the suture is absorbable satisfactory closure can be obtained. All one has to do is to be sure that the absorbable suture does not become absorbed in less time than is needed for adequate tensile strength to develop. The question that cannot be answered, however, is why take the chance? To see how close one can come to failure without actually doing so has never made as much sense as seeing how far

away one can stay from failure. Closure of the abdominal wall is an exercise in maintaining and developing tensile strength of scar tissue. Why not give the patient the greatest possible insurance against loss of tensile strength in a suture before wound healing has produced a safe scar?

Holbrook (1982a) showed that, in order to be of use, an absorbable suture material must retain its tensile strength in body fluids. Chromic catgut in human stomach is destroyed within 24 h and in the biliary tree within 4 days. The polyglycolic acid sutures remain strong for 7 days. Urine, on the other hand, has a particularly powerful destructive effect on various man-made sutures. Polyglycolic acid and polyglactin are rapidly destroyed, especially in infected urine (Holbrook 1982b). Nonabsorbable sutures should not be used in or adjacent to the bladder as stone formation is a common sequela.

We have also studied the suitability of the absorbable sutures for bowel surgery looking at the effect of Gram-negative and anaerobic organisms on suture durability and infectivity (Durdy and Bucknall 1984). Polydioxanone suture (PDS), a monofilament suture, comes out ahead because of its minimal reaction even in the presence of infection and its slower strength loss. This represents a significant step since its long tensile strength retention profile allows it to be used safely in some of the slower healing tissues or where healing is slowed by infection.

Synthetic absorbable sutures have been used in all types of obstetric and gynaecological procedures, including abdominal and vaginal hysterectomies, episiotomy, Caesarean section and various procedures involving the vulval, vaginal and perianal areas. Satisfactory results with few complications were achieved (Laufman and Rubel 1977). It is interesting, moreover, that many surgeons noticed a significant decrease in pain reported by their patients when the synthetic sutures were substituted for catgut.

Rogers (1974) evaluated the occurrence of severity of pain after episiotomy repair using polyglycolic acid sutures in 299 patients and chromic catgut in 301. The incidence and degrees of overall pain and specific stitch pain with polyglycolic acid sutures were half that with catgut. He also noted a trend towards reduced haemorrhoidal pain in patients with polyglycolic acid sutures but no significant differences in the occurrence or degree of abdominal, breast, head, haemorrhoidal or other areas of postoperative pain in the two groups.

Sangines and his colleagues (1969) performed vaginoperineal procedures in 100 patients and noted in the immediate postoperative period that the patients with polyglycolic acid sutures were less incapacitated with respect to walking and sitting than were the controls in whom catgut was used. Livingstone et al. (1974) found significantly less postpartum perineal pain and oedema in 50 patients whose wounds were sutured with polyglycolic acid as compared with catgut. After Richardson and associates (1976) changed from catgut to polyglycolic acid sutures for repair of episiotomy they saw a noticeable decrease in tenderness and induration in the perineal area and have since changed the time of the postpartum examination from the traditional 6 to 4 weeks.

Although the female genital tract is considered potentially contaminated, the obstetric and gynaecological patient most often heals without complication. Vascularity of the tissues, youth and usual good health of the obstetric patient contribute to excellent healing following episiotomy. The occasional wound healing problem may result from hypovolaemia accompanying severe haemorrhage, or an unusually lengthy operation or traumatic delivery.

Absorbable sutures often are used throughout, with the single exception of skin sutures. However, I would recommend a non-absorbable suture for the abdominal fascia. Because the gynaecologist is frequently working in a deep hole, the handling

qualities of the suture become important. The newer absorbable sutures such as Vicryl are finding increasing application in this area (Van Winkle and Salthouse 1975). But I would not use them for large vascular pedicles as the knots do not run home well and the risk of slipping and later haemorrhage is increased. In this instance a braided non-absorbable such as linen as a double tie gives a more secure result.

For fine work, for example tubal reconstruction, monofilament nylon or prolene are very satisfactory sutures although they do need careful knotting. They are however very non-reactive, which is all important in this case.

The comfort and cosmesis of skin wounds have challenged surgeons for many years. We therefore undertook a randomised controlled clinical trial to compare different types of skin closure in an attempt to minimise infection and find the most comfortable and cosmetic method (Bucknall and Ellis 1982). Nylon, steristrips, subcuticular polyglycolic acid and stainless steel staples were compared. Cosmetically, staples and steristrips gave excellent results although the subcuticular stitch was the most comfortable. Experiments in animals have shown that wounds closed with tape (Forrester et al. 1970) or staples (Harrison et al. 1975) are less elastic than when closed with conventional sutures. Taube et al. (1983) have had good cosmetic results with a combination method using subcuticular prolene and micropore.

Suture materials should not therefore be used according to a rigid formula or because a surgeon "always uses this material". Suture selection should be based on a knowledge of the physical and biological characteristics of the material, on a knowledge of the healing rates of various tissues and organs and on factors present in the particular patient, such as infection, debility, respiratory problems and obesity, which can influence the postoperative course and the rate of healing. Usually when all these factors are taken into account there are several choices available. Only then should the selection be made on the surgeon's familiarity with the material, its ease of handling and other subjective preferences (Bucknall and Capperauld 1985).

References

Bucknall TE (1981) Abdominal wound closure: choice of suture. J Roy Soc Med 74:580–585
Bucknall TE, Ellis H (1981) Abdominal wound closure, a com-

parison of monofilament nylon and polyglycolic acid. Surgery 89:672–677

Bucknall TE, Ellis H (1982) Skin closure—a comparison of nylon, polyglycolic acid and staples. Europ Surg Res 14:96–97

Bucknall TE, Teare L, Ellis H (1983) The choice of a suture to close abdominal fascia. Europ Surg Res 15:59–66

Bucknall TE, Capperauld I (1985) Sutures and dressings in wound healing for surgeons. Bucknall TE, Ellis H (eds) Balliere Tindall, London

Capperauld I (1971) In: Mennie AT (ed) Report of the proceedings of the symposium at the Royal College of Surgeons, June 1970, sponsored by David & Geck on polyglycolic acid suture, p 34

Capperauld I (1975) Sutures in wound repair. In: McFarland J (ed) Postgraduate surgery lectures, vol 3. Butterworths, London, pp 9–24

Douglas DM (1952) The healing of aponeurotic incisions. Br J Surg 40:79

Durdy P, Bucknall TE (1984) Assessment of suture materials for use in colonic surgery. J Roy Soc Med 77:472–477

Forrester JC, Zederfeldt BH, Hayes TL, Hunt TK (1970) Tape closed and suture wounds: a comparison by tensiometry and S.E.M. Br J Surg 57:729–736

Forrester J (1972) Suture materials and their use. Br J Hosp Med 11:578–592

Goligher JC, Irvin TT, Johnson D (1975) A controlled clinical trial of three methods of closure of laparotomy wounds. Br J Surg 62:823–827

Harrison ID, Williams DF, Cuschieri A (1975) The effect of metal clips on the tensile properties of healing skin wounds. Br J Surg 62:945–949

Holbrook MC (1982a) The resistance of polyglycolic acid sutures to attack by infected human urine. Br J Urol 54:313–315

Holbrook MC (1982b) Wound healing. J Roy Soc Med 75:820–823

Howes EL, Harvey SC (1929) The strength of healing wound in relation to the holding strength of the catgut suture. New Engl J Med 200:1285–1290

Irvin TT (1981) Wound healing—principles and practice. Chapman and Hall, London

Keill RH, Keitzer WF, Nichols WK, Henzel J, De Weese MS (1973) Abdominal wound dehiscence. Arch Surg 106:573–577

Laufman H, Rubel T (1977) Synthetic absorbable sutures. Surg Gynecol Obstet 145:597–608

Livingstone E, Simpson D, Naismith WC (1974) A comparison between catgut and polyglycolic acid sutures in episiotomy repair. J Obstet Gynaecol Br Commonw 81:245–249

Moynihan BJA (1920) The ritual of a surgical operation. Br J Surg 8: 27–35

O'Dwyer P, Ravi Kumar TS, Steele G (1985) Serum dependent variability in the adherence of tumour cells to surgical sutures. Br J Surg 72:466–469

Richardson AC, Lyon JB, Graham EE, Williams NL (1976) Decreasing post partum sexual abstinence time. Am J Obstet Gynecol 124:416–420

Rogers RE (1974) Evaluation of post episiorrhaphy pain. Mil Med 139:102–104

Sangines AF, Salum MH, Lowenberg EF (1969) Synthetic sutures in vagino-perineal surgery. Gynecol Obstet Mex 26:389–392

Taube M, Porter RJ, Lord PH (1983) A combination of response to subcuticular suture and sterile micropore tape compared with conventional interrupted sutures for skin closure. Ann Roy Coll Surg Engl 65:164–167

Taylor FW (1938) Surgical knots. Ann Surg 107 458–468

Van Winkle W, Salthouse TN (1975) Biological response to sutures and principles of suture selection. Scientific Exhibit: American College of Surgeons Clinical Congress, San Francisco

Williams DF (1971) The reactions of tissues to materials. Biomechanical Engineering 4:152–156

11 · Intestinal Injury and How To Cope

Michael Knight

Accidental injuries to the bowel and its mesentery may occur during the course of any gynaecological procedure but are more frequent during operations for pelvic inflammatory disease, endometriosis and malignancy, particularly if the patient has had previous abdominal surgery. At laparoscopy 0·35% of patients sustain intestinal or mesenteric injuries and these can be particularly serious if the injury is not appreciated at the time and the diagnosis made only when signs of peritonitis are obvious.

An injury to the intestine may be minor, such as a serosal tear of the small bowel, which is easily repaired with a few catgut sutures, or major and colonic necessitating large bowel resection and colostomy. The consequences of the injury will therefore depend upon the site and extent of the laceration, the adequacy of the blood supply to the injured part, the time of its recognition and the institution of early effective treatment.

Pathophysiology

Stomach and Duodenum

The stomach, being thick walled and in the upper abdomen, is rarely injured except during laparoscopy in the chronically scarred abdomen when the organ may be densely adherent to the deep aspect of a previous abdominal wound. Because of preoperative preparation the contents of the stomach would be minimal at the time of injury and this no doubt explains the frequency of missed or delayed diagnosis in this condition. Undetected

and unrepaired, a penetrating laceration of the stomach would result in a severe postoperative peritonitis from leakage of acid gastric juice into the upper abdomen. Similarly, peritonitis would result from an unrepaired duodenal wound, although in some cases the first indication of a duodenal injury may be the appearance of a fistula through the wound. Fluid from such a fistula wound contains not only duodenal juice but also gastric juice, pancreatic exocrine secretion and bile. The result of a duodenal fistula would therefore be rapid dehydration, electrolyte imbalance, acid base disturbance and severe excoriation of the skin.

Small Bowel

The small intestine is at risk from accidental perforation by the laparoscope and during gynaecological surgery if loops of bowel are attached to diseased pelvic organs. Healthy ileum and jejunum are thin walled but with a well-defined serosa, muscular layer, submucosa and mucosa. It has an excellent blood supply from the arcades of the superior mesenteric artery which allows sound healing of suture lines and anastomoses with a very low incidence of leakage. Small bowel contents are fluid and corrosive, particularly in the upper jejunum and an undetected laceration at this level will result in a severe peritonitis and later fistula formation with dense intra-abdominal adhesions and skin excoriation. Approximately 6 litres of fluid are produced each day in the normal adult by the secretions of the stomach, duodenum, small bowel, liver and pancreas. All but 0·5 litres of this fluid is absorbed in the distal small bowel and colon. A high jejunal fistula or intestinal obstruction at this level would therefore result in rapid dehydration and electrolyte imbalance if early and effective treatment was not instituted. In addition to water and electrolytes, the distal small bowel plays an important role in the absorption of fats, bile salts and vitamins. Extensive resection or damage to the lower small intestine will consequently result in diarrhoea, steatorrhoea and malabsorption syndromes.

Large Bowel

The large intestine extends from the ileocaecal valve to the anus to include the caecum and appendix, the ascending, transverse, descending and sigmoid colon, rectum and anal canal. The wall of the colon consists of serosa, muscular layer, submucosa and mucosa. The muscular layer is divided into a complete inner circular coat but an incomplete outer longitudinal coat which is concentrated in three strips, the taenia coli, which fuse at the rectosigmoid to provide a complete longitudinal covering for the rectum. The blood supply of the large bowel, unlike that of the small intestine, is precarious by the nature of its anatomical arrangement. Vessels originating in the superior mesenteric artery supply the ascending and right transverse colon, while those from the inferior mesenteric artery supply the left transverse, descending and sigmoid colon and rectum. The main anastomotic channel between the two systems is the marginal artery of Drummond, which in reality is a series of small communicating vessels and arcades situated peripherally close to the colon. In the elderly atherosclerotic patient, the contribution to this anastomosis from the inferior mesenteric artery may be negligible and great reliance is then placed on the marginal artery to maintain viability of the distal colon (Fig. 11.1). Clearly any suture line, whether anastomotic or reparative, in such a patient will be at risk from ischaemia and poor healing, with a consequently high incidence of leakage.

The nature of the contents of the large bowel, which is always heavily infected with pathogens, changes from a fluid consistency in the right colon to solid faeces in the left colon and rectum. Penetrating injuries of the large intestine will, if not repaired, result in sepsis, faecal peritonitis and faecal fistula. Faecal continence depends upon a healthy rectal mucosa and the integrity of the levator ani muscle and in particular the puborectal sling. Injuries to the levator ani can result from accidents during vaginal surgery or from pressure necrosis during an obstructed labour.

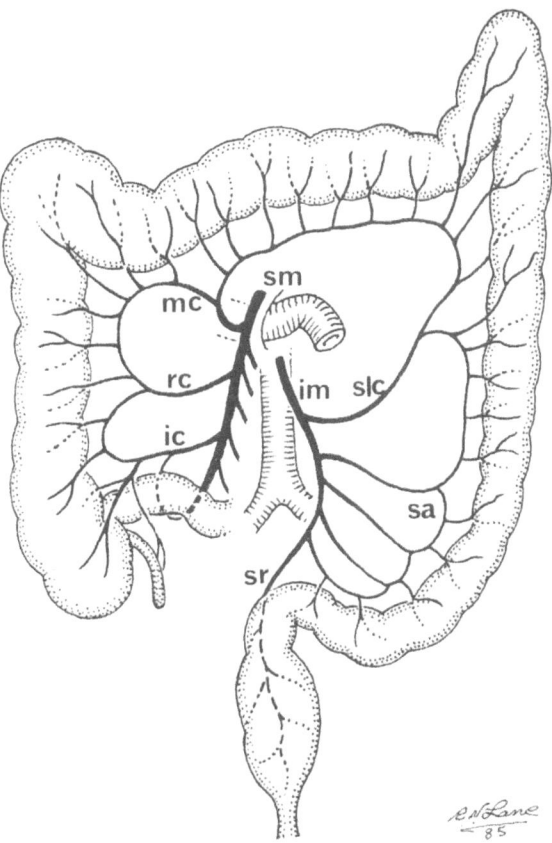

Fig. 11.1. Arterial blood supply to the colon and rectum. *sm*, superior mesenteric artery; *mc*, middle colic artery; *rc*, right colic artery; *ic*, ileocolic artery; *im*, inferior mesenteric artery; *slc*, superior left colic artery; *sa*, sigmoid arteries; *sr*, superior rectal artery.

Sites of Injury and Techniques of Closure

Stomach and Duodenum

A laceration of the seromuscular coat of the stomach or duodenum may pass unnoticed if it occurs during laparoscopy. Penetrating wounds are more easily detected by the odour of the escaping gas, the appearance of digestive juice or by direct visualisation of the laceration through the endoscope. These penetrating injuries should be repaired immediately at open operation using two layers of catgut. A gastroenterostomy is constructed if the gastric outlet or duodenal lumen is significantly compromised by such a repair.

Small Bowel

Serosal tears are repaired by direct catgut suture (Fig. 11.2a,b). Penetrating wounds into the lumen detected by mucosal prolapse and leakage of intestinal contents are first isolated and controlled by the application of non-crushing intestinal clamps and repaired using two layers of continuous catgut, the first through all coats, the second seromuscular and invaginating (Lembert sutures) (Fig. 11.2c,d). To avoid narrowing the bowel lumen, the suture line should lie transversely to the normal axis of the intestine. Injuries to the small bowel mesentery should be carefully inspected to determine whether the vascular supply to the intestine has been compromised. If there is any suggestion of ischaemia, the surgeon is wise to resect the suspect bowel and to carry out an end-to-end anastomosis in two layers of catgut between intestinal clamps, not forgetting to close the defect in the mesentery (Fig. 11.2e-i). Resection is also indicated for extensive or multiple lacerations to a localised segment of small bowel and for some cases of injury to intestine which is the seat of pre-existing disease, e.g. malignant invasion from a pelvic carcinoma, Crohn's disease and radiation ileitis.

Large Bowel

Penetrating large bowel injuries are serious because of the risk of faecal peritonitis, sepsis and the high incidence of poor healing of the repaired wound. A single clean-cut laceration caused perhaps by a scalpel or scissors should be repaired in two layers of catgut and a large rubber drain positioned close to the suture line leading to the exterior through a stab wound in the anterior abdominal wall. The drain is left undisturbed for at least 5 days during which time the patient is treated with broad-spectrum antibiotics, e.g. gentamicin, cephradine and metronidazole. A more extensive wound of the colon, particularly if there is faecal soiling and an ischaemic element from mesenteric injury, will require removal of the affected segment. A decision must then be taken whether to exteriorise the proximal colon as an end colostomy or, in more favourable circumstances (fit patient, no faecal soiling and good blood supply to the remaining bowel), to carry out an end-to-end anastomosis with or without a colostomy. If resection and primary anastomosis are considered appropriate, the lacerated segment is first isolated with intestinal clamps to minimise faecal spillage and mobilised into the wound by division of its peritoneal attachments, taking care

to avoid injury to the ureters and, on the right side, the duodenum. The mesenteric vascular supply is now identified, ligated and divided (Fig. 11.3a). Crushing clamps are applied to each end of the injured bowel while non-crushing clamps are used to occlude the ends of the normal intestine. The injured segment of bowel is removed and an end-to-end anastomosis performed using two layers of catgut, the outer layer being a Lembert suture to invaginate the inner all layer suture line (Fig. 11.3b,c). This technique of anastomosis may be extremely difficult if the distal end is low in the pelvis and in this situation continuity is restored using a single layer of interrupted thread sutures, railroading the upper colon onto the rectum to construct the anastomosis (Fig. 11.3d-f). Mobilisation of the rectum from the sacral hollow with division of the lateral ligaments and dissection from the vaginal wall will allow the rectum to be elevated out of the pelvis for ease of manipulation. Lacerations of the right colon, usually by the laparoscope, are oversewn if minor or treated with right hemicolectomy if complicated.

Injuries to the rectum sustained during operations on the posterior wall of the vagina are repaired directly in two layers of catgut after defining the extent of the rectal wound. This will invariably necessitate increasing the vaginal incision to obtain adequate exposure of the rectum to affect its repair (Fig. 11.4). Unless the laceration is minor and easily repaired without tension, it is wise to divert the faeces from the suture line with a defunctioning transverse colostomy.

Indications for Colostomy, Antimicrobials and Drains

Colostomy

A colostomy provides the means of diverting faeces away from a large bowel anastomosis or repaired colonic or rectal wound. There are two basic types of colostomy, the loop (or defunctioning) and the end colostomy. The end colostomy (Hartmann and Paul Mikulicz) may be temporary or permanent if the pathology or condition of the patient contraindicates its later closure. The construction of a "temporary" end colostomy should therefore be carried out with just as much care as the permanent type.

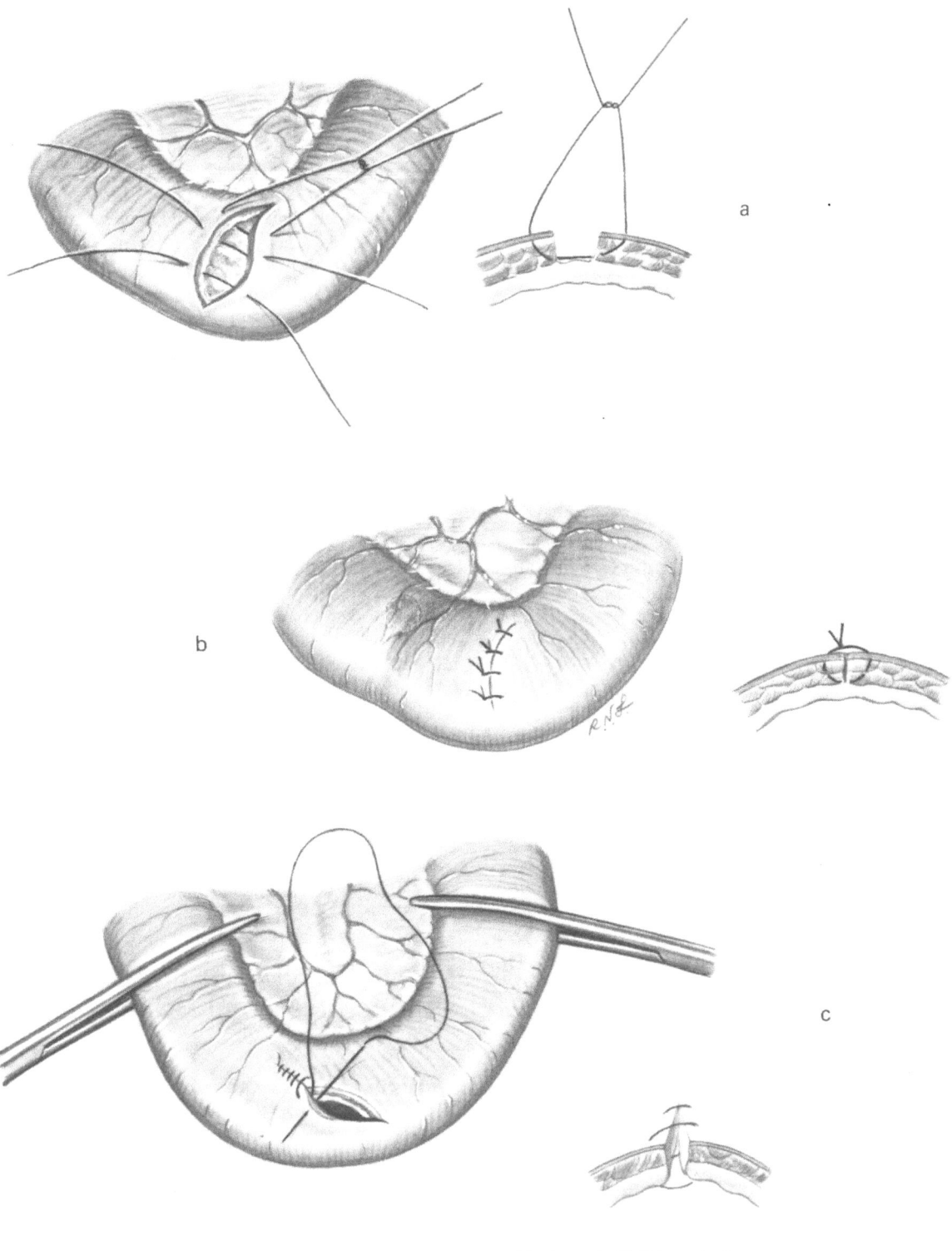

Fig. 11.2. a Repair of seromuscular laceration of small bowel; **b** repair of seromuscular laceration of small bowel—completed; **c** repair of full-thickness laceration of small bowel—first layer; **d** repair of full-thickness laceration of small bowel—second layer; **e** resection of lacerated small bowel—application of clamps; **f** resection of lacerated small bowel—removal of specimen (*continued overleaf*)

Fig. 11.2 (*continued*)

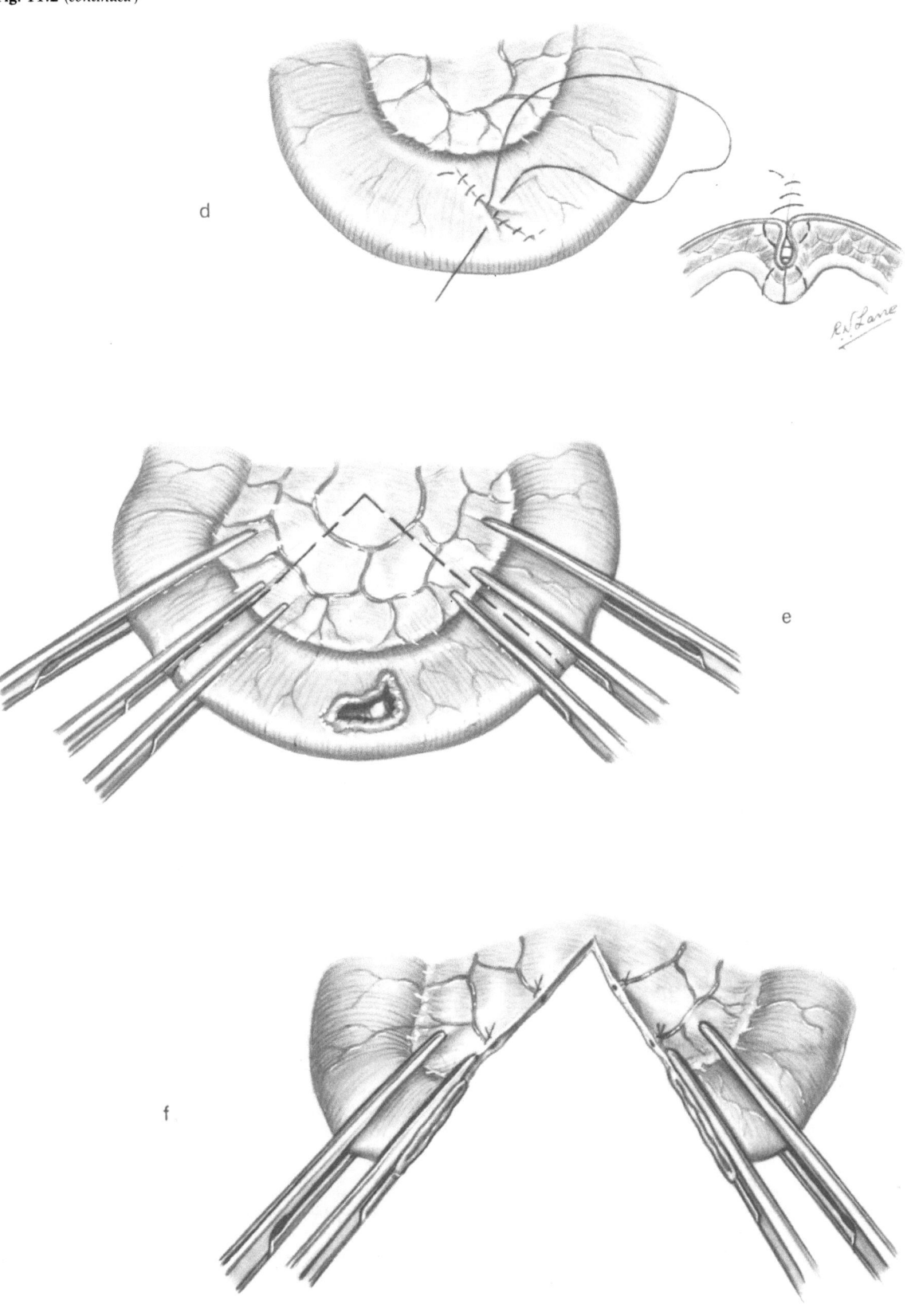

d

e

f

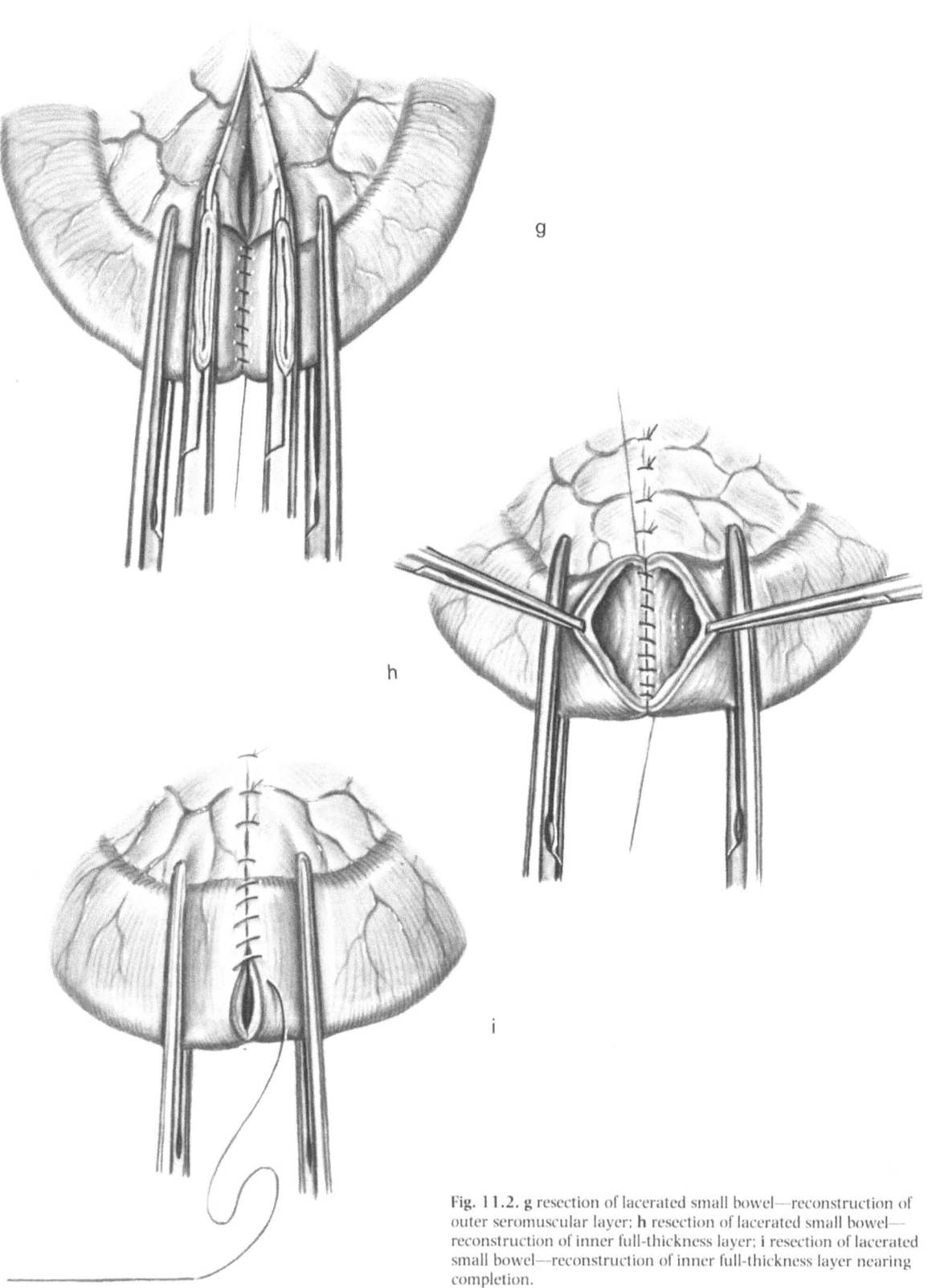

g

h

i

Fig. 11.2. **g** resection of lacerated small bowel—reconstruction of outer seromuscular layer; **h** resection of lacerated small bowel—reconstruction of inner full-thickness layer; **i** resection of lacerated small bowel—reconstruction of inner full-thickness layer nearing completion.

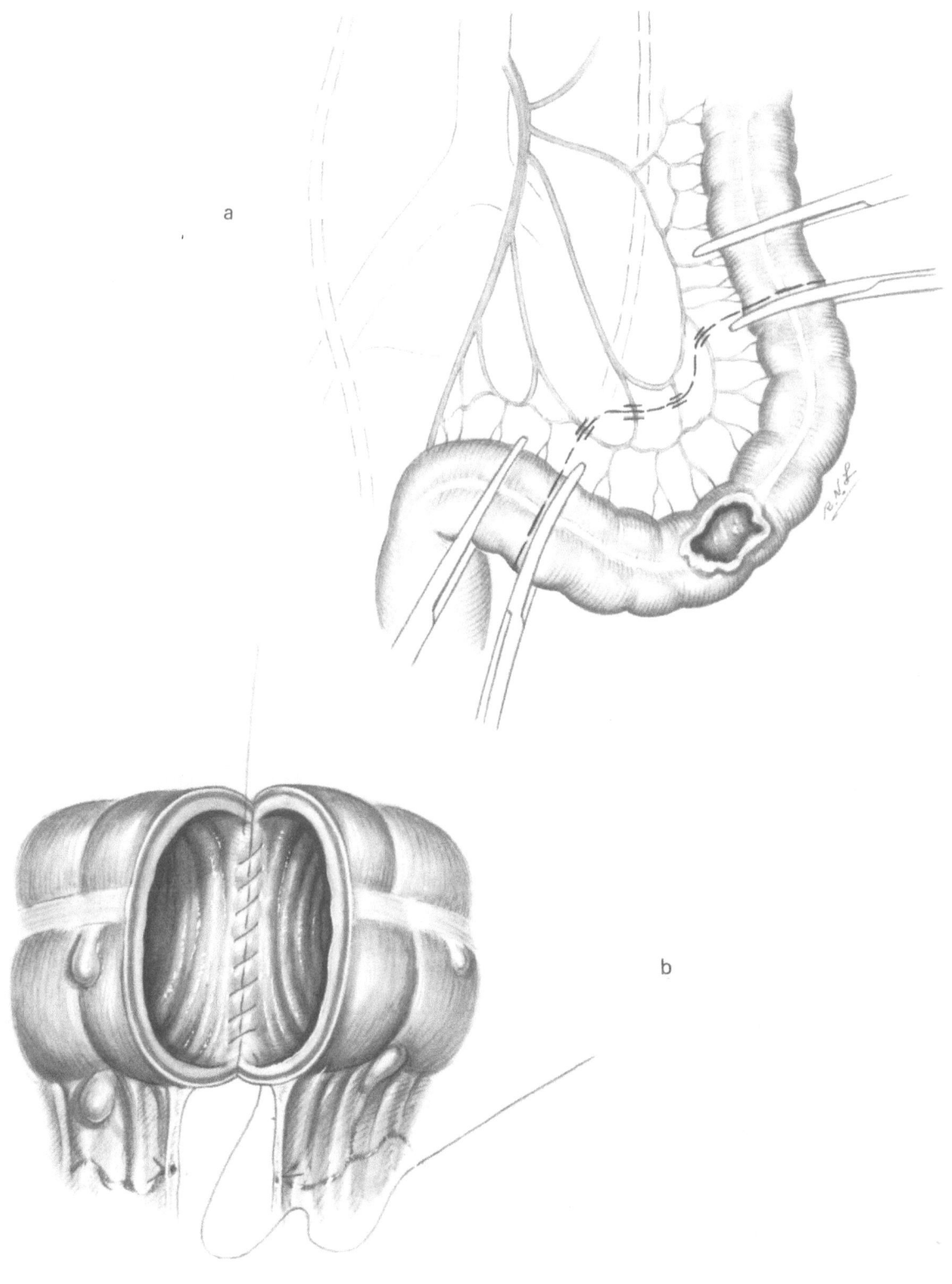

Fig. 11.3. a Extensive laceration of sigmoid colon: ligation of arterial supply and application of clamps; **b** large bowel resection—reconstruction of first layer (*continued overleaf*)

Fig. 11.3 (*continued*)

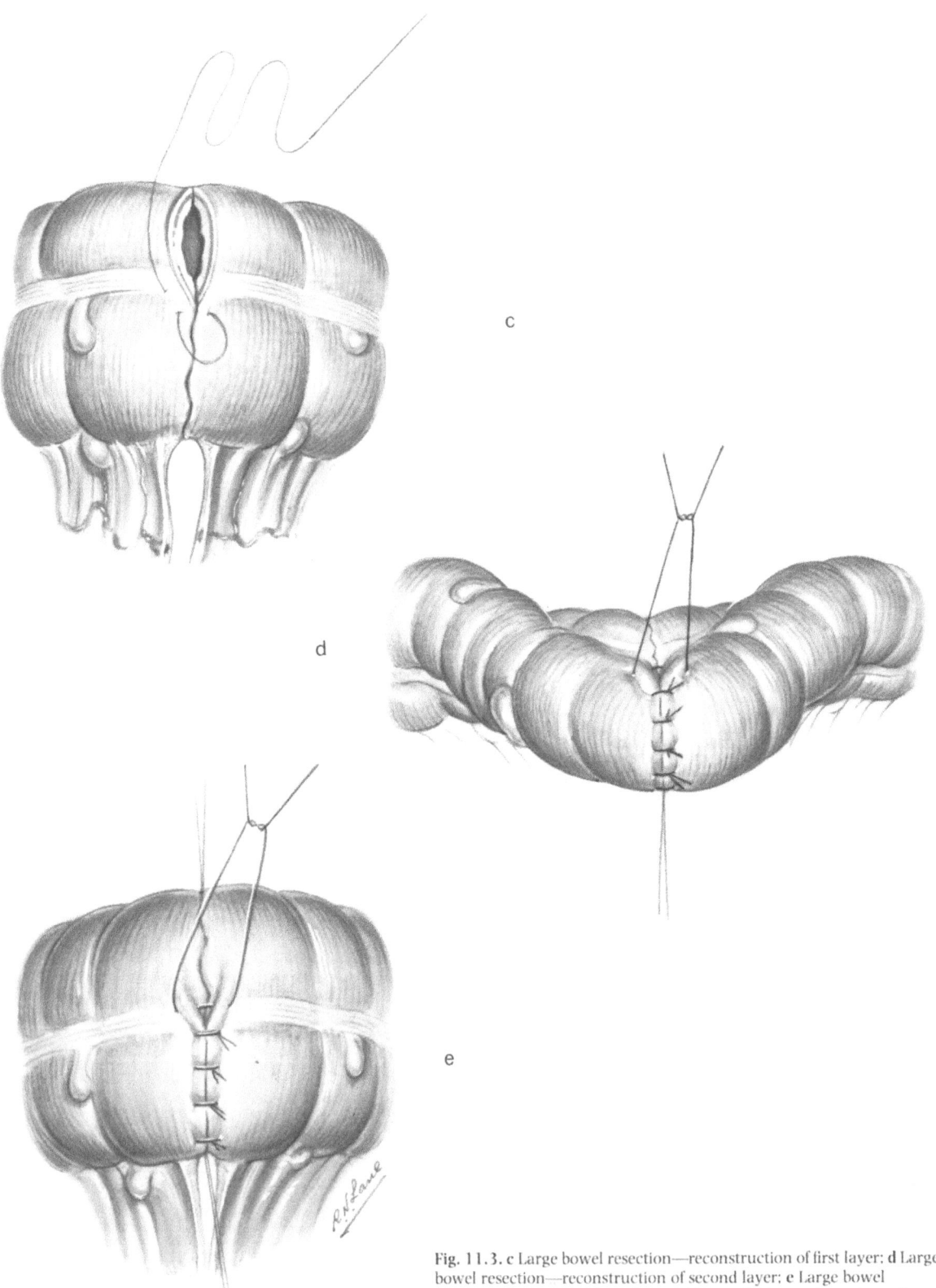

c

d

e

Fig. 11.3. **c** Large bowel resection—reconstruction of first layer; **d** Large bowel resection—reconstruction of second layer; **e** Large bowel resection—reconstruction of second layer; **f** Colorectal anastomosis.

Fig. 11.3 (*continued*)

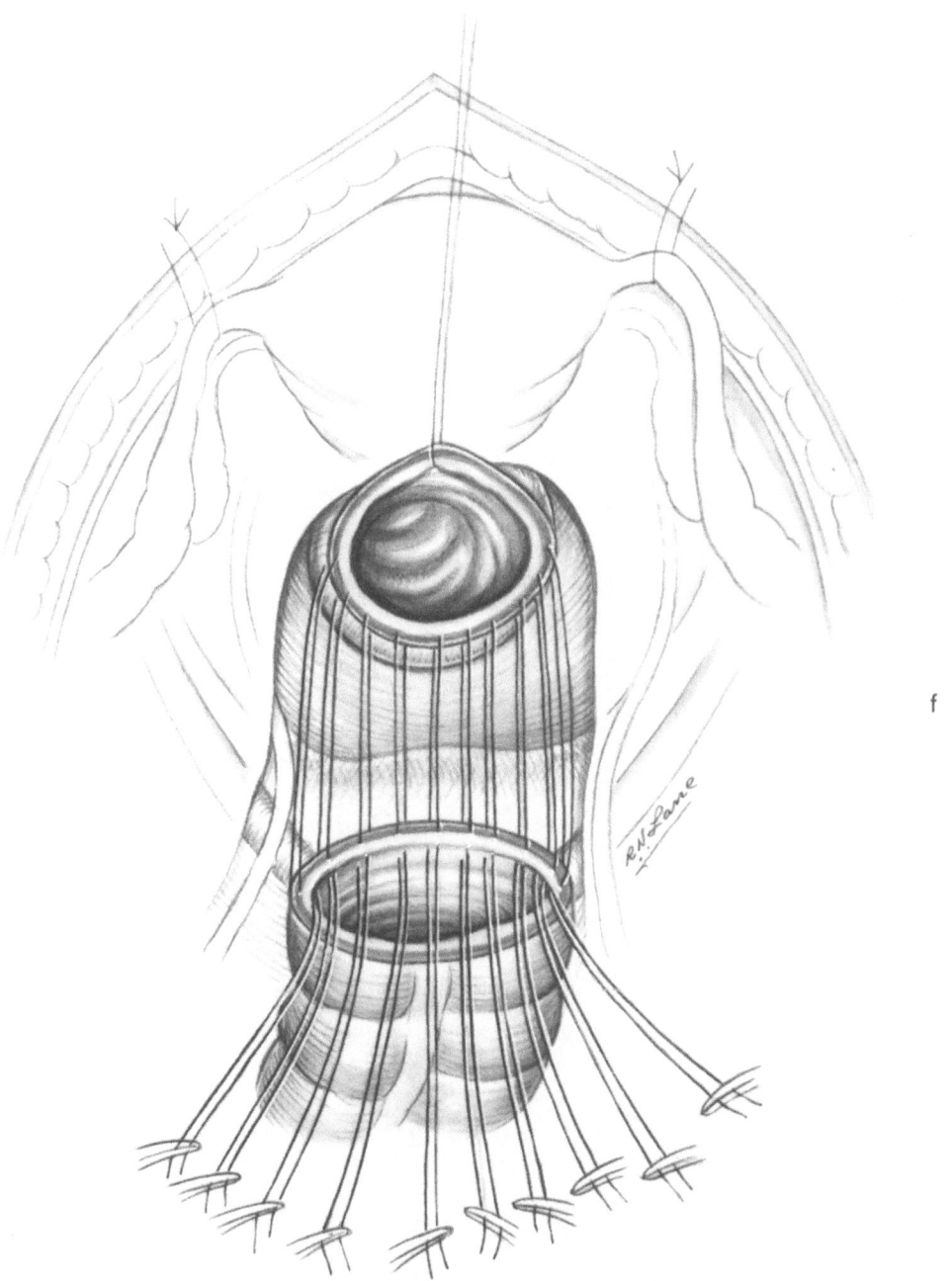

f

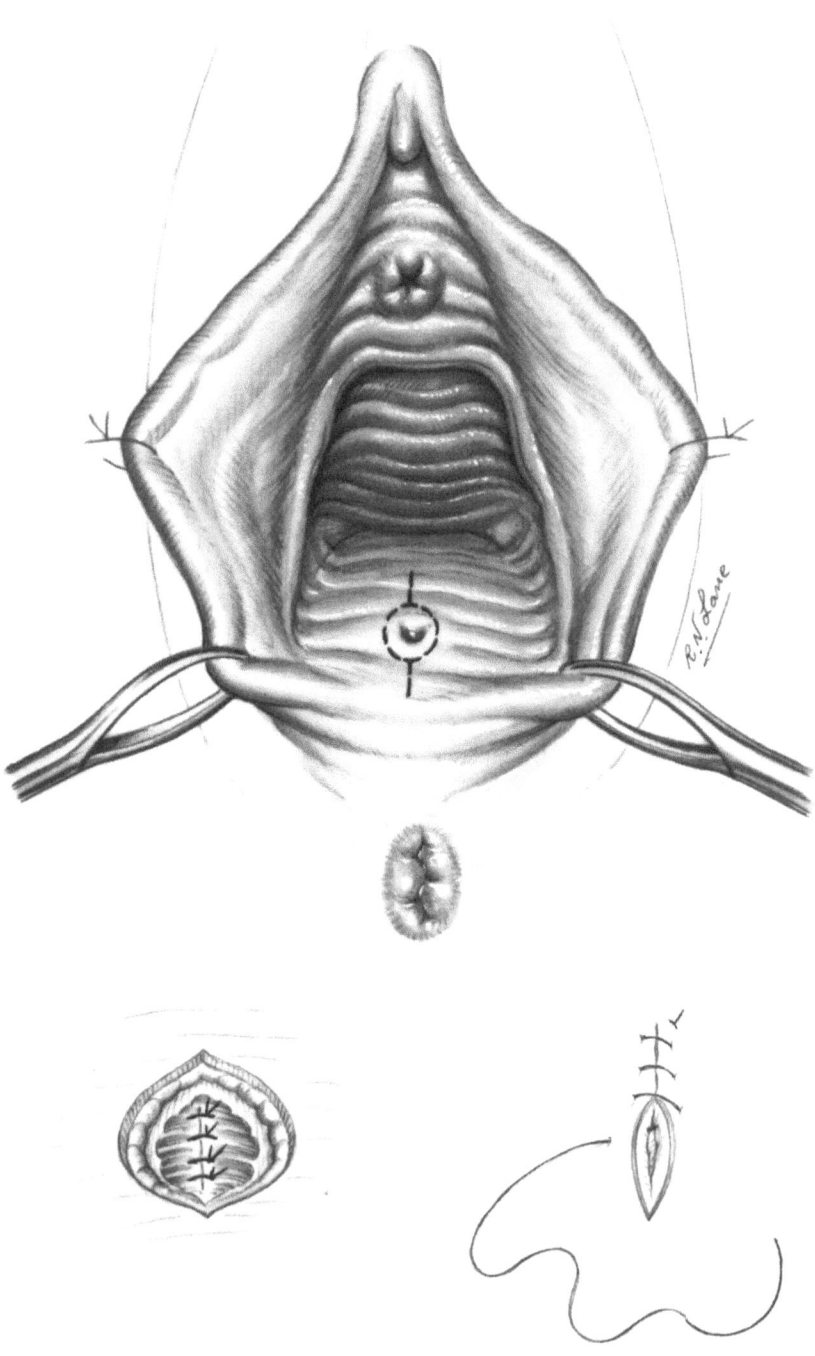

Fig. 11.4. Transvaginal repair of lacerated rectum.

Loop (Defunctioning Colostomy)

The loop colostomy is best sited in the transverse colon and is commonly employed to protect a large bowel anastomosis "downstream". A transverse incision is made over the right rectus muscle 2·5 cm above and to the right of the umbilicus. After incising the anterior rectus sheath in the line of the incision, the rectus muscle is split longitudinally and the posterior rectus sheath incised transversely to gain access to the peritoneal cavity. The most mobile segment of the right transverse colon is then delivered into the wound and a short length of greater omentum detached from the colon at this point. A plastic bridge prosthesis is next inserted through an opening in the transverse mesocolon immediately adjacent to the bowel to maintain the loop of colon on the skin surface (Fig. 11.5a). The wall of the colon is then incised longitudinally with a knife and the cut edges sutured to the skin wound (Fig. 11.5b). An appropriate bag is positioned over the colostomy on its completion. The plastic prosthesis is removed after 7 days and the colostomy is closed as an extraperitoneal procedure a few weeks later after barium studies have confirmed complete healing of the anastomosis without leakage or stenosis.

End Colostomy

The end colostomy is usually sited in the left iliac fossa and may be permanent or temporary.

Permanent. This is usually a planned operation as part of a pelvic exenteration or an abdominoperineal resection of the rectum. As it is an elective procedure there is time to prepare the bowel by prescribing a low-residue liquid diet and enemas for 3 days preoperatively. The site of the proposed colostomy is marked on the skin and should be on a flat unscarred surface equidistant from the

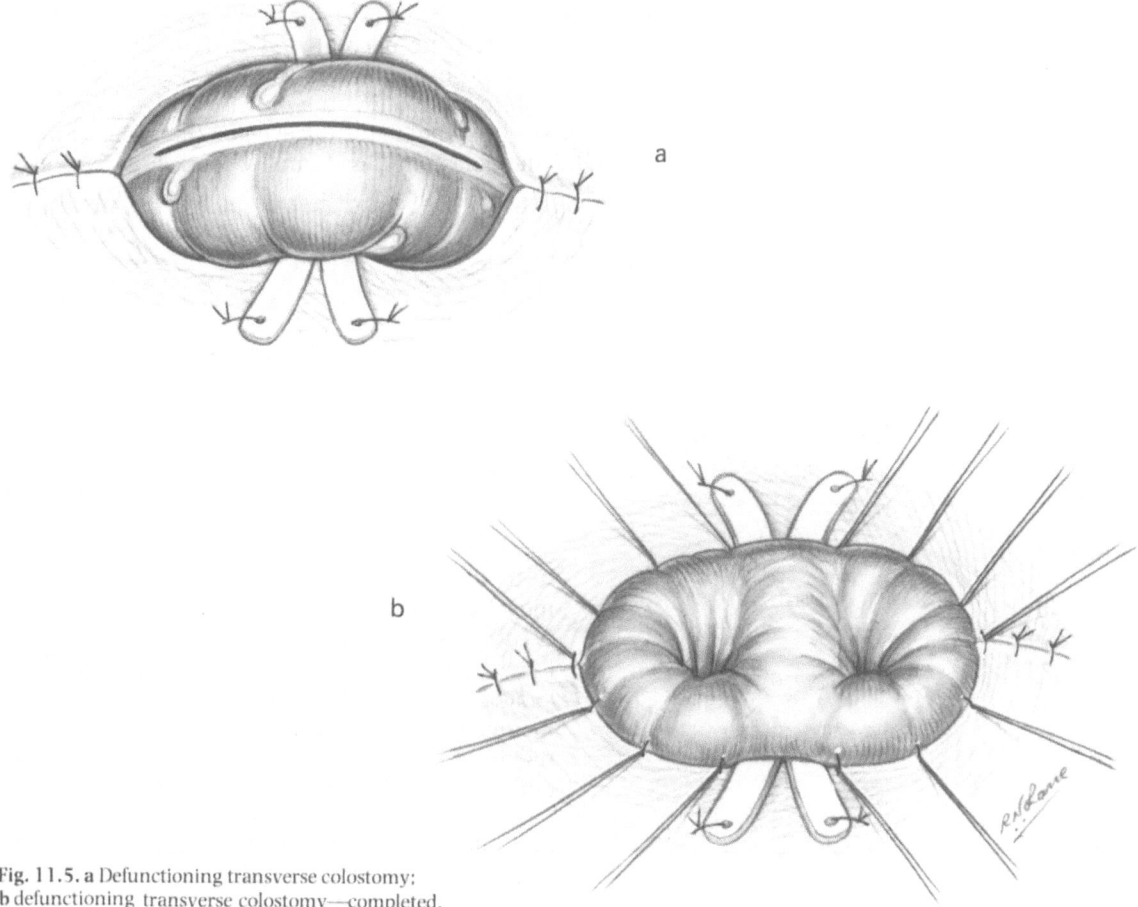

Fig. 11.5. a Defunctioning transverse colostomy;
b defunctioning transverse colostomy—completed.

umbilicus and anterior superior iliac spine. The patient should also be prepared mentally to cope with the colostomy and counselling by a representative of a colostomy Patient's Association is invaluable.

At operation and following bowel resection, a disc of skin and external oblique are removed at the proposed colostomy site and the underlying muscles split in the line of their fibres. The cut end of the proximal colon is then delivered into the wound and the bowel wall sutured with interrupted catgut to the skin. The lateral space between the colon and the parietal peritoneum of the anterolateral abdominal wall is then closed with catgut to avoid the later development of an internal hernia.

Temporary. Hartmann's operation (Fig. 11.6) was originally described as a treatment for carcinoma of the rectum in the poor-risk patient and involves the construction of an end colostomy in the left iliac fossa with oversewing of the distal bowel. The procedure is useful to the trainee surgeon with no experience of large bowel anastomoses and to the experienced surgeon who wishes to avoid leaving a potentially dangerous colonic anastomosis in the peritoneal cavity of a sick patient who would not survive a faecal leak. Included in this group of patients are those presenting with acute large bowel obstruction due to carcinoma of the sigmoid colon

when following resection; the only alternative to a Hartmann's procedure would be the anastomosis of a faeces-laden and dilated proximal colon to a small contracted distal colon or rectum. Closure of the colostomy and restitution of large bowel continuity can be considered at a later date when the patient has fully recovered from the acute illness and this generally speaking is about 3 months from the time of the first operation. At the second restorative operation (Hartmann's II), the colostomy and descending colon are mobilised and anastomosed end-to-end to the distal colonic or rectal stump.

The Paul Mikulicz operation, like Hartmann's procedure, also avoids leaving a potentially dangerous colonic anastomosis in the peritoneal cavity but is applicable only when the injury or other pathology is sited in the easily mobilised mid-sigmoid or descending colon. The operation was originally designed for patients with sigmoid carcinoma but can be useful in cases of sigmoid trauma. Following mobilisation, the sigmoid colon is exteriorised through a left iliac fossa incision (Fig. 11.7a), the lacerated bowel resected and the sero-muscular coat of the afferent and efferent loops sutured together to form a double-barrelled colostomy (Fig. 11.7b). Two weeks later, the spur between the afferent and efferent loops is slowly crushed over the course of a week by a screwed enterome to allow the onward flow of faeces from the proximal to the distal colon (Fig. 11.7c,d). Later the colostomy is formally closed as an extra-peritoneal procedure.

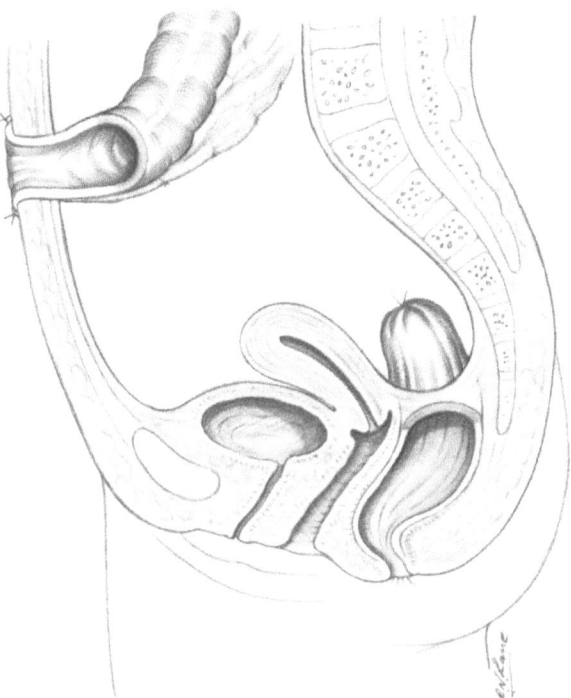

Fig. 11.6. End colostomy and Hartmann's operation.

Antimicrobials

Any patient who sustains a penetrating injury of the large bowel is at risk from faecal contamination of the peritoneal cavity and should receive broad-spectrum antibiotics from the time of the injury until the fifth postoperative day. The organisms most frequently cultured from such a laceration are *Escherichia coli*, enterococci and *Bacteroides*. There is no general agreement about which antibiotics should be used initially, but most surgeons would include a cephalosporin and metronidazole in their regime often in conjunction with gentamicin. These antibiotics can be changed later as a result of culture reports and the patient's renal function. Antibiotics may also be used locally in powder form in the abdominal wound and there is evidence that such a practice reduces the incidence of wound sepsis.

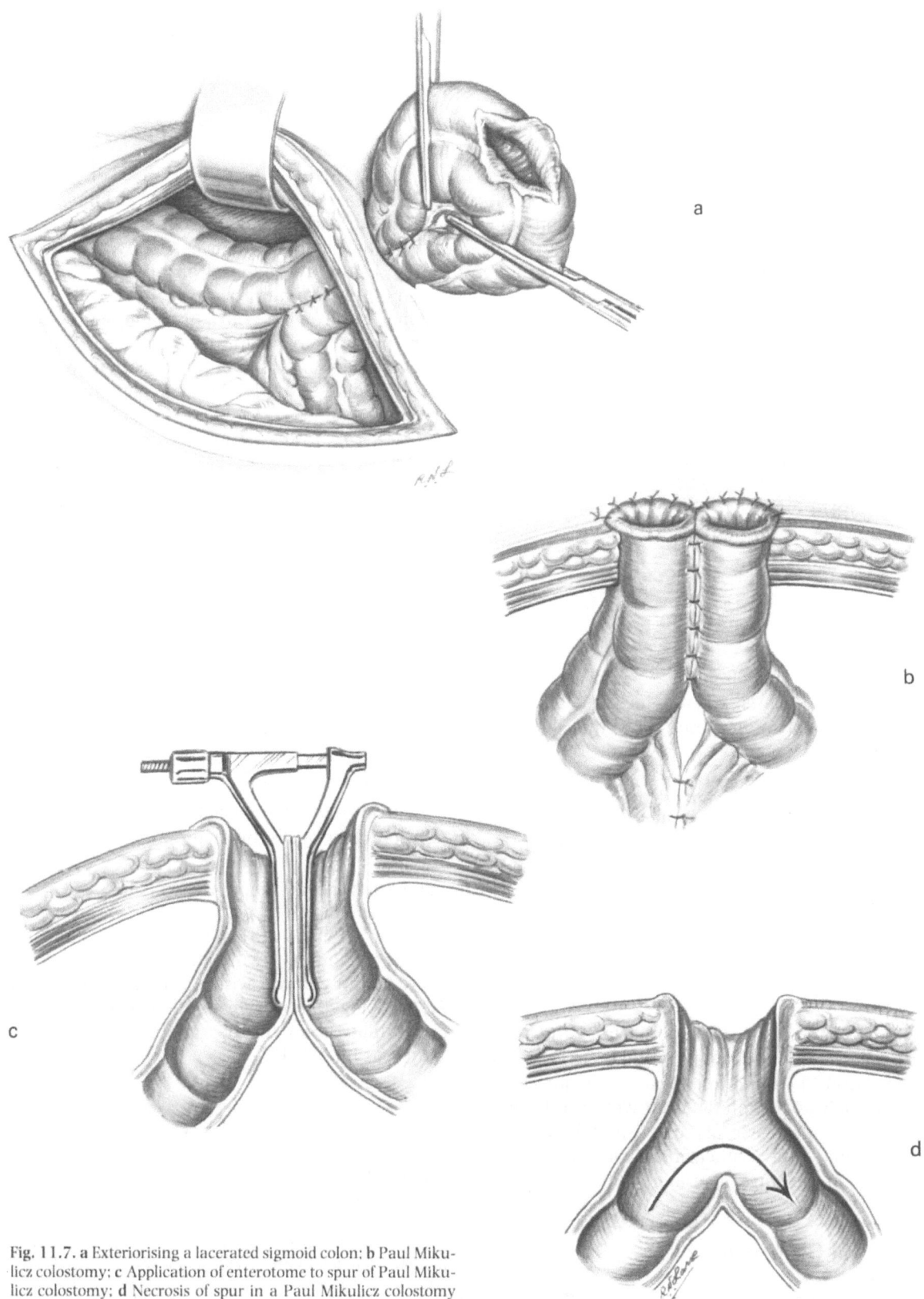

Fig. 11.7. a Exteriorising a lacerated sigmoid colon; b Paul Mikulicz colostomy; c Application of enterotome to spur of Paul Mikulicz colostomy; d Necrosis of spur in a Paul Mikulicz colostomy allowing onward flow of faeces.

Drains

Small bowel anastomoses and suture lines need not be drained to the surface unless there is some doubt about the viability of the intestinal ends. Large bowel anastomoses on the other hand must always be drained to the exterior because of the high frequency of leakage and the serious consequences of faecal peritonitis. The drain employed should be at least 2 cm in width and long enough to extend from the suture line through a stab wound in the anterior abdominal wall to the exterior. Such a drain should be corrugated and made of rubber latex to create a track which will persist even after removal of the drain 5 days later. Finally, the subcutaneous fat layer of the abdominal wound should be drained by a suction catheter, e.g. Redivac, to avoid accumulation of serum and fluid which would otherwise become infected and develop into a wound abscess if the colon had been opened during the operation.

Complications

Haemorrhage

Serious haemorrhage from an anastomosis is rare if proper care has been taken to include all coats of the bowel in the suture line. Those that do bleed usually stop spontaneously and only rarely is it necessary to reoperate to secure haemostasis. It should be remembered that postoperative melaena and rectal bleeding are just as likely to result from stress ulceration of the stomach or duodenum, a bleeding diathesis, undetected large bowel pathology or intestinal ischaemia due to mesenteric vascular occlusion.

Sepsis

Surgical sepsis is particularly likely if the large bowel has been opened and can take the form of a minor surgical wound infection or a major catastrophe such as peritonitis, deep wound infection, subphrenic and pelvic abscesses, portal pyaemia, bacteraemia and septicaemia with metastatic abscesses in the lungs, liver and brain.

Intestinal Obstruction

Intestinal obstruction in the postoperative period can result from a tight bowel anastomosis, extrinsic occlusion by a band adhesion, internal herniae or paralytic ileus associated with intra-abdominal abscesses.

Fistulae

A communication between the bowel lumen and the skin surface or vagina (external fistula) or between the lumens of adjacent loops of intestine (internal fistula) results from an undetected bowel laceration, inadequate closure or ischaemia of an intestinal suture line, intra-abdominal abscesses which rupture into the intestine and also onto the surface or from pre-existing bowel pathology such as Crohn's disease, tuberculosis, malignant disease or radiation change.

Prognosis

The prognosis of any bowel injury sustained during gynaecological surgery depends on:

1. The early recognition of the injury
2. The nature and extent of the injury
3. The part of the bowel affected, i.e. small bowel or large bowel and the degree of preparation of that bowel at the time of surgery
4. The institution of immediate effective treatment
5. The presence or absence of pre-existing intestinal disease
6. The general condition of the patient

In general, an effective repair undertaken immediately after the injury in a young fit patient with a prepared, empty bowel with no pre-existing intestinal pathology, carries very little extra morbidity and mortality than the operation for which the patient was intended.

Suggested Reading

Dudley H, Smith R (1983) Alimentary tract and abdominal wall. In: Rob C, Smith R (eds) Operative surgery, vols 1–3, 4th edn. Butterworths, London
Maingot R (1985) Abdominal operations, 8th edn. Appleton, Century and Croft, Connecticut

12 · Urological Injury and How To Cope

Anthony R. Mundy

The lower urinary tract is at risk of damage during gynaecological surgery, both vaginal and retropubic, but particularly the latter. The commonest cause is the difficult hysterectomy and the commonest organ damaged is the bladder. The prognosis after any urological injury is closely related to the time at which it is recognised and the adequacy of the primary treatment. Immediate peroperative identification of a urological injury and adequate primary treatment should resolve the problem with an excellent prognosis and no complications in most instances. By contrast, failure to recognise an injury until complications have occurred may lead to loss of renal function, septicaemia and death despite the availability of all the trappings of modern medical technology. The crucial factors therefore are to recognise the risk so as to reduce the incidence of injury to a minimum and equally to identify any injury as soon as possible after its occurrence so that appropriate action may be taken.

Causes and Sites of Injury

The commonest cause is hysterectomy either abdominal or vaginal. Caesarian section, colposuspension, sling procedures, anterior colporrhaphy and tubo-ovarian procedures are less common causes (Fig. 12.1).

Hysterectomy

Here the bladder is most at risk because of its relationship to the anterior aspect of the cervix—in all hysterectomies the base of the bladder has to be dissected off the cervix and this is the time when injury most readily occurs; particularly with an extensive cervical malignancy or in the presence of dense inflammatory adhesions.

Their close relationship to the bases of the broad ligaments and to the lateral fornices of the vagina also puts the ureters at risk, particularly when the pelvic anatomy is deranged as in severe pelvic inflammatory disease or endometriosis.

The urethra is rarely damaged.

Caesarian Section

Again the main risk is to the bladder, particularly during an emergency, when the lower segment is being exposed.

Colposuspension

Although urethral injury is a possibility here the main risk is to the bladder (and less so to the ureters) during placement of the sutures that hitch the anterior vaginal wall to the pectineal ligaments. In patients who have had previous retropubic procedures, the bladder may also be damaged whilst dissecting it away from the surrounding adhesions.

Sling Procedures

Here the main risk is urethral injury during dissection between the urethra and the anterior vaginal wall, particularly when the procedure is performed entirely through a retropubic approach and particularly when a non-biological material is used.

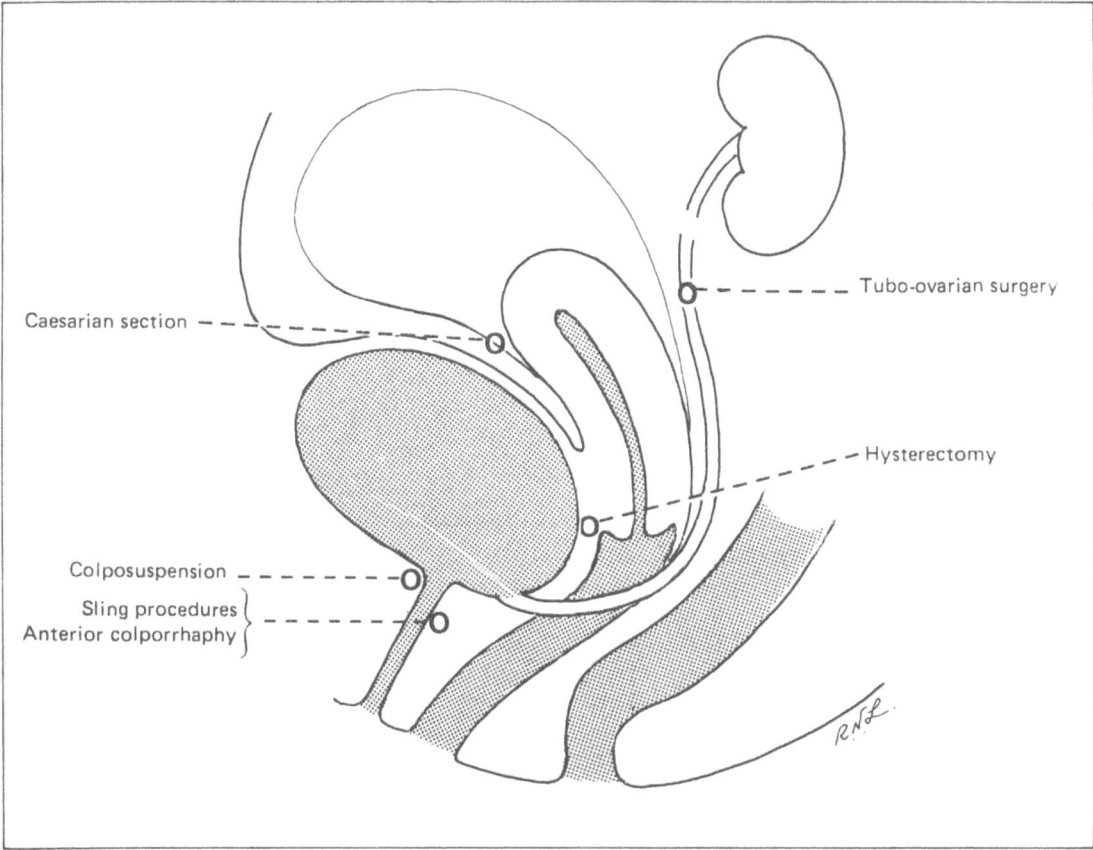

Fig. 12.1. The commoner sites and causes of urological injury during gynaecological surgery.

Anterior Colporrhaphy

Assuming that the exposure has not been high enough to put the ureters at risk (which does happen from time to time) the main risk of urethral damage is in the initial dissection, during placement of the plicating sutures, or because of failure to recognise a urethral diverticulum.

Tubo-ovarian Procedures

The risk here is to the ureter, particularly in relation to the ovary and its vessels on the lateral pelvic wall in patients with ovarian tumours, pelvic inflammatory disease and endometriosis.

In all instances it might be said that there are two types of injury:

1. Direct and immediate—usually due to cutting into a viscus or placing a suture through or around it

2. Indirect and delayed—usually due to devascularisation or a stitch/ligature abscess, especially where the risks are compounded by the effects of radiotherapy or inflammatory fibrosis.

Prevention of Injury

Care and attention to detail in the performance of the procedure are obviously the most important factors in the prevention of urological injury but there are a few sensible precautions that can help to reduce the risks, particularly in complicated cases.

When a difficult hysterectomy or oophorectomy is anticipated a preoperative IVU is useful to exclude a secondary urological complication, and particularly ureteric obstruction. Previous urological symptoms or surgery is another indication for an IVU.

Peroperative catheterisation to keep the bladder empty is useful, particularly during hysterectomy or Caesarian section. A few days of postoperative catheterisation will prevent overdistension of the bladder and therefore reduces the risk of rupture through a partially devascularised area of the bladder.

Finally, if in a difficult procedure the ureter or ureters are liable to be at risk, it is a wise precaution to open the bladder and catheterise the ureters to facilitate their identification, initially up to the point where they are at risk, and subsequently at that point as the dissection proceeds.

Recognition of Injury

The prerequisite for recognition of an injury is awareness that such an injury might occur. If the question—Could I have damaged the bladder, ureter or urethra?—is routinely raised before completing an operation, then any such injury is usually recognised.

Peroperative Identification of an Injury

The presence of urine in the operative field is an obvious indication of leakage and therefore of damage to the urinary tract, but this may be obscured by admixture with blood and may be absent from a catheterised bladder.

Equally, haematuria from an indwelling catheter may be a sign that a stitch has been passed through the bladder wall or that the bladder wall has been breached during the course of dissection.

If there is any doubt a bladder injury may be confirmed or excluded by an incision in the dome of the bladder and direct inspection. Closure of the incision and a few days postoperative catheterisation makes this a safe and therefore perfectly acceptable procedure. Ureteric injury is confirmed or excluded by a similar incision followed by catheterisation of the ureteric orifices with a 4 or 6F infant feeding tube. This type of tube is less rigid than a standard ureteric catheter and is therefore to be preferred.

Retrograde filling of the bladder or the intravenous administration of a dilute solution of methylene blue are alternative ways of identifying leakage from the bladder and ureter respectively.

Neither of these techniques is entirely foolproof but direct inspection and ureteric catheterisation is probably more reliable.

It must be remembered that whenever an injury at one site has been identified, a second injury should be looked for. The commonest example is a ureter that has been transected and ligated a centimetre or two apart.

Postoperative Identification of an Injury

Given that there are two main types of injury—direct damage to the ureter, bladder or urethra, causing leakage of urine, and suture obstruction of the ureter—there are three ways in which such injuries may present in the early postoperative period.

1. External leakage of urine—either through the external incisions or through wound drains.
2. Signs of internal leakage of urine—reduced (external) urine output, signs of a pelvic collection if the peritoneum is intact, signs of urinary peritonitis if the peritoneum was opened and eventual leakage from the wound.
3. Signs of ureteric obstruction—reduced urine output, loin pain and constitutional symptoms if the urine is infected.

Obviously the most sinister features are reduced urine output, loin pain and signs of urinary peritonitis. It would be nice to think that such features would be easily noticed, but in a busy ward following a typical gynaecological operating list, a low urinary output, loin or abdominal pain and mild systemic disturbances may easily go unnoticed in a drowsy patient until a day or two later when the general ward situation is a little less hectic and the symptoms and signs can no longer be ascribed to the usual postoperative course.

Any of the above features and particularly an otherwise inexplicably low urine output should raise the question of a urological injury and urgent investigation should follow. If the patient has not been previously catheterised, this should be the first step. If this is not followed by the prompt drainage of a substantial volume of urine (or if the patient was already catheterised) an ultrasound study of the kidneys and the pelvis should be obtained to look for upper tract obstruction and for urinary extravasation. If a high-quality ultrasound study is not readily available, an IVU is the alternative with a cystogram thereafter if the IVU shows normal upper tracts and a bladder injury therefore seems the most likely explanation.

If either the ultrasound or the IVU shows an upper tract abnormality (Fig. 12.2) a percutaneous

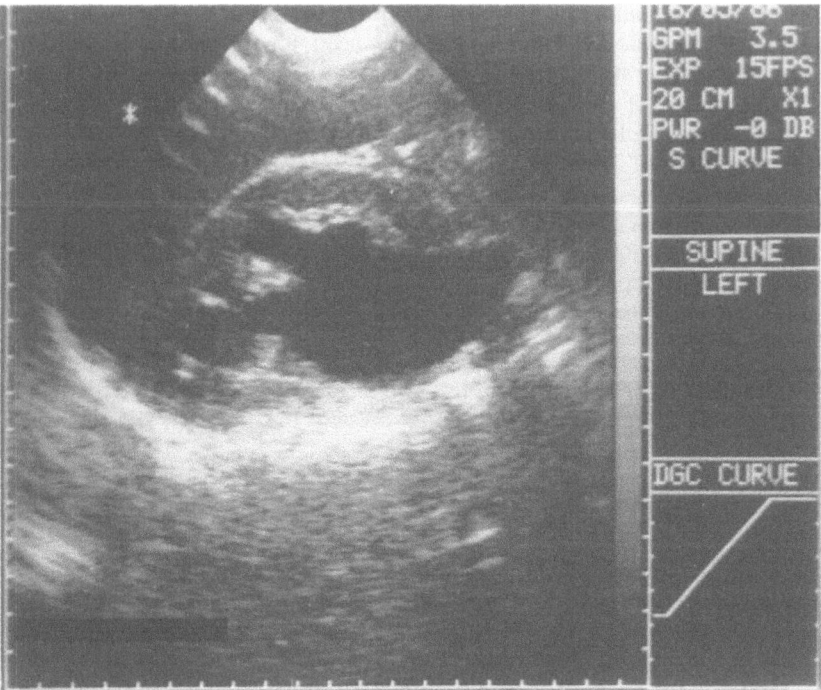

Fig. 12.2. An ultrasound study showing a hydronephrosis due to obstruction of the distal ureter.

nephrostomy is the next step. This is both diagnostic, as it allows antegrade pyeloureterography (Fig. 12.3), and therapeutic, in the short term, as it bypasses the site of injury and provides adequate urine drainage from the affected side until such time as a repair can be attempted.

If there are no facilities for percutaneous nephrostomy the only alternative is cystoscopy and retrograde ureterography both to make an exact diagnosis and, if possible, to pass a ureteric catheter up past the site of injury although in this situation it is much better to proceed directly to exploration and repair of the injury.

Injuries to the urinary tract which have a later presentation are discussed in Chap. 18.

Principles of Management of Injury

Minor injuries can be dealt with by someone without any urological expertise, but more serious injuries will need a urologist's attention. In all injuries the principles are the same.

1. All sutures should be absorbable, chromic catgut, Vicryl or Dexon, and usually the former for the ureter and any of the three for the bladder and urethra (although the author prefers Vicryl for its ease of handling).

2. No suture line should be under tension.

3. Any adjacent suture lines should be kept apart by the interposition of the omentum to prevent fistula formation. This particularly applies to bladder injuries during hysterectomy. Indeed as a general rule the omentum should be tacked over or around any urological repair to facilitate healing and provide support.

4. Ureteric injuries or reimplantations should be splinted by passing a suitable catheter, such as a 6F infant feeding tube, through the ureteric orifice and up the full length of the ureter.

5. Bladder injuries (including intentional cystotomy incisions) should be covered by 5–10 days of catheterisation, preferably with a 14F or 16F suprapubic catheter as this allows a trial of voiding by clamping the catheter before removing it.

6. Urethral injuries should also be covered by catheterisation (urethral or suprapubic and sometimes both).

7. The area of injury/repair should be drained postoperatively using a tubular drain of about 18F calibre. In this way extravasated urine and blood can be collected in a drainage bag. Other types of drain which collect in a sodden mass of swabs on the abdominal wall should not be used.

8. Antibiotic cover is generally advisable. Urinary infection is diagnosed bacteriologically by the presence of greater than 10^6 bacteria/ml urine. Supposedly sterile urine by these criteria may nonetheless contain many organisms and the raw extraperitoneal tissues of the pelvis are an excellent culture medium; thus rampant infection may rapidly supervene.

For minor injuries a single parenteral injection of gentamycin 80 mg peroperatively will usually suffice. In more serious situations, particularly when the diagnosis is delayed, an intravenous cocktail of gentamycin 80 mg tds, ampicillin 500 mg tds and metronidazole 500 mg tds for 5 days is the author's current preference.

Specific Management of the Urological Injury

Peroperative Diagnosis

Ureter

A ureteric injury should always be dealt with by a urologist (that is to say by someone with experience in such injuries) as the penalty for an inadequate resolution of the problem may be loss of the kidney.

The injury itself may be either a cut or an encircling suture or ligature and the site of the injury may be anywhere below the pelvic brim but usually in the terminal 5–7 cm.

If the injury is an encircling suture or ligature it should be removed and the ureter splinted with a 6F infant feeding tube brought out through a suprapubic cystotomy alongside a 14F or 16F suprapubic catheter. If the ureteric wall has been breached or otherwise traumatised it is safer to treat it as if it has been cut.

Theoretically it should be possible to repair a cut ureter by excision of the traumatised area and end-to-end anastomosis, but although this is sometimes possible, it is not always so because either the length of the traumatised ureter precludes this or the site of the injury, close to the bladder, makes this less satisfactory than reimplantation into the bladder.

A ureter injured on the lateral side wall of the pelvis, for instance, during excision of an ovarian tumour, will be amenable to a direct repair. The technique starts with mobilisation of the ureter on either side of the injury, taking care not to damage the blood supply that runs in the thin "mesentery" that surrounds it, particularly on the posterior aspect. If the edges of the cut ureter are not "clean", they should be freshened. The mobilisation of the ureter should allow the two ends of the ureter to be overlapped by 1·5–2 cm *without tension* (Fig. 12.4). When this has been achieved the two ends of the ureter are spatulated by incising along the ureter from the end for 1·5 cm on the opposing sides. This allows an oblique anastomosis (Fig. 12.5), without

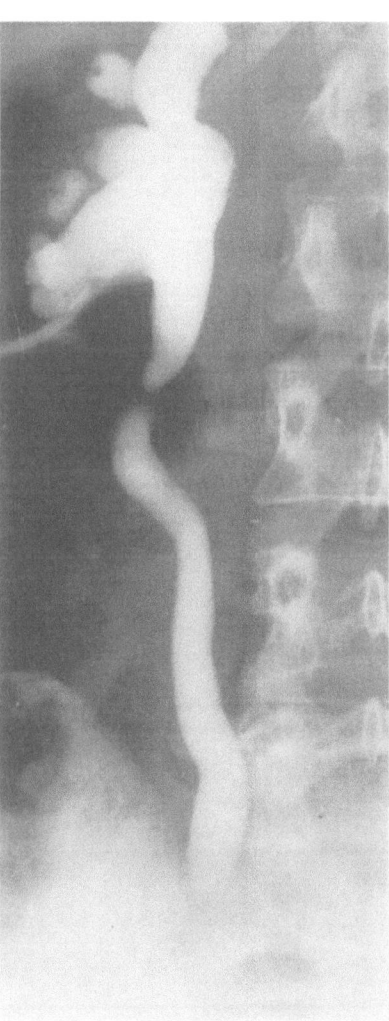

Fig. 12.3. An antegrade pyeloureterogram (performed through a percutaneous nephrostomy) in a patient with obstruction of the distal ureter.

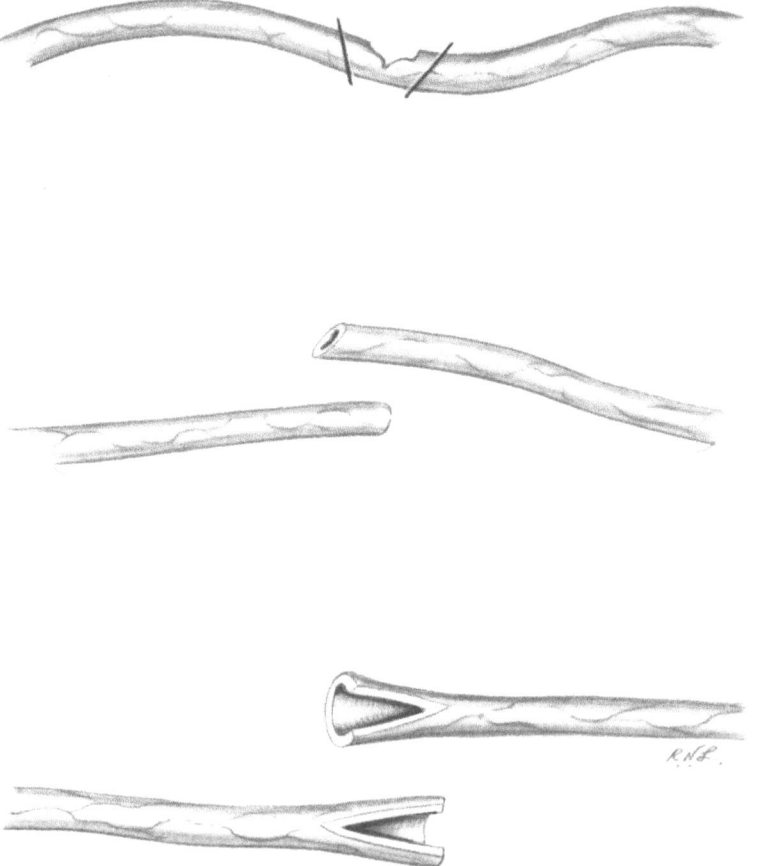

Fig. 12.4. Mobilisation and spatulation of the ureter following an injury near the pelvic brim with sufficient overlap to allow a tension-free anastomosis.

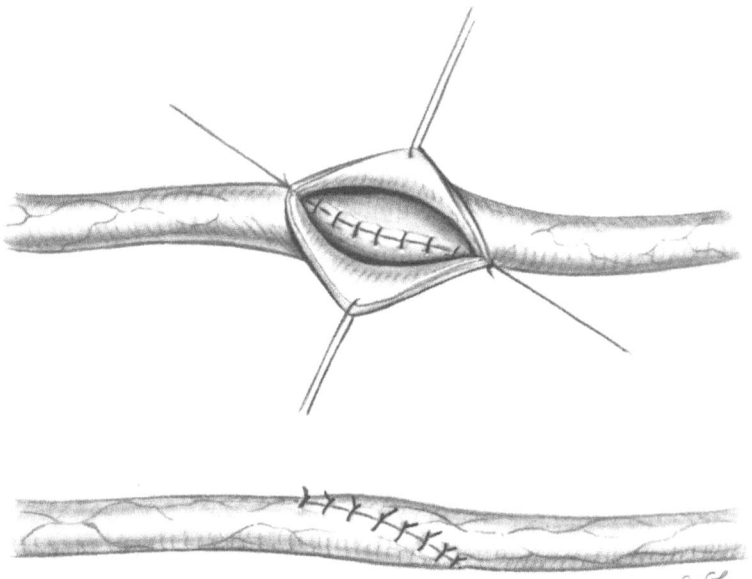

Fig. 12.5. Anastomosis of the spatulated ureteric ends.

tension, that will be far less likely to stricture than an unspatulated anastomosis.

The anastomosis should be performed with interrupted 3/0 chromic catgut sutures placed about 2 or 3 mm apart; about eight sutures will be used in the average case. As always the anastomosis is splinted with a 6F infant feeding tube passed up the full length of the ureter from the ureteric orifice within the bladder and the tube is brought out through the cystotomy alongside a 14F or 16F suprapubic catheter.

The procedure is completed by wrapping the anastomosis with omentum and leaving a tube wound-drain in the area to prevent the accumulation of any extravasated urine which might otherwise lead to fibrosis and stricturing.

For distal ureteric injuries or for any injury of the pelvic ureter where the gap between the freshened ends precludes a direct anastomosis, a ureteric reimplantation is performed. The principle of ureteric reimplantation is to provide a tunnelled ureteroneocystostomy into a stable area of the bladder—tunnelling acts as an antireflux mechanism and reimplantation into a stable area of the bladder prevents kinking of the ureter as the relationship between the ureter and the bladder changes with different degrees of bladder filling.

With distal ureteric injuries just outside the bladder there will be enough ureteric length for a tunnelled reimplantation into the naturally stable area of the bladder base (Fig. 12.6). A finger-sized opening is made in the bladder wall at, or just above, the ipsilateral ureteric orifice and the adequately mobilised ureter is pulled through into the bladder. A submucosal tunnel is then created with McIndoe scissors or a Lahey forceps from this side to a point below or above the contralateral ureteric orifice. It is important that this is a submucosal tunnel and that there are no muscle bundles raised with the mucosa that might subsequently act to compress the tunnelled ureter. The ureter is then passed through the tunnel, spatulated and sutured to the margins of the newly created "ureteric orifice" with five or six interrupted 3/0 chromic catgut sutures. The ureter is splinted and the bladder catheterised as above.

With more proximal injuries of the pelvic ureter there may not be sufficient ureteric length to accomplish this. The ureter must therefore be reimplanted into the posterolateral wall of the bladder and this area of the bladder wall must first be stabilised, for the reasons given above, using the technique known as the psoas hitch. In this procedure the posterolateral bladder wall on the side of the ureteric injury is tacked onto the ipsilateral psoas tendon and the ureter is then reimplanted into the area of the bladder that has thus been stabilised (Fig. 12.7).

First of all the psoas tendon is exposed through the peritoneum just above the common iliac vessels and any overlying fatty tissue is cleaned off the tendon. The bladder is then lifted up to the psoas tendon to see if it will reach without tension. If not, the contralateral bladder wall will need to be mobilised by dividing the wing of peritoneum and underlying fascia that runs from the anterolateral bladder wall to the wing of the pelvis between the anterior midline and the lateral, vascular pedicle of the bladder. If this is still insufficient to allow tension-free apposition of the bladder to the psoas tendon, the obliterated umbilical artery and the superior vesical vessels are divided on the side being mobilised and this will almost invariably allow a satisfactory hitch. The hitch is achieved by three to five interrupted 2/0 Vicryl or Dexon sutures through the psoas tendon and the full thickness of the bladder wall *except* the urothelium. Having fixed the bladder to the psoas tendon the ureter is reimplanted into the bladder using the tunnel technique described above and the usual splint and catheter. A drainage tube is left in the retropubic space at the end of the procedure (Fig. 12.8).

Bladder

A bladder injury is much easier to treat than a ureteric injury and requires, in most instances, no special expertise as long as the basic principles of repair are adhered to.

If the injury is simply due to a stitch passed inadvertently through the bladder wall, as might occur during a colposuspension, all that is required is to remove the stitch, put in a suprapubic catheter for a few days and leave a tube drain in the retropubic space.

If the hole in the bladder is larger then it should be closed with an interrupted or continuous 2/0 chromic catgut or Vicryl suture in one layer, picking up the full thickness of the bladder wall, again leaving a suprapubic catheter and an appropriately placed drain. As always, the drain is removed when it stops draining and the catheter is clamped on about the eighth postoperative day and is removed the next day if satisfactory voiding is promptly re-established. The commonest cause of such an injury is dissection between the bladder base and the cervix/anterior vaginal wall during a hysterectomy and this poses a special problem. This is the close approximation between bladder closure and closure of the vaginal vault. If these two suture lines are left in close contact there is a substantial risk of

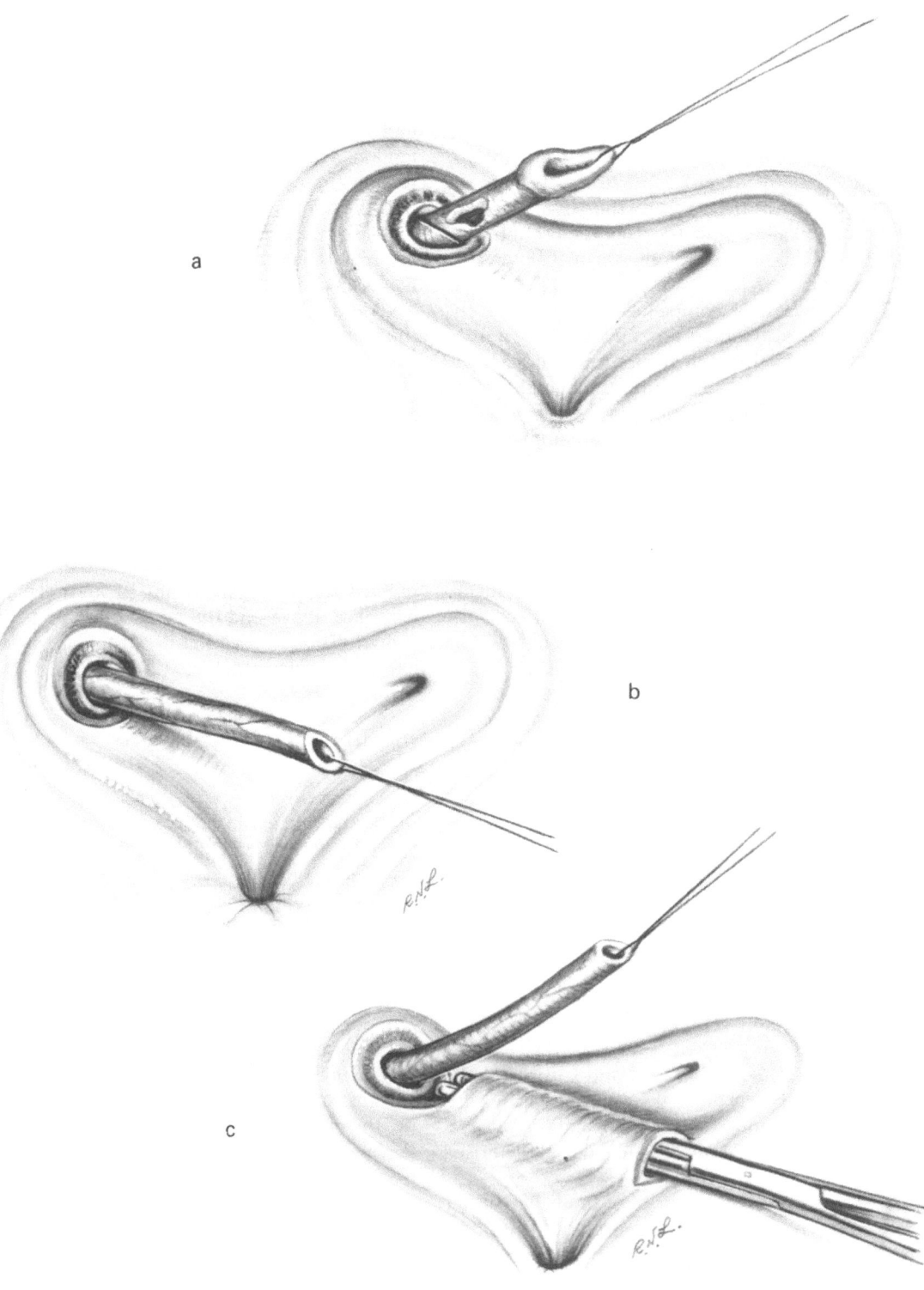

Fig. 12.6a–e. A tunnelled ureteric reimplantation onto the trigone (when the ureteric injury is juxtavesical and there is sufficient ureteric length to allow it to be pulled through into the bladder). **a** The intramural part of the damaged ureter is excised, thereby creating a tunnel through the bladder wall. **b** The ureter is pulled through the bladder wall. **c** A submucosal tunnel is created across the trigone. **d** The ureter is pulled through the submucosal tunnel. **e** The ureteric orifice is spatulated and sutured in place with an indwelling stent.

Fig. 12.6 (*continued*)

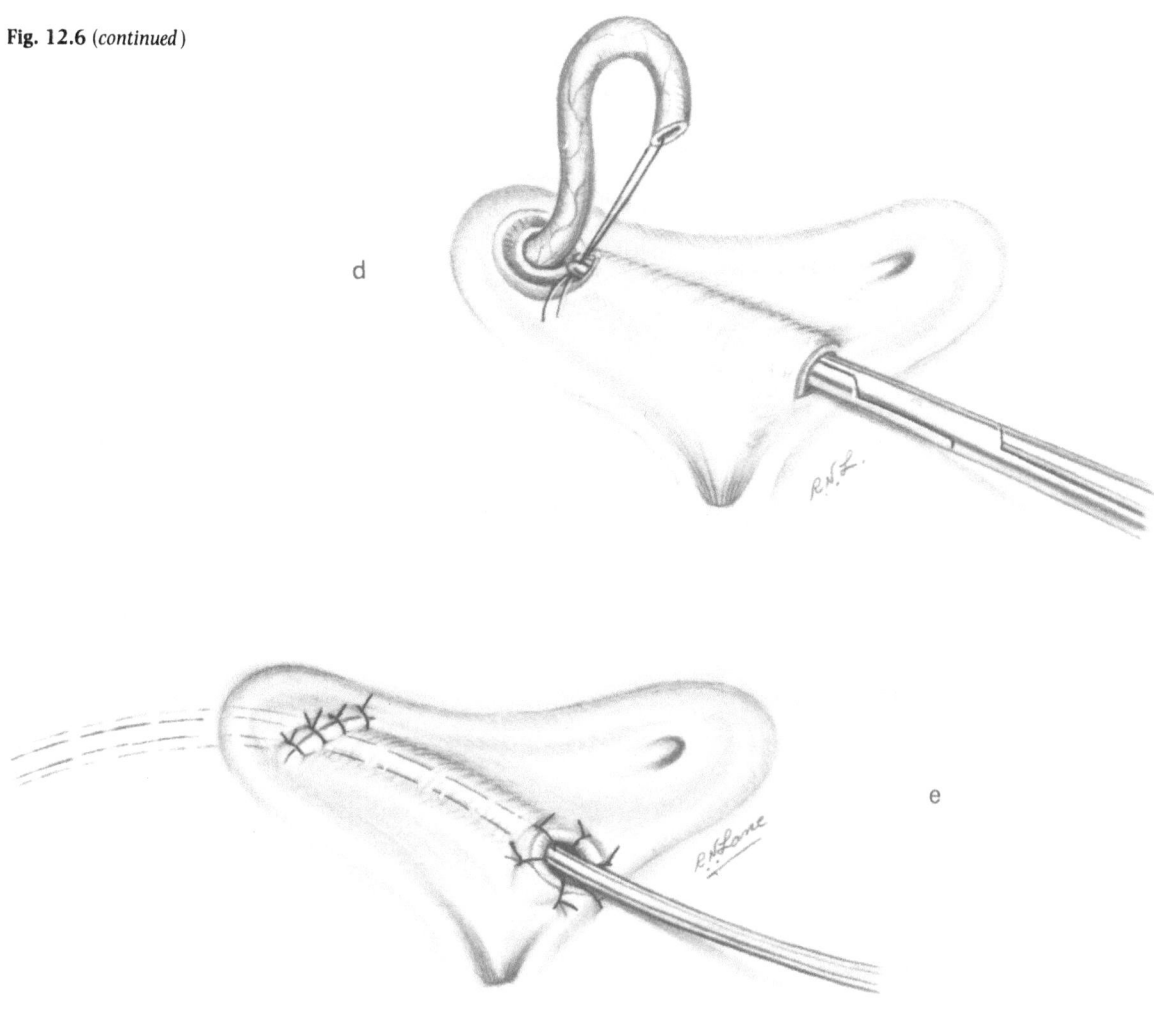

developing a vesicovaginal fistula and it is therefore important to separate these two suture lines by interposing a plug of omentum and holding it in place with a few absorbable sutures to prevent retraction. Omentum is the preferred tissue for this "plug", as it has a good blood supply and therefore predictable viability.

Urethra

Urethral injury is fortunately rare but may occur during a sling procedure or anterior repair (less commonly when an unusually long segment of the vaginal vault is taken during a radical hysterectomy) in which case the posterior urethral wall is the most likely site of injury, or during a col-posuspension in which case the most likely site is through the lateral urethral wall just below the bladder neck

Again it is important not to have a urethral defect, even if adequately closed, in close apposition to a vaginal suture line. The two should therefore be separated either by an omental plug, if this is a retropubic procedure, or by a labial fat pad mobilised on its vascular pedicle if this is a vaginal procedure. Small urethral defects are probably best left to heal without formal closure but larger defects should be closed with interrupted 2/0 chromic catgut, Vicryl or Dexon sutures to prevent the formation of a diverticulum. The most important factor is to provide adequate urine drainage with a 16F or 18F Foley urethral catheter for 2 weeks or so to allow adequate healing before voiding is re-established.

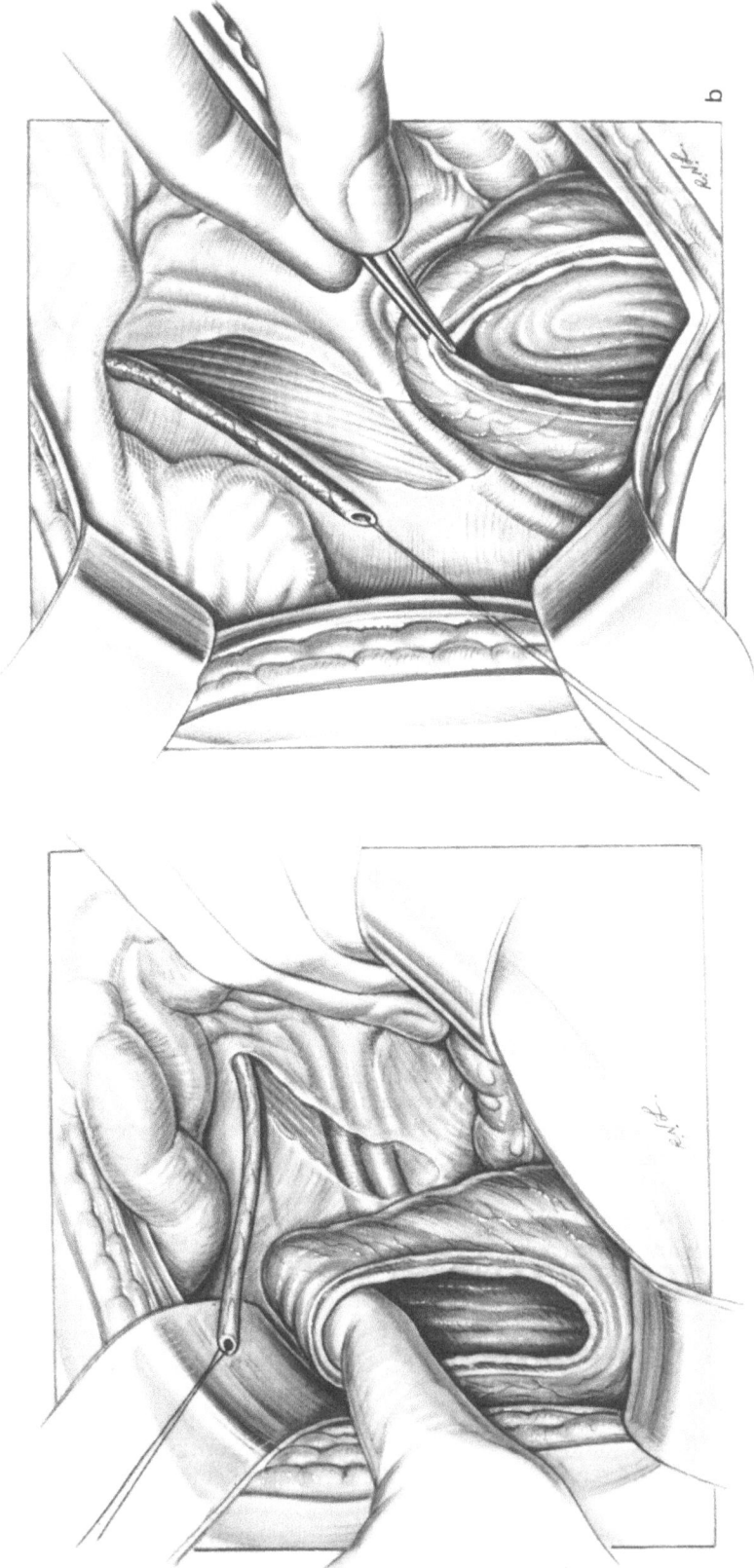

Fig. 12.7a–e. The psoas hitch technique for more proximal injuries of the pelvic ureter: **a** The contralateral bladder wall is mobilised to allow the ipsilateral side of the bladder to be pulled up above the pelvic brim. **b** The psoas tendon is exposed beneath the peritoneum. **c** The bladder is stitched to the psoas tendon. **d** A hole is made through the bladder wall and a submucosal tunnel is created to allow the ureter to be pulled through and sutured in place. A stent is left in the ureter.

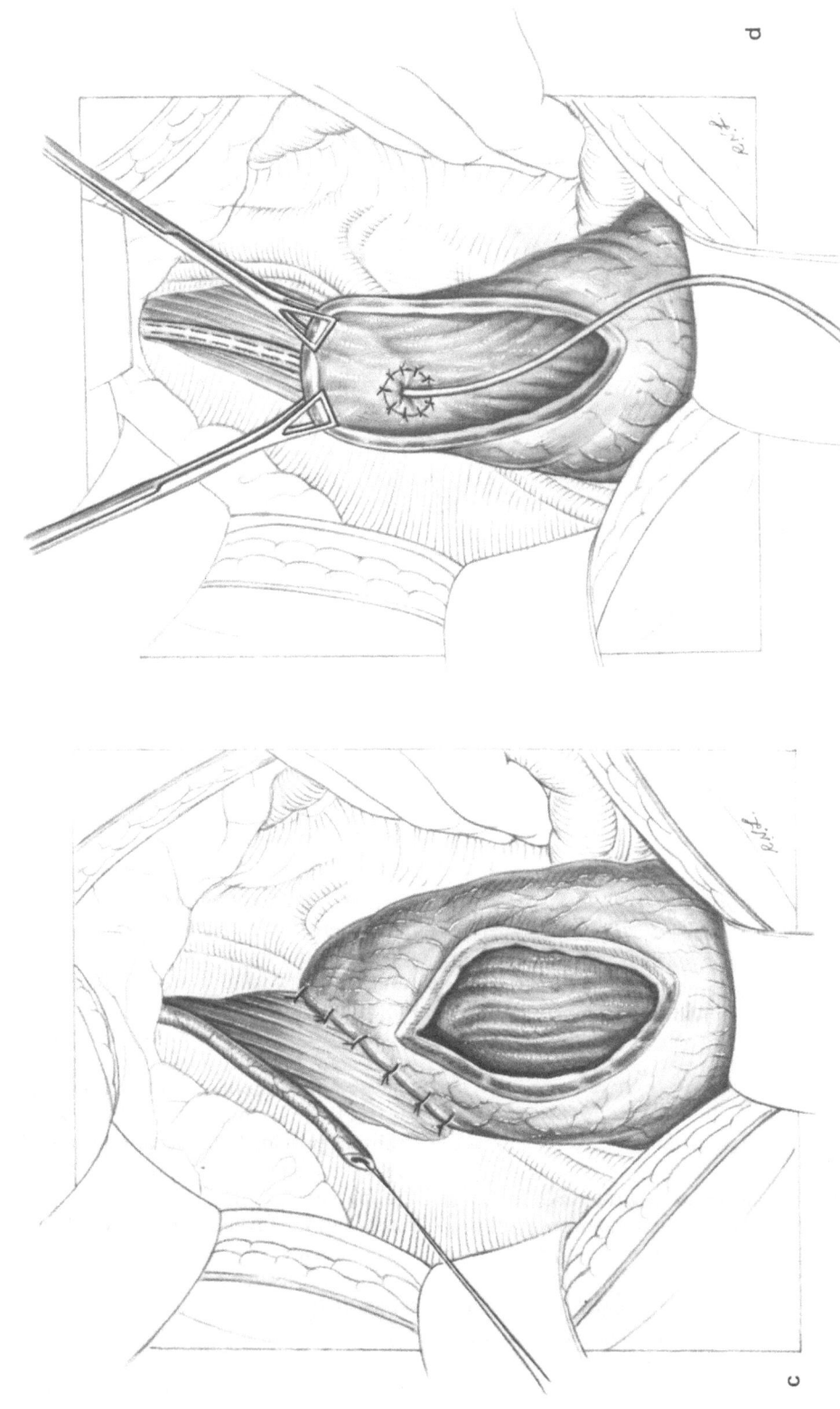

Fig. 12.7 (*continued*)

Fig. 12.7 (*continued*)

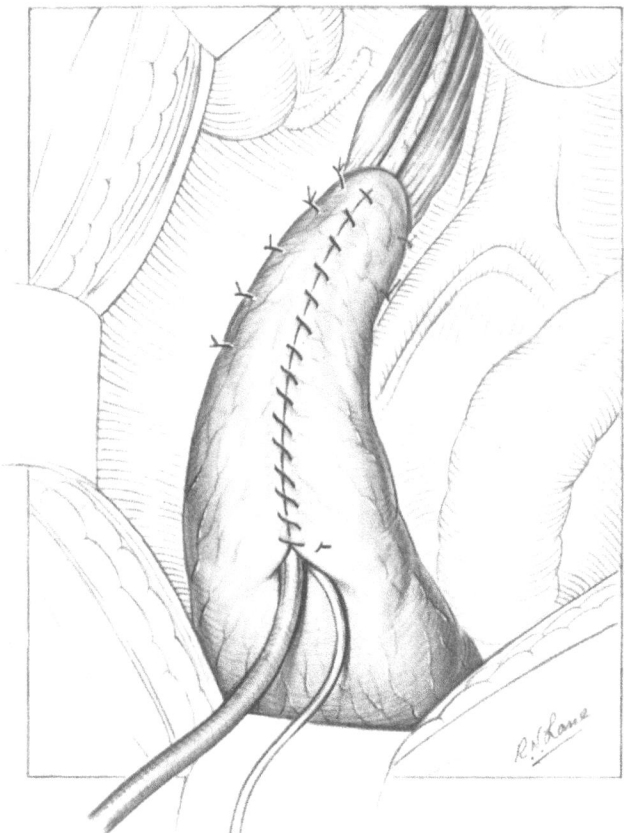

Fig. 12.7e The bladder is closed and a suprapubic catheter is left alongside the ureteric stent.

Postoperative Diagnosis

As mentioned earlier only early postoperative problems will be discussed here. Problems occurring after the first few days will be discussed in Chap. 18.

Ureter

The delayed management of ureteric injuries is largely dependent on the patient's general condition at the time of diagnosis. At one end of the spectrum is the patient with an obstructed or leaking ureter in good general health who can simply be returned to theatre for exploration and repair along the lines described above. At the other extreme is the patient who is practically moribund with either bilaterally obstructed ureters or a peritoneum full of extravasated urine. Such patients can be expected to be

haemodynamically unstable with acute renal insufficiency and Gram-negative septicaemia. This type of situation requires urgent assessment and treatment. If facilities are available promptly then an urgent ultrasound study should be sought to distinguish between extravasation and obstruction (or a combination of the two) and this should be followed by urgent percutaneous nephrostomy if obstruction is diagnosed. With adequate urine drainage provided, the situation becomes a little less urgent and a few hours can then be spent improving the patient's general condition before re-exploration. If such facilities are not available or if clinical or radiological assessment reveals extensive urinary extravasation then re-exploration should be undertaken as soon as possible. Whilst arrangements are being made for the patient's return to theatre the opportunity should be taken to put in a central line (if this has not already been done), restore cardiovascular stability as far as possible, send off blood and urine for culture, send blood for measure-

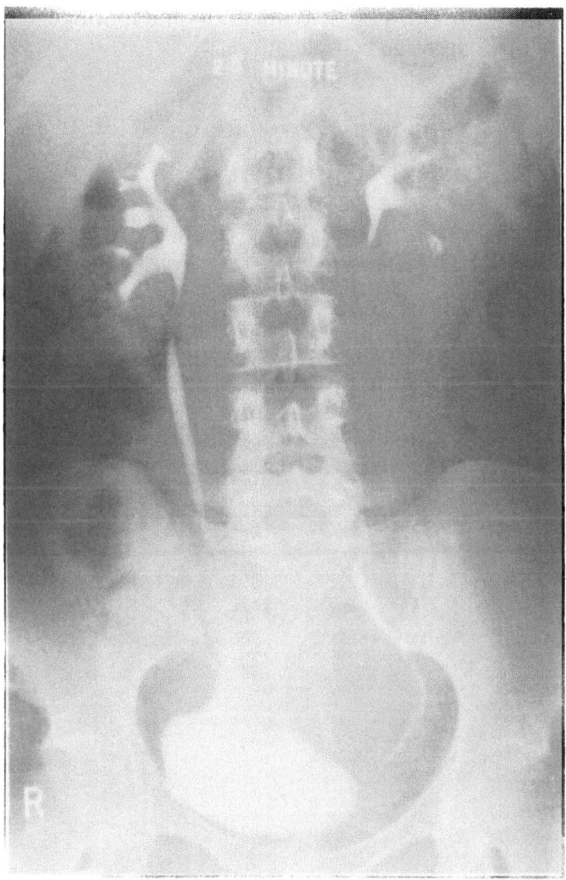

Fig. 12.8. A postoperative IVU film from a patient following a right psoas hitch and reimplantation.

ment of serum creatinine and electrolytes and start parenteral antibiotic treatment with gentamycin, ampicillin and metronidazole.

In the situation described above the patient's general condition precludes the type of definite resolution of the problem as described above, although in less extreme situations this is obviously desirable. In an extreme situation the general principles are to drain extravasated urine, remove any occlusive sutures or ligatures, establish good urine drainage and provide adequate wound drainage. This obviously calls for clinical judgement and considerable urological experience.

Probably the safest solution after dealing with any urine collections, haematomata and obstructing ligatures is to leave the distal ureters alone until a reoperation some weeks later when the acute problem has subsided and simply provide urine drainage by bilateral in situ intubated ureterostomies and then to leave two or three wound

drains (one to each ureterostomy site and one to the pelvis) to prevent reaccumulation of extravasated urine and blood. Intubated in situ ureterostomy is performed by isolating the ureter on each side as it crosses the pelvic brim, making a short longitudinal incision to expose the lumen, and then to pass a 10F Ryle's (or similar) tube up into the renal pelvis. The Ryle's tube is then anchored in place with a stitch around it securing it to the surrounding tissue and is brought out through the skin at a convenient site. This then provides urine drainage until the interval and definitive reoperation to deal with the problem of the distal ureter (along the lines described above), after which the tube is simply pulled out—the ureterostomy incision will then close off around the ureteric stent, which will be placed at the time of reimplantation.

Bladder

This is a much easier problem to deal with. It will usually have been diagnosed either by ultrasound (showing a pelvic collection) or cystography (showing the site of leakage) or both in sequence, in a patient who has been voiding or attempting to void spontaneously. If the volume of extravasated urine per se is not a problem (which usually means if it is sterile) then all that is required is to pass a urethral catheter and leave it in for 7–10 days to allow the defect to heal; the urine collection will reabsorb spontaneously. If the urine is infected, if the collection is large or if simple catheterisation does not resolve the problem then the wound must be reopened and the bladder closed with a suprapubic catheter to provide drainage and a wound drain to prevent any reaccumulation.

Urethra

Again this is only seen in patients who are voiding spontaneously and all that is required is a 7- to 10-day period of urethral catheterisation.

Complications, Prognosis and Follow-up

Prompt adequate treatment should give an excellent prognosis. However, any suture line may stricture and any extravasation may lead to fibrosis or, if two suture lines are adjacent, to fistula formation.

Obviously, stricture formation is mainly a problem related to bladder or ureteric injuries. Fistula formation almost invariably becomes clinically apparent within 3 months of the injury, whereas ureteric obstruction may be silent and follow-up should therefore include clinical assessment at 3 months in all patients who have had a urological injury and radiological assessment at that time in those who have sustained a ureteric injury.

A satisfactory IVU at that time usually carries an excellent prognosis, but any abnormality warrants a reassessment at 6 months or 1 year later. If the IVU is unsatisfactory, then further investigation is necessary. This is discussed further in Chap. 18 with other aspects of the investigation and management of postoperative complications.

Suggested Reading

Mundy A (1983) Injuries of the lower urinary tract. Surgery 1:67–70
Mundy A (1983) Injuries of the upper urinary tract. Surgery 1:96–98
Thompson IM, Carlton CE (1977) Genito-urinary trauma in urologic clinics of North America, vol 4. Saunders, Philadelphia

13 · Haemorrhage and How To Cope

John Dormandy

"The only weapon with which the unconscious patient can immediately retaliate upon the incompetent surgeon is haemorrhage."

Halstead

How To Avoid Unexpected Haemorrhage

Although we may be loathe to admit it, by far the commonest cause of unexpected haemorrhage is a technical error on the part of the operating surgeon. Failure to detect or treat adequately an abnormality in the patient's own haemostatic mechanisms is an exceedingly rare cause by comparison. The three golden rules for avoiding damage to vessels during operation are:

1. Know the anatomy.
2. Be aware of the danger areas and carefully identify all the important structures before proceeding further.
3. Follow meticulous techniques for dealing with minor and expected bleeding.

The same rules apply for avoiding the rarer complication of accidental ischaemia by tying off a vital artery.

Anatomy of the Pelvic Vessels

Figure 13.1 shows semidiagrammatically the arterial blood supply to the female pelvis. The anatomy of the major trunks and the common, internal and external iliac arteries is constant. The common and external iliac give off no significant branches in the pelvis; the occasional anomalous origin of the obturator artery is of no importance. By contrast, the precise pattern of the branches of the internal iliac artery is very variable. The segmental sacral arteries leave the pelvis by passing through the anterior sacral foramina and lie in front of the roots of the sacral plexus. The superior and inferior gluteal arteries, as well as the internal pudendal artery, leave the pelvis through the greater sciatic foramen, the last returning again to the pelvis through the lesser sciatic foramen. The obturator artery usually comes off the inferior gluteal and passes forward along the side wall of the pelvis to leave through the obturator foramen. Of greater importance to the gynaecologist are those arteries which pass medially to supply the pelvic organs. These are the uterine, vaginal, middle rectal and vesical arteries, all branches of the internal iliac. The inferior vesical and middle rectal arteries run in the leash of veins to the posterior border of the bladder. The uterine artery is the largest of the pelvis visceral arteries and descends in front of the ureter to the base of the broad ligament. At the lateral fornix of the vagina it crosses above the ureter. Its branches pass to the vagina, cervix and up the side of the uterus in the broad ligament.

The ovarian artery takes origin from the aorta in the abdomen, crosses medially the external and internal iliac arteries and continues medially in the suspensory ligament of the ovary. The superior rectal artery supplies the upper part of the rectum and is a branch of the inferior mesenteric artery descending in the mesocolon.

It is important to remember that older arteries can become extremely tortuous and dilated. This is especially marked in the bifurcation of the aorta and the common iliacs. It is not unusual for one or other of the iliacs to take such a tortuous course that it actually curves across the mid-line; it may then be mistaken for the internal iliac or one of its

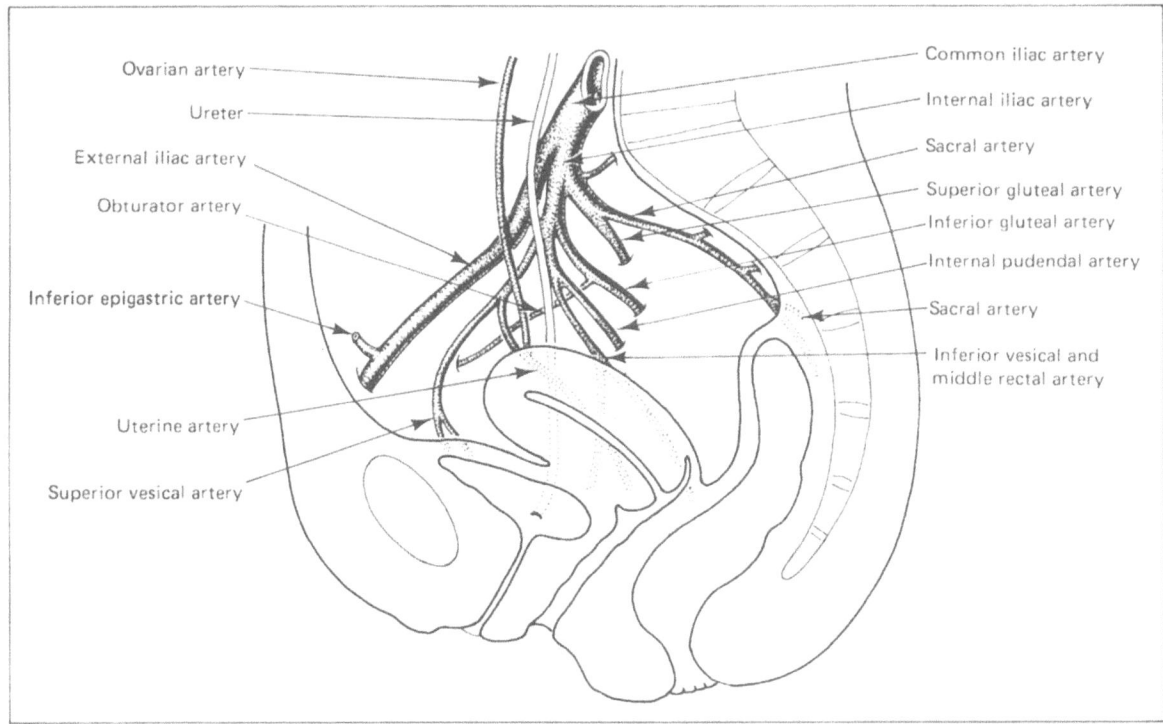

Ovarian artery
Ureter
External iliac artery
Obturator artery
Inferior epigastric artery
Uterine artery
Superior vesical artery

Common iliac artery
Internal iliac artery
Sacral artery
Superior gluteal artery
Inferior gluteal artery
Internal pudendal artery
Sacral artery
Inferior vesical and middle rectal artery

Fig. 13.1. Semidiagrammatic plan of the arteries looking at the right lateral wall of the female pelvis.

branches. If in doubt, the vessels should be traced back to their origin from the aorta. The relationship of the ureter is of paramount importance; it crosses all the arteries medially except the uterine.

Although the venous drainage follows the same basic pattern as the arterial supply, it is much more varied in detail and rich in collateral branches. The veins of the pelvis are best thought of as a series of plexuses draining ultimately through several large branches into the internal iliac vein. Particularly prominent are the presacral plexus and the veins at the base of the broad ligament draining the uterine and vaginal plexuses. The ovarian vein drains into the inferior vena cava or the left renal vein according to the side. The upper rectum is drained through the superior rectal vein to the portal system.

Danger Areas

Figure 13.2 identifies four areas of particular danger, drawn on the same outline as Figure 13.1, but omitting for the sake of clarity details of the vessels. In the floor of the pelvis the uterine artery and the ureter are the two vital structures which must be identified before proceeding to any further

dissection. The uterine artery is usually the largest artery supplying the contents of the female pelvis and normally crosses above the ureter. Like many pelvic arteries, it is frequently very tortuous and a bulk ligature can inadvertently include the ureter. The only really safe rule is to identify both structures at an early stage of any operation in that area.

The other three danger areas are concerned with the venous drainage. Unexpected haemorrhage is more often due to damage to veins than arteries. Veins are more numerous, more variable in their position and thinner. For all these reasons it is inadvisable to dissect and tie them individually. Problems arise in the broad ligament, from an incomplete ligature en masse, and similarly if the ligature is more lateral, where the numerous pelvic veins all drain into the internal iliac vein. Here there is the added danger of inadvertently damaging the common or external iliac artery, an accident reported every year to one of medical defence unions. In the case of the presacral plexus of veins, the problem is due to the vessel walls being held open as they emerge from the anterior sacral foramina. It is extremely difficult to control haemorrhage from veins accidently torn near the exit from those bony channels. As with all surgical complications, it is easier to avoid them than to treat them.

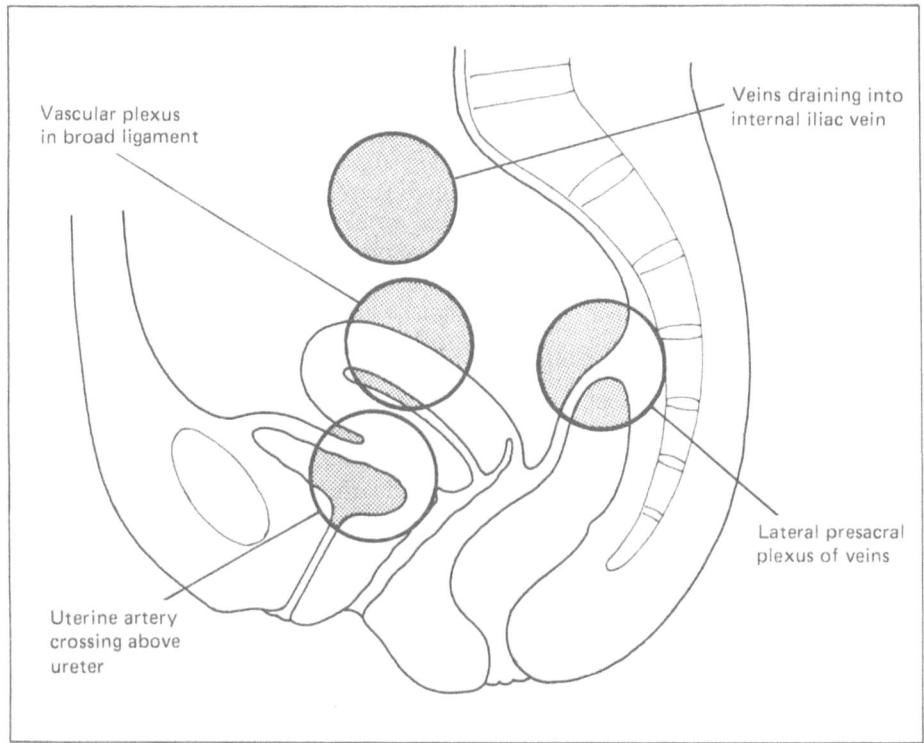

Fig. 13.2. Four vascular danger areas superimposed on the outline of Fig. 13.1.

Planned Control of Vessels

Individual vessels or leash of vessels should be identified and tied before they are divided. There is a dangerous stage in the development of every surgeon, where a particular operation has ceased to be a worrying challenge but the operator has yet to gain the maturity of realising that potentially even the simplest procedure can have serious complications. It is often at this dangerous stage that completing an operation in the minimum time unfortunately becomes the primary aim.

Arteries should be dissected free, identified and securely tied with a non-absorbable suture. 3–0 size ligatures should be adequate as the arterial pressure cannot tear such a suture. Surgeons tend to use heavier material to compensate for insufficient attention to tying knots properly, the commonest mistake undoubtedly being the crossing of knots. In most circumstances there is no place for the suture en masse of arteries. By contrast an attempt to dissect free each vein can be dangerous and ligature in bulk, using catgut, is safer provided all nearby vital structures have been identified.

The indiscriminate use of the diathermy is another common technical error. Arteries, however small, should never be diathermied; nor should

veins of any appreciable size. Diathermy should be confined to dealing with multiple small oozing vessels.

Remarkably often, reoperation for postoperative haemorrhage is required because of insufficient attention to vessels encountered during the approach to the pelvic target organ through the abdominal wall, for instance, haemorrhage from a diathermied or inadequately tied inferior epigastric vessel. This again is probably the consequence of undue haste in getting to the supposed climax of an operation.

Identifying Patients with a Bleeding Tendency

Patients with a significant congenital or acquired bleeding tendency are uncommon and the majority can be identified by a careful history. Failing to enquire whether a patient has had any previous surgical procedures, however minor (for instance a tooth extraction), and whether there were any complications associated with it is indefensible. If the patient is fortunate enough to have escaped all forms of surgical trauma, a direct question should be asked about undue bleeding following accidental trauma. Many patients believe they bruise abnormally easy but in fact have no significant disorder requiring special preoperative treatment. A family history may help identify the significant bleeders. An essential part of the history is enquiring about regular medication or coexisting diseases. Leukaemia, myeloproliferative disorders or liver disease will predispose to abnormal bleeding. A considerable number of patients are also being treated with long-term oral anticoagulants.

Serious bleeding disorders, whether congenital or acquired, may be due to a platelet or coagulation defect. A blood count, blood film examination and simple bleeding time will pick up nearly all platelet abnormalities. Haemophilia (factor VIII deficiency), Christmas disease (factor IX deficiency) and Von Willebrand's disease are the only congenital coagulation disorders at all likely to be encountered. The blood count, blood film and even the bleeding time may be normal. The activated partial thromboplastin time (APTT) will, however, be prolonged in all cases. The precise identification of the disorder and its treatment requires the expertise of a specialist haematologist (Brozovic 1981; Rizza 1981).

In severely ill patients one should be aware of the increasingly frequent condition of disseminated intravascular coagulation (DIC), which is associated with abnormal bleeding. The cause is essentially the widespread deposition and consequent consumption of fibrin and platelets. It may result from a variety of conditions such as haemolytic transfusion reactions, widespread mucin-secreting adenocarcinoma, endotoxaemia, Gram-negative septicaemia and some virus infections. The diagnosis is suggested by a low platelet count and plasma fibrinogen level. (DIC is also encountered in obstetric complications like intrauterine death or amniotic fluid embolism.)

Although congenital bleeding disorders are rare, most surgeons will sooner or later encounter one previously undiagnosed case of a congenital bleeding disorder. Abnormal bleeding due to medication or concomitant disease is commoner and an example is likely to present most years to every surgeon.

Practical Management of Uncontrolled Bleeding

All bleeding can be temporarily controlled by pressure. Above all, avoid applying clamps or sutures blindly.

Pressure can best be exerted over firm packing with large abdominal packs or even a gauze roll. Not only will this gain valuable time, while help can be sought and facilities prepared for rapid blood transfusion, but in many cases of venous bleeding pressure may stop the haemorrhage by giving time for the injured vessel to constrict spontaneously and for the blood to clot. The operator should wait at least 3 min before removing the packs and inspecting the area of damage. (The habit of some surgeons to ask for packs soaked in hot saline to stop bleeding is more for the surgeon's benefit than the patients'. If heat does anything at all it dilates vessels and denatures clotting factors. It does not simulate the effect of the diathermy.)

Even if the bleeding has stopped with pressure the source of the unexpected haemorrhage must be identified and secured. The bleeding may only have stopped temporarily because the vessels have gone into spasm or the blood pressure fallen. Generally, arterial bleeding is far easier to identify and ligature. To control venous bleeding mass sutures may be necessary, but these must only be applied after identifying any adjacent vital structures such as the ureter. Metal clips (as frequently used by neurosurgeons) may be useful to control bleeding from the sacral foramina or other bony channels where any attempt at placing a ligature or suture would only make the bleeding worse.

Proximal control of arteries may be useful in decreasing haemorrhage. Tying an internal iliac artery at its origin will never cause dangerous ischaemia of the pelvic contents, provided the contralateral internal iliac is patent. For the same reason ligature of the internal iliac on the side of the arterial bleeding may not altogether stop it, although it will probably decrease the rate and pressure of the haemorrhage. Although tying even both internal iliac arteries may not produce total ischaemia because of the rich collateral supply of the pelvis, it is probably wiser only to occlude temporarily one of the vessels with a rubber sling or arterial clamp while the bleeding is controlled. By contrast, occluding the common or external iliac artery is very likely to produce disastrous ischaemia in the leg. (How to cope with accidental occlusions or damage to these arteries is described in the next section.)

A large number of systematically administered drugs have been claimed to be haemostatic. In the past none have stood up to critical evulation (Verstraete 1977), with the possible exception of the antifibrinolytic agents, epsilon amino caproic acid (EACA) and the safer and more potent tranexamic acid. The latter has been shown to decrease blood loss in menorrhagia and after cervical conisation in two double-blind randomised trials (Rybo and Westerberg 1972). Of the topical haemostatic agents, gelatine sponges (for instance, Gelfoam and Sterispon) and oxidised cellulose (Oxycel) are the most widely available. There are theoretical reasons why these materials could work and both are absorbed within a few weeks. Definite beneficial effect has not yet been proven in double-blind randomised trials measuring blood loss, but their use in controlling oozing from raw surfaces is logical and appears to carry little or no risk.

Very rarely bleeding from multiple vessels cannot be controlled and continuing efforts to apply ligatures appear to be counterproductive. The solution is then to pack the bleeding areas with one or even several gauze rolls; vaginal packs can be used for this purpose. The ends of the rolls should be brought out through the wound or a separate incision and gradually removed starting on the first postoperative day. Alternatively, the packs can be removed at a formal laparotomy under optimal conditions.

How To Deal with Accidental Damage to Vital Arteries

The common and external iliac arteries are most likely to be injured in older patients where the vessels may be atherosclerotic and take an unusual and tortuous course. Older iliac arteries are not infrequently also dilated to two or three times their normal diameter. (Such aneurysmal dilatations rarely require treatment in themselves.) Accidents most commonly arise as a result of large, partly blind, sutures placed in an attempt to control a haemorrhage. As usual, the injury can be easily corrected provided it is recognised and disasters occur only when the operator is unaware of the possibility of such injury. If in doubt, not only should the pulse be felt in the femoral artery below the inguinal ligament, but the whole extent of the common and external iliac artery should be checked. The presence of a femoral pulse does not exclude a suture involving part of the arterial wall, possibly leading to intravascular thrombosis after the operation.

If one of these vital arteries has been injured it should be isolated proximal and distal to the injury and controlled with a rubber sling. Ideally, arterial clamps should then be applied and the injury repaired. If arterial clamps are not readily available the rubber sling (a thin catheter will serve this purpose) can be looped around the vessel twice, pulled tight and held in place with an ordinary clamp. This alternative procedure, for which no special instruments are required, is illustrated in Fig. 13.3.

A clean cut or puncture of the artery can be simply repaired with a few interrupted sutures. Lacerations and more extensive damage, particularly in atherosclerotic arteries, require wide excision of the damaged segment with reconstruction using either a synthetic (commonly Dacron) tube graft or, if the damage is not circumferential, a vein or Dacron patch. The decision whether to attempt a primary repair or excision with grafting is difficult; if in doubt the later course should be followed as the damage to the inside of

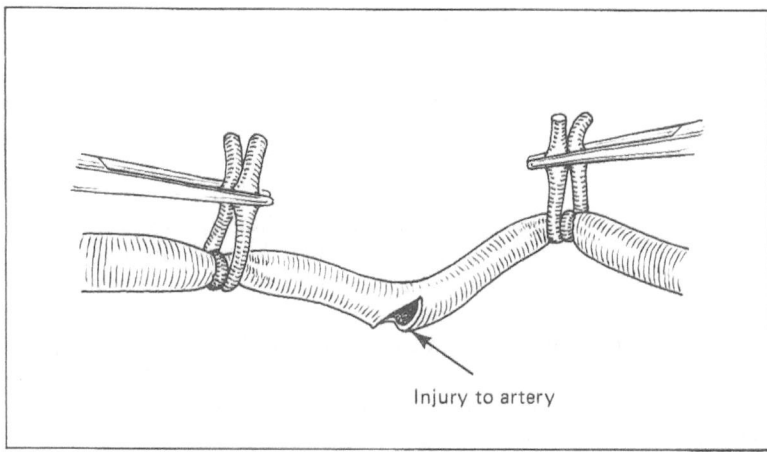

Injury to artery

Fig. 13.3. An alternative method for controlling an injured artery if arterial clamps are not available.

an atherosclerotic artery is always more extensive than is apparent from the outside. Atraumatic 4–0 Prolene sutures are recommended for all forms of arterial repair. Although elective arterial reconstructive surgery is usually performed with total heparinisation, in the circumstances of accidental damage to an artery it is probably wiser not to heparinise the patient. Complete occlusion of the vessel need not last longer than 5–15 min and the danger of continuing haemorrhage due to anticoagulation outweighs the slight risk of thrombosis in the artery during the period of occlusion. Patients requiring arterial repair under these circumstances need to be monitored particularly carefully postoperatively. An arteriogram within the first few days is a wise precaution.

Replacement of Blood Loss

Adequate volume replacement is as important a part of coping with unexpected haemorrhage as identifying and controlling the bleeding vessels. Unless the source of bleeding is obvious and can be easily controlled, it is safer simply to stop the bleeding by pressure until facilities for rapid transfusion have been established and any major blood loss replaced by some fluid.

The magnitude of a "major" blood loss varies from patient to patient. Whilst a previously fit young patient can sustain a blood loss of 20%–30% (approximately 1 litre) of her total circulating blood volume, a patient with impaired myocardial function or significant coronary, carotid or renal artery stenosis may sustain irreversible damage to a vital organ following the loss of only 10% of her total blood volume. It should be remembered that anaesthesia dampens the normal homeostatic baroreceptor reflex designed to maintain central arterial blood pressure so that in the absence of treatment an unconscious patient is less able to compensate for a blood loss than a conscious patient.

Choice of Fluid Replacement

The decision whether to cross match blood before operation depends on the type of planned surgery and the usual expected range of blood loss. If the total blood loss is likely to be less than 500 ml then it is probably unnecessary to cross match blood although it may be prudent to send blood preoperatively for grouping and save serum for cross matching later if necessary.

Maintaining circulatory volume and cardiac output is more important than maintaining a normal red cell concentration. Indeed, normovolaemic haemodilution has some theoretical and practical advantages which will be considered later. Therefore, unless the patient's haemoglobin concentration was already low before surgery, the first 500–1000 ml blood loss can be safely replaced with fluids other than blood. Saline or another electrolyte solution will suffice, but it must be remembered that the half-life of these fluids in the vascular compartment is only $\frac{1}{2}$–1 h. Low molecular weight dextran (Rheomacrodex), which has a half-life in the circulation of approximately 6 h, may therefore be preferable. There is no indication for using blood or plasma in the early stages of blood loss.

With massive blood loss every effort should be made to transfuse blood after the first litre. If blood has not yet been cross-matched plasma or plasma protein fraction (PPF) should be given instead. It will conserve the circulating volume better than saline or dextran, although it will not help to maintain oxygen-carrying capacity. Full cross-matching of blood takes approximately 1 h. If there is some urgency the appropriate tests can be carried out more quickly using a spin technique instead of the longer usual incubation. The use of uncross-matched universal donor (group O rhesus negative) blood should virtually never be necessary.

Rate of Fluid Replacement. Importance of the Central Venous Pressure

How quickly should blood loss be replaced? It should be replaced as quickly as possible, provided one can be certain to avoid overloading the heart. The most appropriate way to avoid overloading the heart is by monitoring the central venous pressure (CVP), and not by replacing the fluid slowly thereby increasing the period of dangerous hypovolaemia. It should be remembered that the haemoglobin level and haematocrit are absolutely useless in estimating acute blood loss. They will, however, change over several hours if red cell replacement is inadequate.

As with all physiological measurements, it is important to be certain that the results are completely reliable. Too often doctors ignore the results of such measurements if they do not fit in with their expectations, on the grounds that the measurements are probably inaccurate. The proper response should be to make sure that the results are reliable. Ideally, problems of fluid exchange should be anticipated, patricularly in patients with limited cardiac reserve, and a CVP line established before the operation begins. A large CVP catheter needs to be inserted making sure that it lies in or near the right atrium and that there is free flow of fluid in both directions. Because the exact level of the right atrium and the tip of the catheter is unknown, absolute measurements of CVP are less accurate than measurements of changes in the CVP. Provided the same zero point is taken for successive readings, zero errors with be constant and the error of any measurement of change in the CVP should be no more than 1 cm of water pressure.

The CVP does not assess the volume of blood loss or the venous return; it assesses the ability of the heart at a given moment to cope with the existing venous return, which is much more useful information. A rise of CVP beyond 5 cm of water indicates that the heart is beginning to find difficulty in coping with the venous return and further expansion of the circulating volume may begin to precipitate congestive cardiac failure. This information is much more important than an accurate estimate of blood loss. During a period of hypovolaemia, hypotension and decreased coronary flow, a damaged myocardium may well sustain further ischaemic impairment so that the heart may no longer be able to cope with the circulating volume and venous return that it could deal with before the operation. Although an estimate of blood loss is obviously necessary and a useful guideline for the approximate volume of necessary fluid replacement, an accurate continuous recording of the CVP is a finer guide to the maximum safe rate of fluid replacement.

Dangers of Blood Transfusion in General

Massive blood transfusions which may be necessary if unexpected bleeding is difficult to control carry some special dangers which will be considered in the next section. But any blood transfusion however small is associated with some well-recognised dangers. These should be avoided if possible and treated promptly if they occur (Mollison 1979).

1. Major mismatch. This is not easy to recognise in the anaesthetised patient. It may present with sudden unexplained hypotension, cyanosis or possibly massive bleeding due to DIC. The first sign may be an urticarial rash. If suspected, the transfusion should be stopped immediately and if an error is confirmed 100 mg hydrocortisone given intravenously. Increased infusion of other fluids may be necessary to maintain blood pressure. Symptoms and signs may come on after operation and include skin rash, chest and back pain, dyspnoea, restlessness, headaches, rigors

and fever. Tubular necrosis may lead to acute renal failure.

2. Minor mismatch is far commoner and may be early or delayed. It may be due to hypersensitivity to donor plasma proteins or HLA antibodies. The signs of urticaria, pyrexia and rigors usually appear after the operation and can be controlled in most cases with antihistamines. Rarely the only sign of a delayed transfusion reaction may be a progressive anaemia with or without jaundice.

3. Transmission of disease, hepatitis and AIDS are the most feared. Hepatitis is usually due to the B virus, but is getting much rarer with routine testing of all blood donors.

4. Cardiac overload has been discussed in the previous section.

5. Air embolism is fortunately extremely rare since the introduction of plastic bottles.

6. Local thrombophlebitis.

Dangers of Massive Blood Transfusion

These are largely due to the changes which occur in stored blood, such as an increase in extracellular potassium, acidosis or depletion of haemostatic factors, which may produce important complications in the recipient if large volumes of stored blood are transfused over a short period. The surgeon and anaesthetist should be aware of these possibilities if 2 litres or more are transfused within a few hours:

1. Hypothermia. This can be avoided by routinely inserting a heating coil in the donor line.

2. Hyperkalaemia due to the movement of potassium from inside the red cell during storage. This may increase myocardial excitability and cause fibrillation. It is best monitored by observing the height of the T-waves of the electrocardiogram. Hyperkalaemia can be corrected by the infusion of 10 ml calcium chloride, which should be routine after four units of blood.

3. Acidosis, due to the production of lactic acid by glycolysis in stored blood, may also increase myocardial excitability as well as decreasing contractility. It can be avoided by infusing 100–200 ml 8·4% sodium bicarbonate for every unit of stored blood after the fourth unit.

4. Hypocalcaemia due to the infusion of anticoagulant in stored blood (citrate toxicity). Again the danger is the effect on the myocardium. In addition, the patient's blood may become less coagulable. It will be avoided by the

routine infusion of calcium cholride mentioned already.

5. Decrease in function and quantity of platelets. Although stored blood will be deficient in most clotting factors, particularly the labile factors II, V and VIII, normally there is such an abundance of all clotting factors in the recipient's blood that dangerous dilutional effects will not occur until at least 30% of the patient's blood volume has been replaced by other fluids. Even then the only likely cause of a haemostatic problem will be the hypocalcaemia already mentioned and possibly the decrease in functioning platelets. After 3 days' storage whole blood has virtually no useful platelets. A simple platelet count will not necessarily assess a depletion in normal platelets and if there seems to be an abnormal tendency to generalised oozing after transfusing four or more units of stored blood, it is reasonable to request fresh platelets or fresh whole blood. There should also be an attempt to keep the total platelet count above 70×10^9/litre. Following platelet transfusion approximately 50% of the platelets become trapped in the spleen for a few hours and then return into the circulation.

6. Decreased concentration of clotting factors is only likely to reach dangerous levels after the transfusion of about 3 litres of fluids in an average sized patient. At this stage, the patient will probably have received approximately four units of stored blood. This should then be followed by one unit of free frozen plasma (FFP) and two units of cryoprecipitate.

Surgeons should remember that the greatest risk in massive blood transfusions is that it was either not massive enough or too massive, that is the rate of infusion was incorrect.

Changing Attitude to Optimal Haemoglobin Level

Over the past 10–20 years there has been a general movement away from the older attitude that the higher the haemoglobin level before operation the better. This shift has been caused by an increased awareness of the dangers of a high red cell concentration due to its effect on the flow or rheological properties of blood. The viscosity of blood is now recognised as an important determinant of blood flow in vivo and there is no doubt that the concentration of red cells is the single most important

determinant of blood viscosity. The total blood flow in the normal leg has been shown to be related to the changing blood viscosity resulting from changing red cell concentration. There is also now a large body of accumulated epidemiological and clincial evidence that a red cell concentration at the upper end of the normal range is a significant primary and secondary risk factor for a number of circulatory complications including myocardial and cerebral ischaemia as well as venous thrombosis (Dormandy 1984).

On the continent of Europe this new attitude has resulted in the increasingly routine use of preoperative normovolaemic haemodilution. It is applicable to all patients undergoing majory surgery except in those with overt clinical evidence of myocardial damage. Approximately 1 litre of the patient's blood is removed in the 48 h preceding elective surgery or in the anaesthetic room and it is replaced with an equal volume of low molecular weight dextran. The total circulating volume must be maintained. The advantages of this procedure are:

1. If the patient bleeds unduly during surgery she loses diluted blood and more important she can be retransfused with her own fresh blood. This avoids many of the dangers and complications of transfusing somebody else's old blood.

2. The decreased red cell concentration and blood viscosity increases cardiac output and peripheral flow velocity. This will not only decrease the risk of thrombosis, particularly in the leg veins, but may actually increase the oxygen delivery to vital organs, like the brain and the kidney.

3. There is an overall saving in the quantity of blood required from public donations. This is a more important consideration in some countries than others, depending on the organisation of the blood transfusion services.

Despite these significant advantages and the absence of any important disadvantages it must be said that at the moment preoperative normovolaemic haemodilution has not yet become routine practice in the United Kingdom or North America (Haemodilution 1981). Nevertheless, the increasing awareness of the importance of haemorrheology in the normal and pathological circulation has already led to two definite changes in the general attitude of surgeons in all countries. Firstly, patients are no longer transfused with blood routinely before operation unless their red cell concentration is below 35%–40%. Secondly, in patients with a preoperative haematocrit above 45%, the first 500 ml to 1 litre of blood loss is not replaced with stored blood. It must, however, be emphasised that the total circulating volume must be maintained at all times. These changes in general surgical practice are probably partly responsible for the decreased incidence in peroperative venous thrombosis as well as other cardiovascular complications.

References

Brozovic M (1981) Acquired disorders of blood coagulation. In: Bloom A L, Thomas D P (eds) Heomostasis and thrombosis. Churchill Livingstone, Edinburgh

Dormandy J (1984) The dangerous red cell. Clinical haemorheology 4:115–132
Haemodilution Symposium (1981) Bibliothca Haematologia 49. Karger, Basle
Mollison P L (1979) Blood transfusion in clincal medicine, 6th ed. Blackwell Scientific, Oxford
Rizza C R (1981) Management of patients with inherited blood coagulation defects. In: Bloom AL, Thomas D P (eds) Haemostasis and thrombosis. Churchill Livingstone, Edinburgh
Rybo G, Westerberg H (1972) The effect of tranexamine on postoperative bleeding after conization. Acta Obstet Gynecol Scand 51:347–350
Verstraete M (ed) (1977) Haemostatic drugs. A critical appraisal. Martinus Nijhoff Medical Division, The Hague

14 · Microsurgery

Robert M. L. Winston

Microsurgery is now the standard method used for reconstructive operations in infertile patients. It also has a place during incidental laparotomy in young women, who may become infertile following adhesion formation after surgical damage.

Strictly speaking, microsurgery means surgery performed under magnification, although sometimes only the principles of a refined atraumatic technique are required. The primary reason for magnification is the small size of the tubal lumen. At the narrowest part of the fallopian tube, the interstitial portion (which commonly becomes blocked) is usually less than 0·5 mm in diameter. This is not possible to join accurately with the unaided eye. The reason for using microsurgery is not just because these organs are very small. Few surgeons have such feeble vision that they cannot see the ovary; yet microsurgery is just as important when operating on the ovary. An essential feature of microsurgery is that it avoids microscopic damage of delicate serosal and coelomic surfaces. Handling the tissues under some magnification gives immediate awareness of any trauma that may be caused.

History

The first surgeon to employ a microscope for tubal surgery was Walz (1959) from Germany. He described what would now be regarded as a relatively crude technique to improve tubal implantation and suggested that the microscope be used for salpingostomy. He made the important observation that the microscope would reduce iatrogenic damage. He also pointed out that improvements in technique alone would not greatly improve the results of tubal surgery; this, he stated, would be achieved with more careful selection of patients. Magnification with loupes was used by Swolin (1975), who introduced the important concept of electrosurgery for tubal operations. Gomel (1977) also used loupes but remained rather unconvinced of the value of the microscope until after 1977 (Gomel 1978). Refined microsurgical methods were introduced in animal work by Paterson and Wood (1974) and by Winston and McClure Browne in 1974. These workers also used microsurgery for clinical work and by the late 1970s it was apparent that magnification, whether by loupes or by microscope, gave improved surgical results. Tubal microsurgery became increasingly widespread for all infertility surgery.

Indications

The main indication for tubal microsurgery is tubal block. The commonest cause of blockage is inflammatory tubal disease. Lesser degrees of scarring are equally common and if the tubes are not actually blocked, surgery may not be always justified. Usually either the fimbrial end or the intramural portion is the site of blockage. Mid-tubal block is comparatively rare and is usually associated with very severe scarring, or tuberculosis. Endometriosis may occasionally cause tubal blockage—most frequently at the cornual end of the tube. Congenital anomalies are an important cause of tubal block. They may result in hydrosalpinx formation, though cornual block can also be congenital. Blockage may also follow iatrogenic damage—the most common cause, of course, being previous sterilisation.

Terminology

Operations on the Tubes

A. Blockage at the fimbrial end leads to hydrosalpinx formation. Hydrosalpinges have a better surgical prognosis if thin-walled. Thick-walled fibrous and hypertrophic hydrosalpinges do not lend themselves to a microsurgical approach and may reocclude even after careful surgery. When a hydrosalpinx has been long-standing, the mucosa tends to become flattened and the ciliated epithelium lost. This is associated with a poor prognosis (Vasquez et al. 1980a) and some surgeons therefore feel that patients with hydrosalpinges should not be left indefinitely on waiting lists.

These are the standard operations for fimbrial damage.

Salpingostomy (Salpingoneostomy). By international agreement (FIGO 1978), this term is used for surgical procedures to open a totally blocked fimbrial end. The block may be either *"terminal"*— if no part of the tube is resected and the opening is made at the most terminal part of the tube, or *"ampullary"*—if some tubal tissue is removed or if the end is so damaged that the ostium has to be fashioned in the ampullary side-wall. *"Isthmic"* salpingostomy refers to similar operations on the isthmus, when the whole ampulla has been removed.

Fimbrioplasty. This term refers to procedures similar to those above but should be used only if the tube is already partly open. Typically, fimbrioplasty will be employed for fimbrial phimosis or when there is a fibrous ring partly obstructing the fimbrial end. It is important that fimbrioplasty is not confused with salpingostomy. Fimbrioplasty carries a generally better prognosis. Unless proper terminology is used when publishing results, there is a risk of giving misleading information.

Salpingolysis. Division of adhesions around the tube. Occasionally, it may be used in conjunction with *fimbriolysis* if the adhesions involve the fimbrial end. The term *"tuboplasty"* is a loose description of tubal surgery and is best avoided. It simply refers to plastic operations on the tube and its use in

publications makes it impossible to evaluate reported results.

B. Blockage at the uterine end is usually in the interstitial portion itself, in the wall of the uterus— or in the first part of the isthmus. Most blocks are due to old infection, usually following miscarriage or pregnancy. The great majority of cases of cornual block can be treated by joining the healthy isthmic or ampullary segment onto the cornu, having first resected the blocked segment. The following terminology is widely accepted:

Cornual Anastomosis. This may be *"deep"* if the whole of the intramural tube requires excision, or *"superficial"* if little of the interstitial tube is damaged. Cornual anastomosis may be either *isthmocornual* or *ampullocornual*, depending on the amount of distal tube that requires resection.

Tubal Implantation. In about 10% of cases there is no tissue on the uterine side for anastomosis—in which case implantation may be indicated.

Tubal Anastomosis is the term for operations such as reversal of sterilisation, when the tube may be blocked somewhere between cornu and fimbria. The term *"reanastomosis"* is generally wrongly employed and should be reserved for those patients undergoing a repeat attempt at joining the tubes, after failed surgical reconstruction.

C. An exploratory operation on the tube may also be indicated, the commonest being conservative surgery for ectopic pregnancy. The most important of these procedures (apart from *salpingectomy*) is:

Salpingotomy. This refers to incision in the tube wall and inspection of the lumen, usually with evacuation of its contents. This is a better procedure for eccyesis than expressing the tubal contents through the fimbrial ostium as it creates less mucosal damage and the implantation site can be resected if necessary.

Operations on the Ovary, Uterus and Supporting Structures

Microsurgery is also valuable when the tubes are intrinsically healthy, but there are adhesions around the ovaries, ovarian cysts, ovarian or peritoneal endometriosis, or uterine disease. Many of these procedures do not require the use of a microscope, but application of microsurgical principles is usually sufficient.

Instruments

Microscopes and loupes

A decision has to be made whether to use a microscope or loupes (magnifying spectacles). In my view, the advantages of a proper operating microscope are really overwhelming. For certain procedures, particularly cornual surgery, a microscope is essential; loupes will not give sufficient magnification. Loupes may be an advantage for simple ovarian surgery when low magnification only is helpful.

Features of a Suitable Operating Microscope

The operating microscope should give variable magnification and high optical resolution; good, preferably coaxial, illumination is also necessary. Most modern microscopes are reasonably adequate in these respects. A major decision is whether to buy a single- or two-man microscope (diploscope). Diploscopes give the surgical assistant a stereoscopic view of the same field as the first surgeon but are more cumbersome. This disadvantage may outweigh the advantages; but if surgical training is to be an important part of the unit's work, a diploscope is invaluable. The various types of microscope (Figs. 14.1–4) include:

Manually Operated Single-Man Microscope. Examples include those made by Carl Zeiss (West Germany), Wild (Switzerland), Applied Fibroptics (Boston, United States) and Olympus (Japan). The best buy in this category is perhaps the Zeiss OPMI-1, or the rather overpriced Wild. The Applied Fibroptics machine is excellent but not mounted quite as rigidly as the two European microscopes.

The advantages of manual microscopes (especially that of Zeiss) are that they are easily moved in and out of the operating field, are very robust and not given to tremor, are quick in use and are relatively cheap. Little can go wrong as they can be focused even if there is a total power failure. I prefer a simple hand-operated microscope for most routine surgery. Their main disadvantage is that the surgeon has to take his hands from the operative field for adjustment. This can lead to inadvertent contamination of the operative field, unless care is taken. It is also difficult to attach cameras, assistant's viewing arms and other accessories to most manual microscopes without causing loss of stability.

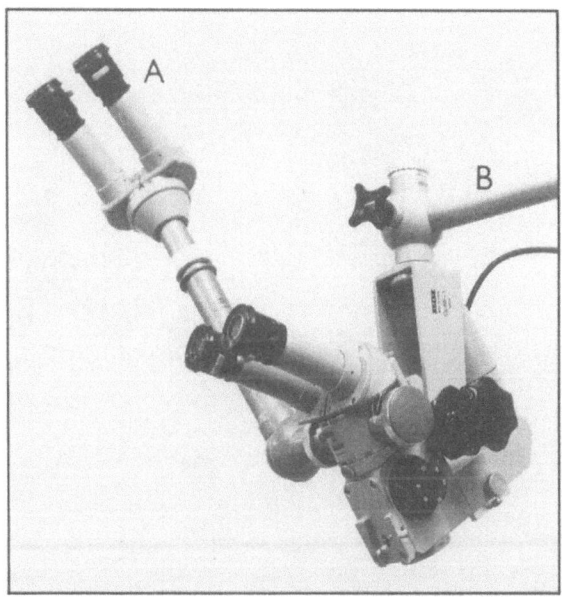

Fig. 14.1. Zeiss OPMI-1 hand-operated microscope. This is lightweight and highly manœuvrable. A beam splitter is fitted with an assistant's viewing binoculars at *A*. The extension to the carriage arm is at *B*.

Electrically Controlled Single-Man Microscope. Perhaps the best microscope of this sort is the Zeiss OPMI-6, though recently Wild have produced a microscope which is, in many respects, its equal. Most electrically driven microscopes are controlled remotely by either a foot pedal or by switches on the microscope body. They allow the surgeon to change magnification without removing his hands from the surgical field; most of them also have electrically controlled focusing as well. The great advantage of these microscopes is that there is less risk of wound contamination. I am not convinced that they make surgery much faster, though this is widely claimed. It is far easier to take good photographs through an electrically driven microscope and if closed circuit videophotography is envisaged, these machines are almost indispensable.

However, they are bulkier and more cumbersome than manual microscopes. The microscope body tends also to be longer so that the working distance may be less (there is a risk that a long surgical instrument may momentarily touch the microscope). The biggest disadvantage is that most of these microscopes cannot usually be focused or adjusted if there is a power failure or if the switching gear fails. Failure of switches is not uncommon. Switches in foot pedals are particularly vulnerable and tend to collect dirt or get damp. These microscopes are also more expensive.

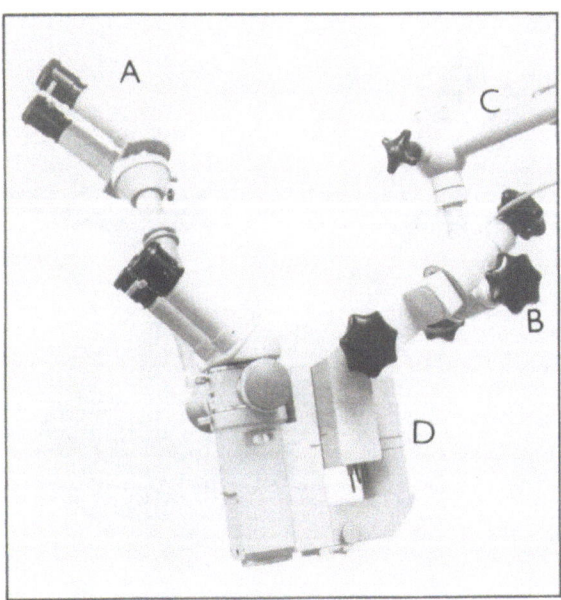

Fig. 14.2. Zeiss OPMI-6 electrically driven single-man microscope. Assistant's binocular at *A*, geared-angled coupling for lateral tilt at *B* and extension arm at *C*. The coaxial illuminator is at *D*. Note that the body of this microscope is considerably longer than that of the manual microscope, which makes it slightly more cumbersome.

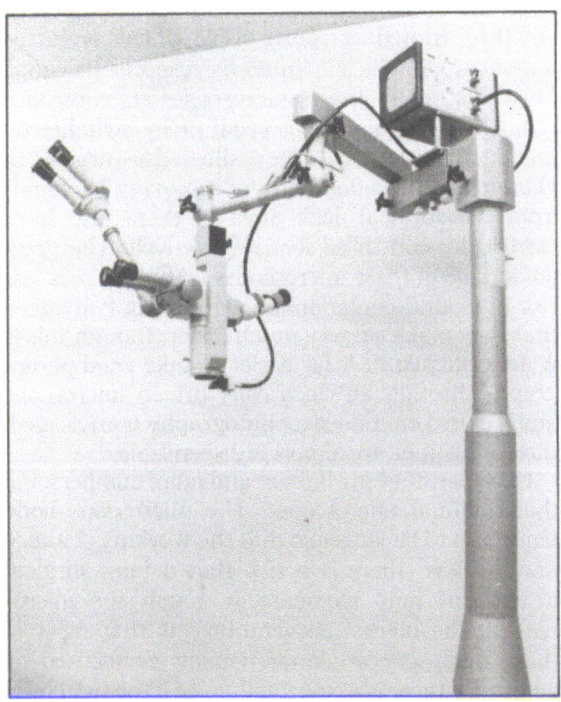

Fig. 14.3. Zeiss diploscope. This is the OPMI-7, which is the most basic of the range. The illumination is mounted distally on top of the microscope stand and brought coaxially under the objective by means of a fibreoptic cable.

Two-Man Microscope (*Diploscope*). All these are electrically controlled, by foot pedal. The most successful of these are made by Zeiss, the OPMI-7 and the OPMI-6D. The surgeon and his assistant can sit opposite each other and view the same field stereoscopically. This is helpful for teaching and if an "active" assistant is required to cut sutures to take some of the strain of operating.

The disadvantage is that these machines are all large. Moreover, the height of one set of binoculars is often most comfortable for one surgeon when the height of the eyepiece opposite leads to the other surgeon (usually the assistant!) being very uncomfortable. Because all these microscopes are vertically mounted, lateral tilt is limited and none of them is as mobile as a single-man microscope. In order for two people to have the same field of view, a beam-splitter must be employed. This means that the available light is halved. This may be a problem if closed-circuit television or photography is being used, as yet another beam-splitter will be needed. This can lead to quite dim images and rather poor visual acuity.

Important General Features

Whatever microscope is used, it is important that it has certain accessories:

1. An objective of a focal length between 200 and 300 mm. Lenses with a shorter focal length give greater magnification. If the focal length is too short there is a risk of instruments being contaminated. Lenses with longer focal length give weaker illumination.
2. Low-power eyepieces. Usually ×10 eyepieces are best.
3. An extension to the carriage arm. This allows the microscope stand to be well away from the microscope body which gives better access to the pelvis. An alternative is to have a ceiling-mounted microscope but this is costly to install.

The Zeiss range are probably the best buy. They have interchangeable accessories but are rather expensive. The Wild microscopes give rather better illumination and a very flat field of view but are bigger and clumsy to use.

Features of Loupes

Loupes are magnifying eyeglasses. They are attached to a headband or a pair of spectacles. Many people regard loupes as an alternative to

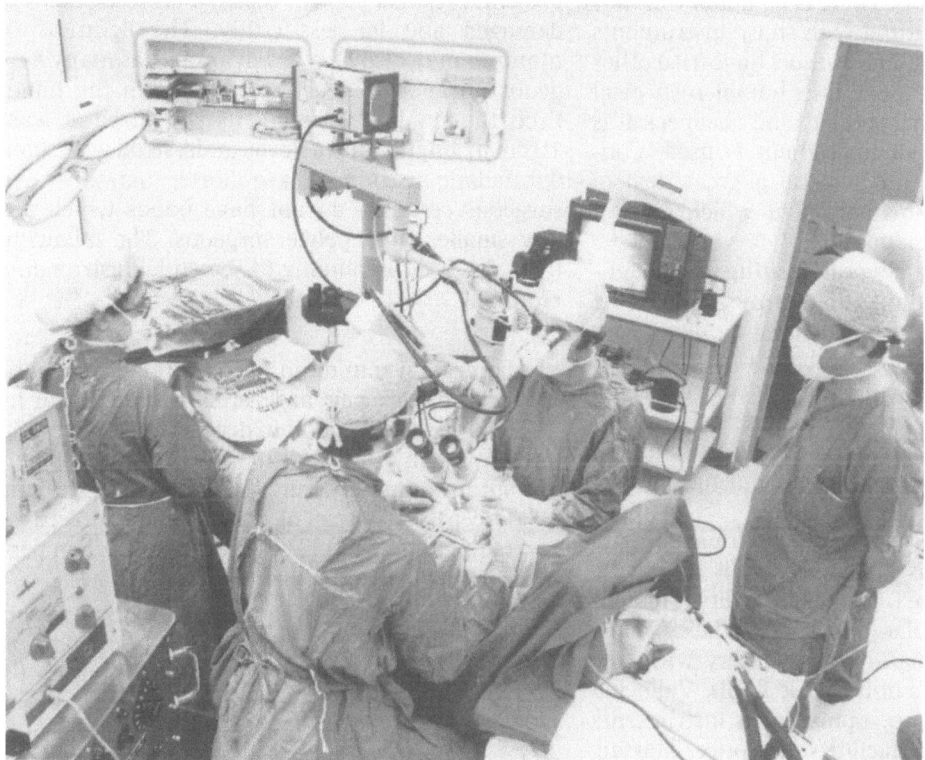

Fig. 14.4. The diploscope in use with a closed-circuit TV camera and monitor attached for teaching purposes. A microsurgical diathermy unit (Siemens Radiotom) is at the *bottom left* of the picture.

the microscope. They should be used rather as an adjunct, when the higher magnifications offered by a microscope are a disadvantage. Loupes are ideal for ovarian cysts, endometriosis and for adhesiolysis—especially in preparation of the pelvis for in vitro fertilisation (IVF). They give inadequate magnification for most tubal surgery, such as anastomosis or salpingostomy.

Loupes are portable and relatively cheap, costing about £500. They are easier to learn to use as they have a fixed focus and magnification. They also give a wider field of view than some low-power microscopes and this is a considerable help when working in a badly distorted pelvis.

Loupes have disadvantages. Their optical resolution is not as good as the microscope. They do not provide coaxial illumination, so the image is rather dim. This can make identification of pathological tissue impossible. High-power loupes magnify up to eight times but are very difficult to use. Because loupes have a fixed focal length, the surgeon has to keep his head static, which is tiring. Moreover, the telescopic lenses themselves tend to obscure normal vision and this can be infuriating.

In spite of these various shortcomings, loupes are useful, providing they are employed for the most appropriate procedures. The cheapest good loupes are manufactured by Keeler of London. Better, lighter loupes are made by Carl Zeiss of West Germany and by Designs for Vision of the United States. Designs for Vision also manufacture a headband, to which can be fixed a fibreoptic light. I personally find these restricting and uncomfortable. These companies can all make a pair of loupes which are permanently fixed to spectacles with lenses according to your prescription, if needed. If you decide to order loupes, it is wise to buy a pair with no more than $2\frac{1}{2}$ times magnification. An ideal focal length for most people is about 28–34 cm.

Diathermy

It may seem strange to emphasise diathermy, but this is a crucial instrument. Fine electrosurgery has proved to be one of the most important innovations in infertility surgery. Diathermy dissection of pelvic tissues and adhesions gives very clean results and can be largely bloodless. There is no doubt that it is greatly superior to cutting with sharp instruments or blunt dissection. Various authors have tried other instruments such as the CO_2 laser but microsurgical diathermy is definitely superior (and cheaper). It is essential that the right instrument is used. Conventional diathermy units cause a great deal of tissue damage and an instrument which gives a very weak output is mandatory.

Suitable units must generate cutting and coagulation current. Cutting diathermy should be unipolar, through a fine needle used for dissection. As little as 4–5 W must be reliably given. It is useful if the cutting current can be blended with some coagulation current for better haemostasis. A unit with added bipolar coagulation is also useful, for dealing with larger blood vessels during cornual surgery.

There are a variety of good instruments. The Valleylab Surgistat is cheapest and is adequate, though unsophisticated. The blend facility is limited and there is no bipolar outlet. Nonetheless, it is possible to achieve high-quality surgery with this machine, which costs only about £650. Valleylab also make much more sophisticated instruments having a full range of facilities at a price. Martins of West Germany also make a satisfactory machine, though I have found a certain amount of charring with the cutting output. The best machine, which is also very expensive (currently about £3000), is made by Bard of the United States. This is by far the best microsurgical diathermy made so far and has the advantage that its output can be increased for conventional surgical requirements so that over 300 W can be delivered. It can be used when a powerful diathermy unit is needed, for transurethral prostatic work and for cutting through thick muscles.

Although laser surgery has the reputation of being very valuable, there is virtually no evidence that the laser offers any significant advantage. Haemostasis is better with fine diathermy and dissipation of the burn is minimal. Diathermy is much quicker to use and the clinical results which have been published are the equal or better than those achieved with lasers. The most expensive microsurgical diathermy costs less than one-tenth of the cost of a laser and the running costs are only those required to replace the hand switch and the electrode needles periodically.

Microsurgical Instruments

These must be high quality and simple. Stainless steel is preferable although titanium is in vogue at present. Steel is easier to repair if an instrument is damaged and far less costly. The lightness of titanium may also be a disadvantage, as many surgeons prefer some feeling of weight in the hand. Even the smallest instruments should be at least 10 cm in length; I have never understood why some ophthalmic instruments are shorter than this—eye surgeons certainly do not have hands which are any smaller than pelvic surgeons. The following (Figs. 14.5–8) are among the essential instruments required:

1. Forceps. A minimum of two straight pairs are needed. One pair at least should be 18 cm in length, for dissection in deeper places. One pair should have a platform at the tip, to grasp fine suture material easily. In addition to straight forceps, one pair of fine toothed forceps is required to get hold of fibrous tissue when performing cornual surgery.

2. Scissors. Two pairs are needed, one of which should have curved blades. The best length is about 18 cm. Microsurgical scissors must be able to cut along the length of their blades. It is very important that the blades close with using uniform pressure, or fine dissection will be impossible.

3. Needleholders. One fine microsurgical pair is required which should be reserved only for microsurgical needles, i.e. needles less than $150\,\mu m$ in diameter (a fine 6/0 needle). If bigger needles are grasped the blades will deform, and they will not hold fine suture during knottying. Needleholders with a round grip are easier to use for long periods without getting cramped fingers. A second microvascular needle-holder is also needed for large 6/0 or 4/0 needles.

4. Probes and splint material. Fine metal probes are useful during anastomosis. Splinting helps to approximate cut tubal ends during anastomosis, though splints should not be left in the tube after surgery. Much thicker probes, made of Teflon, plastic or glass are useful for handling tissues and supporting them during dissection. They reduce abrasion or trauma that would be caused by handling with gloved fingers.

A set of fine lachrimal probes may be used to dilate the narrowed intramural tube. If the isthmic segment requires probing, for example, to introduce a splint, the probe should be no thicker than 0·5 mm in diameter, otherwise there is a risk of damaging the tube. An ideal probe is made by Spingler-Tritt (S & T; see below). They also manufacture a probe for the

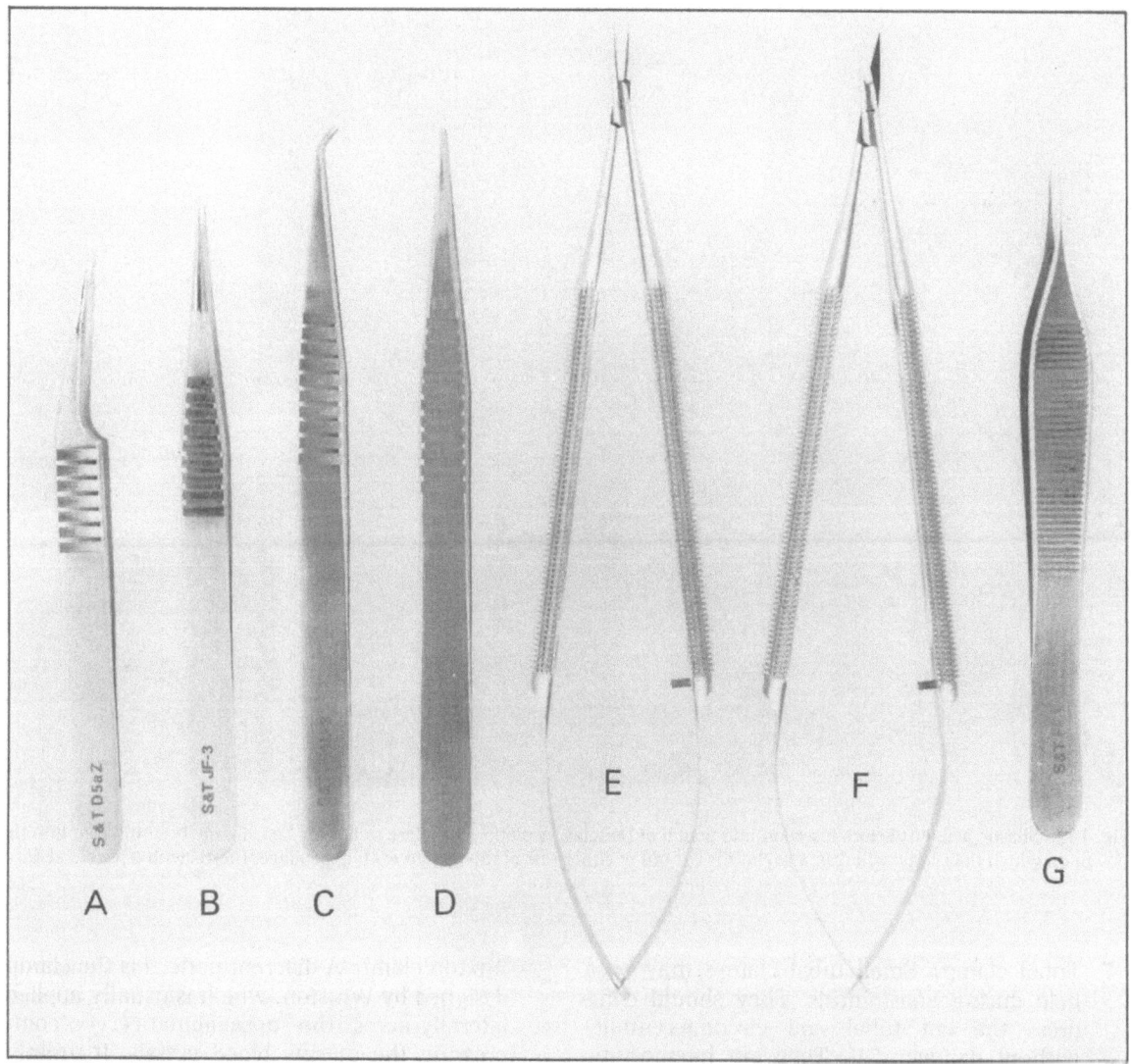

Fig. 14.5. Basic microsurgical instrument set, suitable for most tubal surgery. *A* Very fine forceps, used mainly for gentle dilatation of the lumen of the isthmus before difficult anastomoses. The polished tips of the closed forceps are gently inserted into the lumen and are allowed to open, thus dilating the tube. *B–D* Standard microsurgical forceps for knot-tying, tissue handling, etc. They should be a minimum of 12 cm in length. *E* Needle holder with round grip. The well-made pair illustrated are from Spingler-Tritt, catalogue no. B-18, and represent excellent value for money. *F* Fine scissors with lightly curved blades (Spingler-Tritt SDC-18). These are 18 cm in total length and the blades cut accurately throughout their length. *G* Toothed forceps. The teeth are fine so that tissue damage is minimised. These are valuable for cornual anastomosis.

ampullary end of the tube which is introduced through the fimbrial end.

5. Fine scissors. Although most dissection will be with needle diathermy, microsurgical scissors are helpful for fine dissection when initiating cleavage of tissue planes, when dissecting near the cut end of the tube before anastomosis (excessive diathermy may cause undue fibrosis subsequently) and for cutting sutures. Castro-viejo scissors are most suitable; there are many variations of this design on the market.

6. Silicone operating pad. This is a pad, available from S & T, which can be slid into the pouch of Douglas, over a damp swab, for supporting the uterus and appendages. It keeps the appendage in a fixed plane under the microscope. The pad should be a natural colour and should not cause glare.

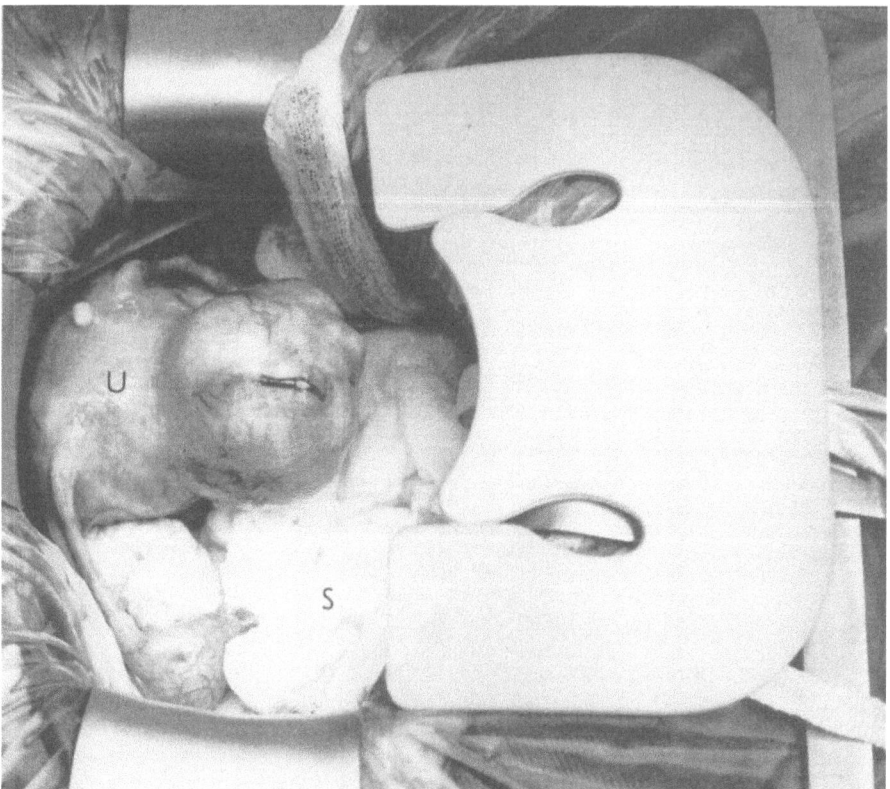

Fig. 14.6. Silastic pad, just before insertion into pouch of Douglas. A platform of loose swabs (S) has already been inserted into the pouch on which the silastic will rest; a keyhole is cut out of either side of the pad for each appendage. Uterus with a fibroid at U.

7. Tubal clamps. Small tubal clamps may be a help during anastomosis. They should compress the cut tubal end circumferentially without damaging it. They are haemostatic and aid identification of the tissues during suturing.

8. Suture material. Non-absorbable suture is generally preferable for fine work. 8/0 nylon on a thin 3/8 needle is ideal fine work. The needle should be about 140 μm diameter. The most suitable is made by S & T; Ethicon and Davis & Geck make satisfactory alternatives, though their needles may be somewhat thicker and less well fixed onto the thread.

   Thicker sutures of polypropylene amide (Prolene) are also needed. This material is ideal because of its lack of tissue reaction. The 6/0 or 4/0 Prolenes made by Ethicon on different needle sizes are suitable.

9. Cervical clamp. A standard clamp is the Shirodkar pattern, which is applied over the uterine fundus. It is rather bulky and tends to get in the way; a similar alternative is the Buxton clamp. A different pattern is the clamp designed by Winston, which is usually applied laterally across the supravaginal cervix, compressing the uterine blood vessels. It greatly aids haemostasis during cornual surgery and helps elevate and steady the uterus from behind without getting in the surgeon's way.

10. Retractor and plastic Steridrape. The best retractor has four blades. The biggest exposure is gained with a modified Kirschner retractor, which compresses the wound edge very effectively, maintaining haemostasis. This is better than the O'Connor-O'Sullivan pattern more commonly used by gynaecologists. It can be obtained from Down's Surgical, UK.

    The Steridrape with a 5-inch plastic ring (3M's; catalogue no. 1074) can be inserted inside the wound at the start of laparotomy. It prevents leakage of blood into the abdominal cavity from the wound edge and keeps the peritoneal edge moist and free from trauma. It reduces the risk of serious peritoneal abdominal wall adhesions after surgery.

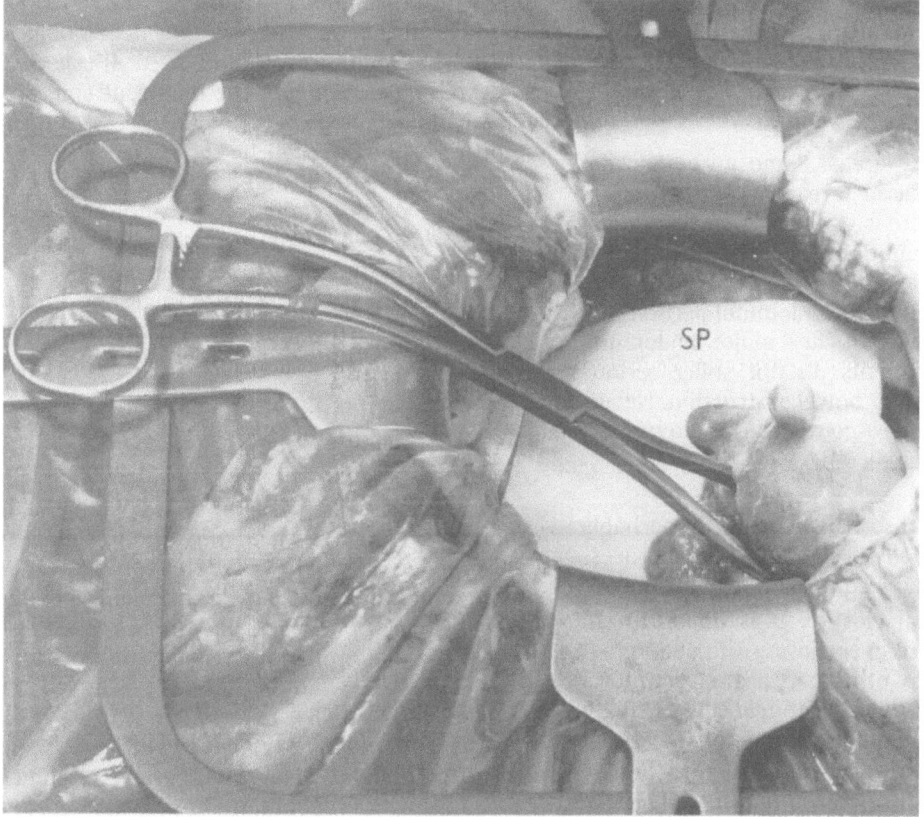

Fig. 14.7. Cervical clamp in place. This is behind the cervix and occludes it to facilitate transfundal dye injection for cornual anastomosis. This clamp is made by Spingler-Tritt. A silastic pad is in situ at *SP*.

Surgical Principles

The avoidance of wanton surgical damage is of key importance. Too often, clumsy surgery can make matters worse. It is worth remembering that the use of magnification is not sufficient in itself—it is perfectly feasible to perform gross surgery under a microscope.

Secondly, microsurgery is designed to reconstruct tissues in the best possible anatomical relationship. This requires a knowledge of tubal physiology and anatomy as well as an understanding of pathology, particularly the pathology of pelvic inflammatory disease. It simply is not enough to think of tubal disease in terms of tubal blockage. Merely unblocking the tubes does not produce good surgical results. The important principles are:

1. Good exposure. Inadequate surgical exposure leads to unnecessary trauma because of the need to grasp tissues to pull them into view.
2. Good haemostasis. Excessive bleeding prevents the surgeon obtaining a good view of what he is doing. Persisting blood clot and fibrin leads to adhesion formation after abdominal closure.
3. Constant irrigation. Irrigation with isotonic fluids, such as Ringer lactate, keeps tissues moist

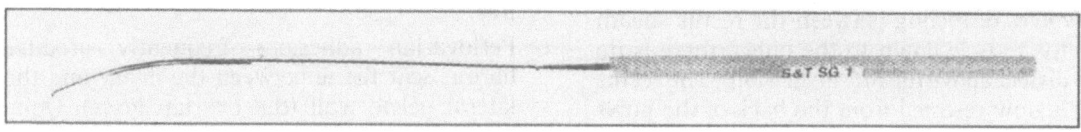

Fig. 14.8. Grooved probe for inserting splint material into tubal ampulla (Spingler Tritt catalogue no. SG 1).

and free of clot. Dry tissue is easily traumatised.

4. Avoidance of tissue trauma. Raw areas, bruising and necrotic tissue all can lead to adhesion formation or fibrosis. Avoid causing unnecessary peritoneal damage.

5. Avoidance of raw areas. Some authors claim that deperitonealised areas will heal spontaneously but there is good evidence from laparoscopic examinations performed after microsurgery that the fewer raw areas, the better. It is true that the abdominal peritoneum can be left unsutured after major abdominal surgery—most patients do not suffer serious consequences such as bowel obstruction. Nevertheless, check laparoscopy clearly shows that healing is more predictable with thorough peritoneal closure.

6. The use of non-absorbable suture. Absorbable sutures are gradually broken down by a process of rotting. This can lead to excessive fibrosis.

7. Careful abdominal closure. It is important to take as much care over closing the abdominal peritoneum as any other part of the procedure. It is worth everting cut peritoneal edges using a mattress suture. Relatively thin suture material should be employed.

8. Avoidance of infection. Infection is a real enemy because it encourages poor healing, adhesion formation and fibrosis. Care should be taken not to lengthen procedures unduly. Antibiotic cover should be considered if surgery has taken longer than usual. Never operate if there is any suspicion of active inflammatory disease; this must be treated first.

Abdominal Incision

Although a midline incision used to be favoured by many tubal surgeons, perfectly adequate exposure can be achieved with a transverse suprapubic incision. This heals better and looks more sightly, important considerations in young women.

Although the Pfannenstiel is the most popular transverse incision, it tends not to give really adequate exposure unless extended laterally or unless the rectus muscles are at least partly transected. I now prefer a modified Cherney incision. This involves dissecting between the rectus sheath and rectus muscle down to the pubis (there is no need to dissect above the line of incision). The rectus muscle is now resected from the back of the pubis and reflected upwards. Once the fundus of the bladder has been exposed, the peritoneal cavity can

be entered through a transverse incision. The advantage of this approach is that it is bloodless, particularly if diathermy is employed. If especially wide exposure is required, the recurrent epigastric vessels can be ligated.

Closure of this incision needs care. It is wise to use interrupted sutures and it is important that the anaesthetist gives full relaxation until the rectus sheath is closed. The rectus muscle should not be sutured back to the pubis, as this can cause osteitis. All that is necessary is to suture the rectus muscle into the fibrous aponeurosis above the pubic symphysis.

Adhesiolysis

Although salpingolysis and oophorolysis are the simplest microsurgical procedures, there can be considerable damage if done badly. Like all tubal surgery, the first operation has the best chance of success. The main principles relevant to most tubal surgery include:

1. Whenever possible avoid picking up tissues with the fingers. Never grasp any peritoneal surface with crushing instruments.

2. Use a glass or plastic probe to dissect adhesions. Adhesions are best elevated on the tip of the probe and then divided using fine diathermy.

3. It is usually best to leave adhesions slightly "long" on the tubal serosa, so as not to leave a raw area. They can always be trimmed once division is competed; cut adhesions will tend to roll back on themselves making further resection unnecessary.

4. Suture raw serosa on the tube with 8/0 nylon. The ovarian capsule usually requires a slightly thicker suture, such as 6/0 Prolene.

5. Try to secure a good relationship between the fimbria and the ovary. This may necessitate vigorous dissection between the end of the tube and the ovary, particularly if there are fibrous adhesions in this region. The fimbrial blood supply must not be damaged; scissors may be safer for this part of the operation than diathermy. Raw area on the ovarian capsule should be excised and sutured once the tube is free.

6. Periovarian adhesions frequently produce fibrous scar tissue between the ovary and the lateral pelvic wall (the ovarian fossa). Quite vigorous dissection is usually needed and it is often necessary to create a large raw area

before the ovary can be freed. One should not be nervous about this, providing the ureter has been carefully identified. Raw peritoneum can be sutured vertically using 4/0 Prolene to cover the lateral pelvic wall. The raw ovarian surface can be excised before carefully suturing the capsule.

7. Adhesions in the pouch of Douglas should be removed if possible. This seems to improve the chance of an egg being picked up from the pouch.

8. It is a mistake to divide adhesions which do not appear to be interfering with tubal mobility or egg pick-up. Extra dissection carries extra risk of recurrent adhesion formation.

9. Ventrosuspension or shortening of the round ligaments is generally unnecessary and may cause more problems. It is best reserved for those cases where there is a high risk of dyspareunia after operation.

10. Steroids seem to be the most effective adjunctive treatment. An insoluble suspension of hydrocortisone acetate (between 1·0 G and 1·5 G) can be left in the pelvis before closure of the peritoneum.

Salpingostomy

It has been suggested that salpingostomy has been made redundant by in vitro fertilisation. This is not the case; providing patients are selected carefully, good results—certainly better than those currently achieved with IVF—can be achieved. If the tubes are thin-walled, with little muscle fibrosis and reasonable mucosa, over one-third of patients will achieve a live birth afterwards. Moreover, about half those conceiving will have a second spontaneous conception and live birth.

Salpingostomy is not easy. Although it is not at all difficult to open a closed ampulla, a good deal of experience is needed if a functional tube is to be obtained. Generally, the best instrument for actual incision in the tube is the fine needle-point diathermy, which should be used at just sufficient intensity to allow cutting without charring (Fig. 14.9). Once the tube is opened, a very few sutures—preferably of 8/0 nylon—are all that is needed to keep the margin of the tube everted (Fig. 14.10). If the walls are fibrotic or hypertrophied, a somewhat thicker suture (say 6/0) may be required. Very often, if the salpingostomy has been made properly, the tubal end everts itself and suturing is unnecessary.

There are ten points to be born in mind during salpingostomy:

1. Wherever possible, the anatomical relationship between the ampulla and the ovary should be restored before opening the tube. This will require identification of the ovarian end of the mesosalpinx and careful dissection so as not to damage the tubal blood supply.

2. The tube should be opened at its most terminal part. Usually a fibrous line can be clearly seen at this point—very often where little blood vessels run radially away from a so-called "pucker point". Any incision made elsewhere is an incision in the wall of the tube and not where the fimbrial end was originally; it may heal spontaneously so that the tube may become blocked again within a few weeks.

3. When opening the tube, one should try to avoid cutting across any residual mucosal folds. Transection of the epithelial folds may damage the blood supply. Moreover, as egg transport is likely to be mediated by interaction of two ciliated epithelial folds, the integrity of these folds may be an important factor in the success of surgery. Adhesion between mucosal folds should be deliberately divided.

4. Evert the tubal mucosa just enough to achieve a stable ostium. Too much eversion may devitalise the fimbrial lip by reducing venous drainage.

5. Tubal tissue should not be resected unless it is obviously redundant. It is common to find that involution of even very large and 'floppy'' hydrosalpinges occurs after salpingostomy.

6. The reconstructed ostium should be positioned so that it is capable of movement over the whole ovarian surface.

7. The fimbria ovarica should be reconstructed whenever possible. It may be an important channel of communication between the tube and ovary.

8. It is all too easy to damage the tubal blood supply in the region of the fimbria ovarica. These vessels should be identified before putting any stitches in this region.

9. All raw areas near the newly constructed fimbria should be carefully repaired, usually with 8/0 nylon. It may be necessary to place a free peritoneal graft in this region if dissection is extensive.

10. Maximise the amount of the surface area of the ovary available for ovulation. Good tubal surgery also usually means ovarian surgery.

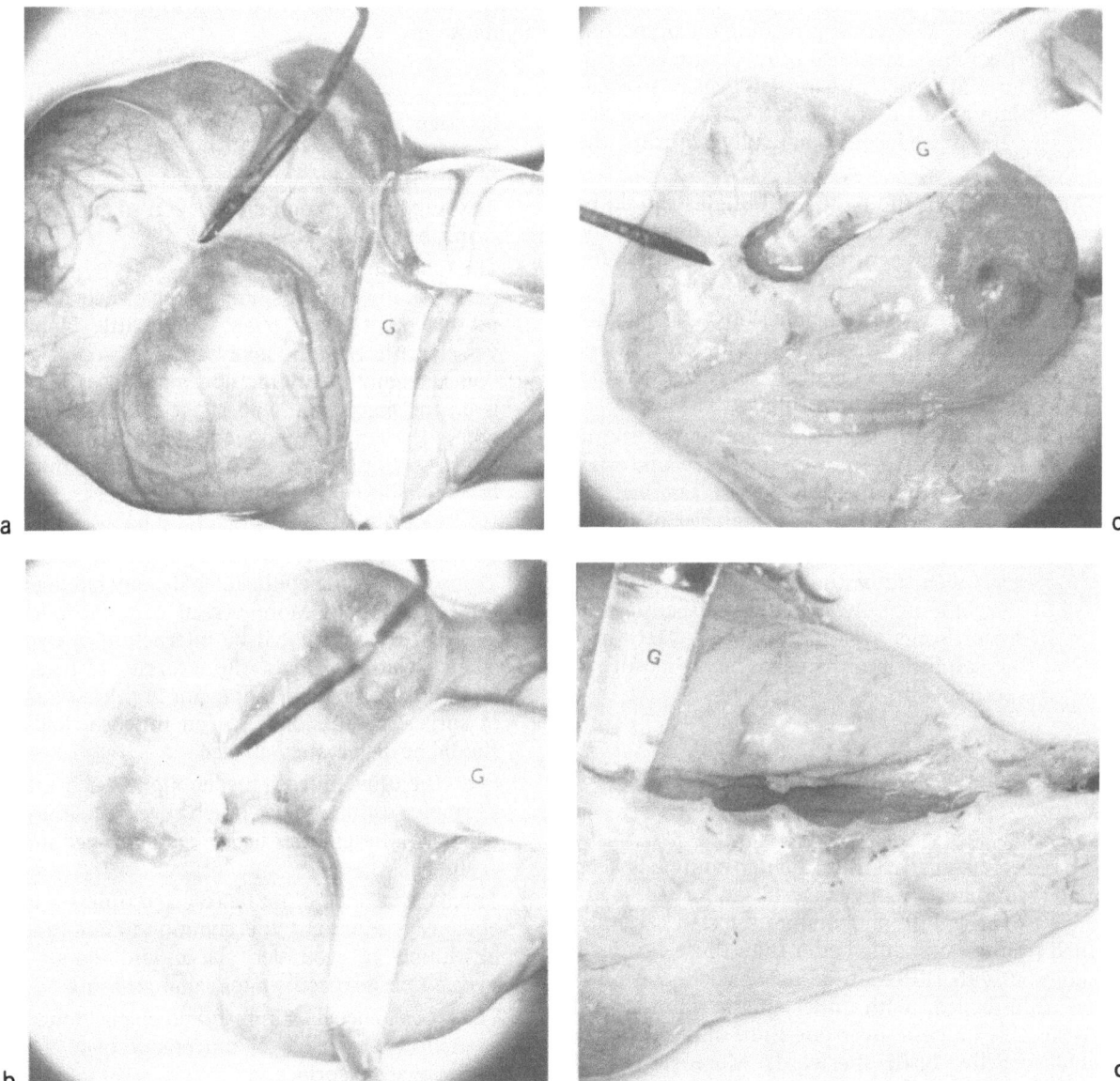

Fig. 14.9a–d. Salpingostomy. **a** The pucker point is clearly delineated by the fibrous indrawn line and by radial blood vessels. Glass rod at G. **b** A small incision is made bloodlessly using a diathermy needle. **c** The tip of the glass rod (G) is inserted into the incision, which is then enlarged with the diathermy needle in **d**.

Cornual Anastomosis

Cornual anastomosis after inflammation is highly successful. When the ampulla is not diseased between 50% and 60% of patients have a live birth. A microscope is essential, because of the small diameter of the lumen of the tube in this region. The surgery can be very demanding indeed, particularly if there is much fibrosis in the uterine muscle, considerable nodularity and expansion of the cornu or if the block is deep in the myometrium. If the whole isthmus is diseased and needs excision, the surgeon has the difficult job of joining two segments of tube with widely disparate luminal sizes.

It is often more comfortable to sit down for cornual surgery. This is because quite high magnification is needed and the hands are steadier when operating in a seated position with the forearm supported. The surgeon should operate on the side of the table corresponding to the tube being repaired, changing sides when one tubal anastomosis is finished.

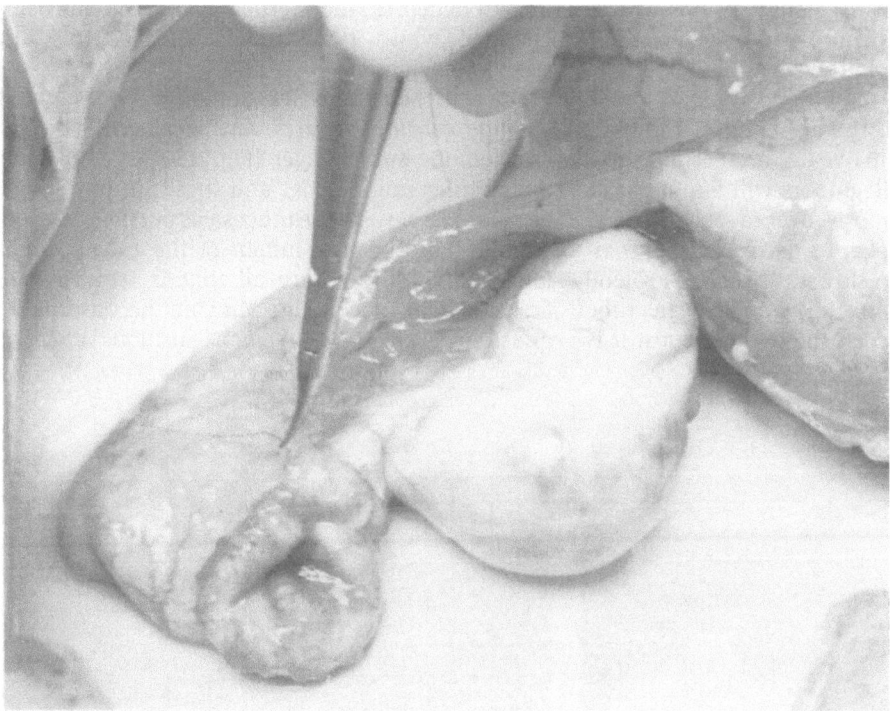

Fig. 14.10. Completed salpingostomy. The everted margin is sutured with 8/0 nylon to hold it in position.

The first stage is to free the tubes from adhesions. The cervix is now secured from above using a Shirodkar or Winston clamp. The Winston clamp is preferable because bleeding will be controlled by the clamp's position across the uterine arteries. Dye should now be injected—preferably transfundally, using a 19-gauge needle attached to a plastic tube and a 20-ml syringe. This confirms that the cornua are blocked; they will expand under the pressure of the dye in the uterine cavity, which will help dissection of the interstitial portion.

The microscope is now positioned. The isthmic portion of the tube should be dissected from the cornu. Using magnification, the isthmic portion should be inspected and all blocked or pathological tissue carefully resected. The vascular arcades in the mesosalpinx must not be damaged. The subtubal artery bleeds vigorously when cut across and can be controlled with diathermy or possibly a tubal clamp. If diathermy is used to make the initial cut across the tube, this should be "freshened up" with a fine scalpel blade, so that no charred, compromised tissue is included in the anastomosis.

Diseased tissue is now sliced away from the cornu. It is important to remove all pathological tissue, otherwise there is a risk of reocclusion. Mere patency is insufficient. The signs that all diseased tissue have been removed are:

1. Four or five mucosal folds can be seen in the cornual lumen.
2. There are no mucosal polyps visible.
3. Fine blood vessels can be seen running in the epithelium close to its cut edge.
4. The circular muscle coat shows regular striations around the tube.
5. All white, gritty, fibrous tissue has been resected.
6. There is no extravasation of dye and no diverticula are present.

Care must be taken not to denude peritoneum by making the cornual incision too broad. Diathermy is extremely helpful to control bleeding and an injection of oxytocin (20 i.u.) will also reduce bleeding.

The block may be deep in the myometrium and access to the patent interstitial portion difficult. Under these circumstances it may be very helpful to "open up" the cornu. A vertical incision can be made for about 2 cm above the cornu, towards the midline of the uterine fundus. This will be sutured at the end of the procedure in an inverted "Y". If access is still a problem, two stay sutures of 6/0 Prolene can be placed behind and in front of the interstitial portion, to hold the edges of the vertical incision apart.

Once all pathological tissue has been removed and interstitial patency to dye has been established, repair can commence. Beginners will find it easier to perform the anastomosis over a polyethylene splint. Certainly this helps to get rough approximation of the cut ends. A stay suture of 6/0 Prolene placed in the mesosalpinx just beneath the tube will relieve tension between the two cut ends. It is

helpful to depress the uterus towards the side being operated whilst tying this suture, as this also relieves tension.

Once the cut ends are roughly approximated, the fine cardinal sutures can be placed. The first anastomotic suture layer (Fig. 14.11) should join the circular muscle coat and these sutures should be placed as close to the mucosa as possible, without actually entering the lumen of the tube. Usually four or five sutures are all that is required, the first stitch in place being that at the base of the anastomosis at the "six o'clock" position. Wherever

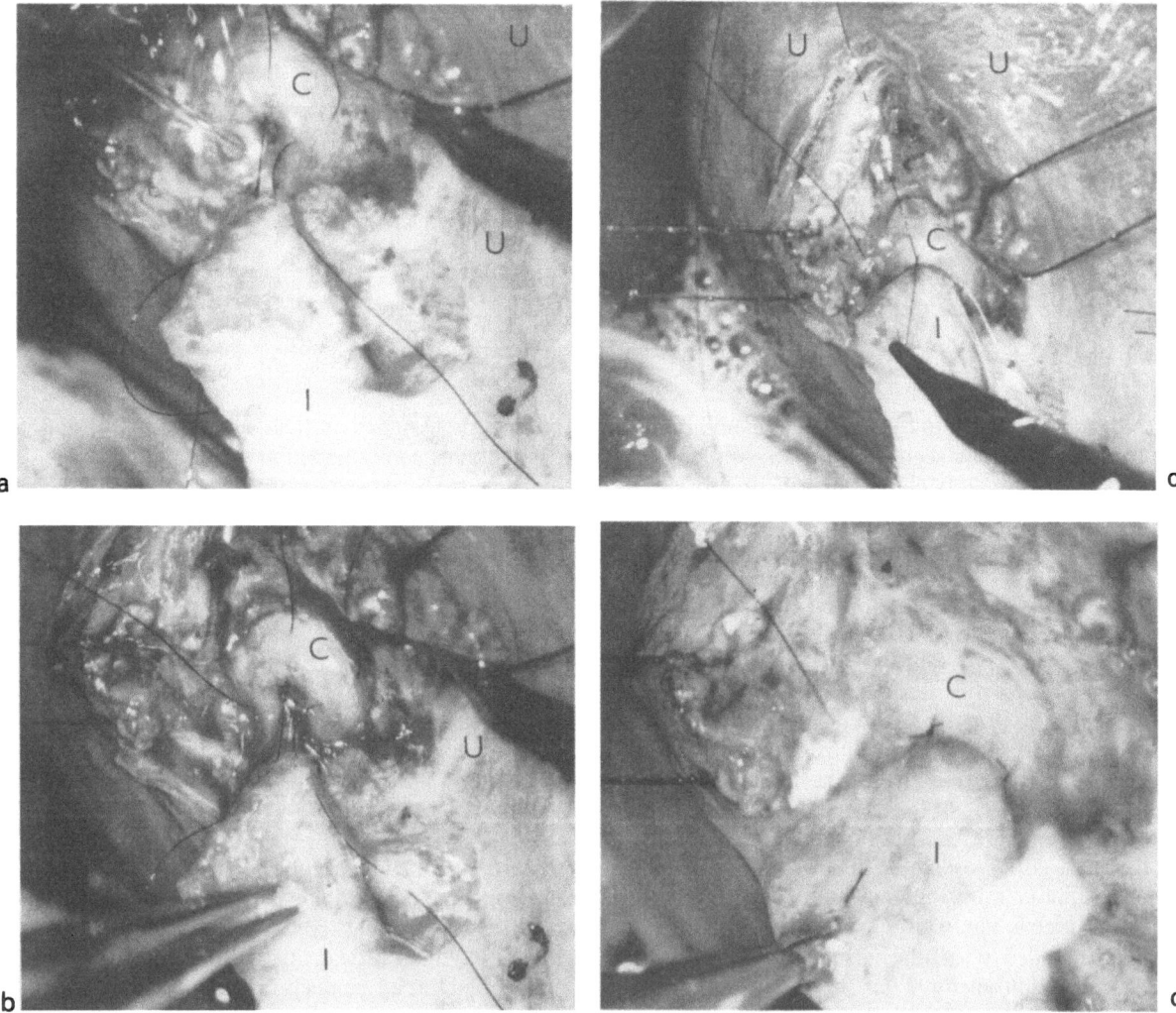

Fig. 14.11a–d. Cornual anastomosis. **a** The isthmus (*I*) is approximated to the cornu (*C*) over a fine polyethylene splint in the lumen. Two fine 8/0 nylon sutures are left untied at the 3 and 9 o'clock positions. Uterus is marked *U*. A jet of Ringer's lactate can be seen in *top left-hand corner of picture*, × 15. **b** The 12 o'clock suture is now in position, following which all the inner layer sutures will be tied. This is a good method for suturing when there is marked luminal disparity, × 15. **c** The 12 o'clock and 3 o'clock sutures have been tied. Note the thicker stay sutures of 6/0 Prolene laterally which help to hold the cornu apart for better access. These will be removed at the end of the procedure, × 15. **d** Tying the 9 o'clock suture at completion of the inner layer of the anastomosis, × 25.

possible, 8/0 nylon should be used; sometimes there is too much tension for such fine needlework and 7/0 or 6/0 Prolene will be required. It is a matter of preference whether these sutures should be tied as they are placed, or all tied at the end. If the anastomosis is deep, it may be easier to tie them when they are all in position.

At this stage it is wise to test the join. The splint in the tube should be pulled out via the fimbria and dye injected into the uterus with the cervix still clamped. The tube should be patent and retrograde spill should occur without much leakage at the join. If there is excessive leakage or if the anastomosis is not patent, the sutures should be unpicked and a fresh start made. Once the surgeon is satisfied that the join is functional, a second anastomotic layer can be placed. This layer should take the longitudinal muscle coat together with a bite of serosa. If the anastomosis is very deep in the myometrium and stay sutures have been employed, these should be removed. It may also be necessary to remove a little of the peritoneum from the isthmic end of the tube, so that peritoneum is not buried in the join. The second layer of sutures can be continuous or interrupted; the need is to give some strength to the join without kinking it—at the conclusion of the second layer, there should be no raw surfaces. If an inverted Y incision has been made, it can be closed at this stage and dye injected once again to confirm patency.

One beauty of this operation is that healing is usually good. The cornu is quite strong enough to maintain a growing pregnancy and rupture is unknown. Caesarean section is usually not indicated. Follow-up is important. Although it is felt unnecessary to perform a check hysterosalpingogram on patients after cornual surgery, a check laparoscopy should certainly be undertaken if conception has not occurred after 1 year. It seems that rather a high proportion of pregnancies miscarry after cornual anastomosis—the reason for this is unclear. Because reocclusion after pregnancy is not uncommon, it is important that these patients should have broad-spectrum antibiotic cover in the event of a threatened miscarriage.

Reversal of Sterilisation

Reversal of female sterilisation is usually the most straightforward of all tubal operations. The principles and technique are very similar to cornual surgery but more simple. This is because access to both ends of tube is easier and dissection into the muscular intramural portion of the cornu, which has many blood vessels, is seldom needed.

Even when the tubes are quite short, reversal can produce good results. Providing there is at least $2\frac{1}{2}$ cm of adhesion-free ampulla with healthy fimbrial mucosa, at least 50% of patients will conceive. The length of residual isthmus seems unimportant. The method of sterilisation is not in itself important, though excessive diathermy can cause quite severe fibrosis—particularly in the region of the cornu.

Because the basic technique needed for reversal of sterilisation is very similar to that used for cornual anastomosis, a detailed description of the microsurgical technique would be repetitive. Attention is confined in this chapter to methods for dealing with common problems.

Excessive Scarring of the Tubal Stumps

When the tubes have been ligated for more than about 5 years, the segment medial to the ligation often becomes dilated and the isthmic stumps become replaced by small fibrous hydrosalpinges. Sometimes this dilation extends into the intramural portion of the tubes; quite often this may be associated with endometriotic changes in the medial tube (Vasquez et al. 1980b) possibly because endometrial fragments are regurgitated through an incompetent uterotubal junction repeatedly into the blind tube.

This can complicate tubal anastomosis because, unless all the fibrotic and scarred tubal tissue is removed, the join may not allow ovum transport. Alternatively, an ectopic pregnancy may follow conception. Consequently, the microscope must be used to ensure that all fibrotic tubal tissue, especially that overlaid with flattened or avascular epithelium, is resected. Resection of the isthmus up to the dilated intramural segment may lead to the necessity of joining two segments of disparate luminal diameter—the narrower lumen being that on the lateral side of the anastomosis. This usually requires extra sutures in the inner layer to achieve a watertight join.

Joining Segments of Tube of Widely Disparate Diameter

Some authors have advocated artificially widening the "mouth" of narrower segment of tube by fishtailing it. This is not very satisfactory. Others plicate the wide ampullary lumen, reducing its diameter with several circumferential sutures of 8/0 nylon. Prolapsed mucosal folds can be trimmed if they get between the cut edges of the tube.

A better method is described in Brosens and Winston (1978). These authors use a grooved probe of 1 mm diameter (S & T catalogue no. SG1), which is inserted through the fimbrial end of the tube, towards the blind end of the ampulla. The tip of the probe—which is smooth and bulbous—is gently pushed into the blind end, stretching the tissue. The peritoneal coat of this segment is circumcised 4–5 mm from the tip of the tube and is then stripped from the muscle coat at this point. The very tip of the tube is then transected and the end of the probe advanced through this hole. This small incision leaves the diameter of the cut ampulla about that of the transected isthmic portion. The probe is advanced a little further, a polyethylene splint is placed in the groove of the probe and the probe is then withdrawn through the fimbria. This movement cannulates the ampullary segment. The other end of the splint is now passed into the isthmus and the anastomosis can be made over the splint without difficulty. This method is very simple unless there has been much scarring of the ampullary side of the anastomosis.

Preparation of the Ovaries Before In Vitro Fertilisation

A recent indication for surgery is when there are many adhesions around the ovaries and the tubes are so badly damaged that reconstructive tuboplasty alone is unlikely to benefit the patient. Many of these women may be suitable for egg collection for IVF by ultrasonically guided follicular puncture. At the time of writing, however, this method seems less successful than laparoscopic egg collection. A comparatively high success rate has been achieved in some centres by preparing the pelvis for egg collection by preliminary oophorolysis (Winston et al. 1984). This may be particularly indicated if the ovaries are cystic or damaged by old endometriosis, or if bowel is plastered firmly over the ovaries.

The principles of this surgery have been fully described elsewhere (Winston et al. 1984) and include careful lysis of omental adhesions, often combined with partial omentectomy, elevation of the ovaries with wedge resection of raw areas from the ovarian surface, repair of all raw peritoneal surfaces with Prolene suture, free peritoneal grafting of the larger damaged peritoneal surfaces and sometimes ventrosuspension of the uterus. Oophoropexy, using 4/0 Prolene suture to attach the ovaries up to the cornu, is also helpful in many cases, and in our experience in no way interferes with the view of the ovaries subsequently seen using ultrasound. It is a moot point whether salpingectomy should also be undertaken. This may

not be a good idea, as even the most severely damaged tubes may work occasionally and a surprising number of spontaneous pregnancies have been reliably recorded after such "last ditch" surgery when it was thought that IVF would be the only possible chance for the patient. Moreover, total salpingectomy may have bad psychological implications for the infertile patient and it does not even guarantee freedom from ectopic pregnancy; eccyesis can still occur in the residual intramural portion of the tube following extracorporeal fertilisation and embryo transfer.

Manufacturers

Bard Electro Medical Systems, Bard Ltd, Pennywell Ind. Estate, Sunderland, SR4 9EW, UK. Telex 537092.
Carl Zeiss (Oberkochen) Ltd, PO Box 78, Woodfield Rd., Welwyn Gdn. City, Herts. AL7 1LU, UK.
Designs for Vision, Inc. 120 East 23rd St, New York, NY 10010, USA. Tel 212–674–0600.
Down's Surgical, Church Path, Mitcham, Surrey CR4 3UE, UK. Telex 927045.
Keeler Instruments, 21–27 Marylebone Lane, London W1M 6DS, UK. Telex 847565.
Spingler-Tritt (S & T), Surgical Needles and Instruments, Allmendweg 2, D-7893 Jestetten, Postfach 1104, FRG. Tel 07745-7027.
Valleylab Instruments Inc., Boulder, Colorado, USA.
Wild Instruments, 48 Park Street, Luton, LU1 3HP0, UK. Telex 825475.

References

Brosens I, Winston RML (1978) Reversibility of female sterilisation. Academic, London
FIGO (1978) Conference on classification of tubal disease, chaired by R. Palmer, Miami, USA
Gomel V (1977) Tubal anastomosis by microsurgery. Fert Steril 28:59–66
Gomel V (1978) Salpingostomy by microsurgery. Fert Steril 29:380–388
Paterson P, Wood C (1974) The use of microsurgery in the reanastomosis of the rabbit Fallopian tube. Fert Steril 25:757–765
Swolin K (1975) Electromicrosurgery and salpingostomy: long-term results. Am J Obstet Gynecol 121:418–423
Vasquez G, Boeckx W, Winston RML, Brosens IA (1980a) Human tubal mucosa and reconstructive microsurgery. In: Crosignani A, Rubin BL (eds) Microsurgery in female infertility. Academic, London, p 41
Vasquez G, Winston RML, Boeckx W, Brosens IA (1980b) Ultrastructural changes in the tube following sterilisation. Am J

Obstet Gynecol 138:86–95

Walz W (1959) Fertilitäts Operationen mit Hilfe eines Oper-
ationenmikroskopes. Geburtshilfe Gynakologie 153:49–58

Winston RML, McLure Browne JC (1974) Pregnancy following
autograft transplantation of the Fallopian tube and ovary in
the rabbit. Lancet ii:494–496

Winston RML, Margara RA, Hillier SG (1984) Technique and
results of ovariolysis in preparation for in vitro fertilization.
Eur J Obstet Gynaecol 18:381–389

Suggested Reading

Chamberlain G, Winston RML (eds) (1984) Tubal infertility.
Blackwells, London

Lees DH, Singer A (eds) (1983) Color atlas of gynaecological
surgery, vol. 5. Infertility surgery. Year Book Medical
Publishers, Chicago

15 · The Role of Laser

Joseph Jordan

Historical

The word LASER is an acronym for Light Amplification by Stimulated Emission of Radiation. The principle of stimulated emission of radiation is not a new one for it was first described by Albert Einstein in 1917 in his publication *The Quantum Theory of Radiation*. However, it was not until 1954 that Gordon et al, described how stimulated emission of radiation could be achieved in the microwave range of the spectrum. This was known as the MASER (Microwave Amplification by Stimulated Emission of Radiation). In 1958 Schawlow and Townes extended the principle of the maser into the optical frequency range and in 1960 Maiman created the first working ruby laser. In 1961 Bennett et al, produced the first gas laser, the helium-neon (He-Ne) laser and also in the same year the neodymium-yttrium-aluminium-garnet (Nd-YAG) laser was developed. In 1968 Patel created the CO_2 laser for Bell Laboratories as a means of rapid communication using the 10·6-μm new wavelength as the carrier signal. In 1968 at the American Optical Laboratories, Pulanyi and Bredemeier (1973) modified the CO_2 system to be used in conjunction with an operating microscope for the destruction of lesions of the vocal cords. Bellina (1974) was the first to describe its use in gynaecology.

To date, several types of laser are currently used in surgery. The individual properties of each laser depend on the wavelength of the substance used to produce the laser beam (Table 15.1).

The applications of laser microsurgery in gynaecology are increasing year by year and will continue to do so. However, while the surgeon can be taught to use a knife relatively quickly, the same cannot be said of the laser. Before embarking on laser microsurgery it is imperative that the surgeon understands the basic principles of laser physics, the bioeffects of laser beam, the principles of laser treatment and the safety aspects of laser microsurgery. It is beyond the scope of a chapter such as this to describe these aspects of laser microsurgery and those who wish to practice this technique are urged to consult a basic reference work such as *The Principles of Practice of Gynaecological Laser Surgery* (Bellina and Bandieramonte 1984) and a report by

Table 15.1. Surgical lasers in use

Laser type	Wavelength (μm)	Power output (W)	Penetration depth (skin) (mm)	Main applications
CO_2	10·6	$\leqslant 500$	0·05	Cutting and vaporising
Argon	0·488–0·514	$\leqslant 20$	0·2	Coagulation of retinal vessels and superficial skin lesions; neurosurgery
Nd-YAG	1·06	$\leqslant 100$	0·8–2·0	Coagulation of gastrointestinal tract bleeding
Ruby	0·6943	> 10		Ophthalmology; dark skin lesions
HeNe	0·633	0·8–2·0	–	Finder beam

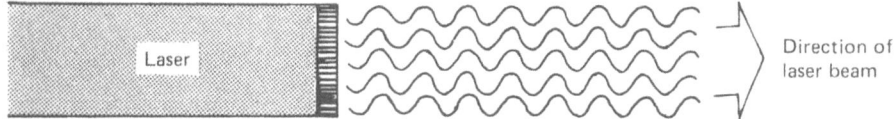

Fig. 15.1. Laser light is coherent, i.e. all of the light waves are in phase with each other.

the 1985 Study Group of Royal College of Obstetricians and Gynaecologists *Gynaecological Laser Surgery* (Sharp and Jordan 1986).

Properties of the Laser Beam

All lasers produce laser light, which has the following unique characteristics:

1. It is coherent, i.e. all of the light waves produced by the laser are in phase with each other (Fig. 15.1).
2. It is highly collimated, i.e. all the rays are virtually parallel with each other (Fig. 15.2). This is a unique characteristic of laser light and even over very long distances the laser beam exhibits minimal divergence as compared with light from an electric torch or light bulb.
3. It is monochromatic, i.e. all the waves have the same wavelength and energy.

4. It is the brightest existing light.

The laser beam itself produces very little power as measured in watts but the energy density or intensity of the beam is extremely high. If the beam is focused by an appropriate focusing lens the energy can be concentrated into an extremely small area. At the focal point of the beam, the laser is capable of releasing enormous amounts of energy (Fig. 15.3) and it is this property which is utilised in using the laser for surgical procedures. The distance between the lens and the focal spot is variable and depends on the focal length of the focusing lens. The energy released in this way can be likened to using the same focusing lens to focus the sun's rays. On a hot day prolonged exposure to the sun will result in a generalised burn, but if the sun's rays are focused by a focusing lens then at the focal point of the lens the energy or heat will be so strong as to actually burn the skin in a very short period of time.

The amount of power produced by the laser can be controlled very easily by the operating surgeon. The power is measured in watts (W) and the

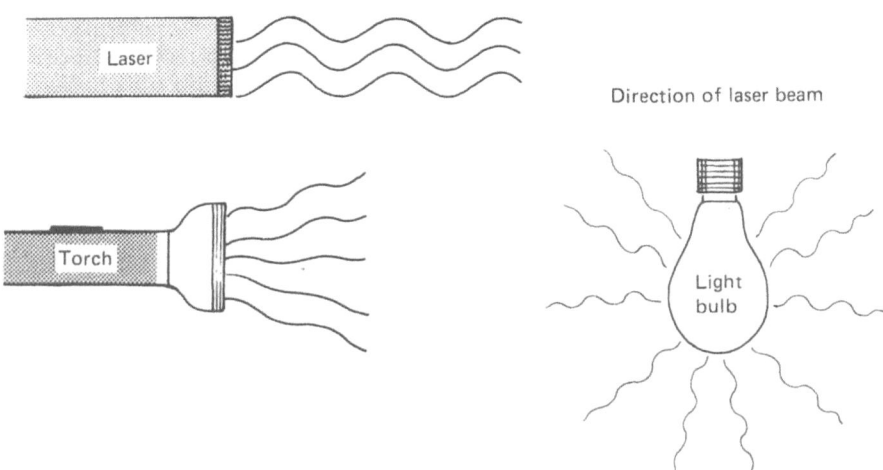

Fig. 15.2. Collimation—laser light is highly collimated, i.e. all the rays are virtually parallel with each other. Compare this with the divergent rays from a torch or light bulb.

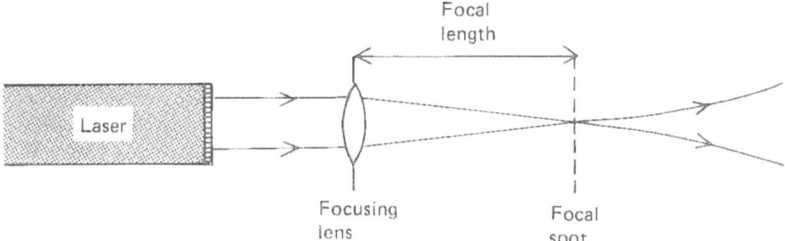

Fig. 15.3. The laser beam is parallel (collimated) as it leaves the laser but it can be focused, so concentrating all of its energy into a very small area.

amount of power released at the focal point of the laser beam is referred to as the power density (PD). It is important that the laser surgeon understands the concept of power density for it will dictate exactly what he can do with the laser beam. The power density of any given laser is measured in W/cm^2 and can be calculated quite simply by checking the power output of the laser (in watts) and measuring the spot size of the focal point of the laser. The following formula allows a quick estimation of power density:

$$PD = \frac{W \times 100}{\text{Spot size in mm}^2}$$

Power density is the single most important factor in understanding laser surgery and the range of power density employed determines whether the laser will coagulate, vaporise or cut. Reference to the above formula will make it clear that the power density will vary according to the wattage output of the machine and the size of the spot. For a given wattage over a set exposure time a small spot size will give a very much higher power density than a larger spot size, i.e. a spot size of 1 mm will produce

a power density which is four times higher than a spot size of 2 mm. It is imperative that the operating surgeon understands this concept and that the power density is affected not only by the wattage of the machine, but by the diameter of the spot.

Carbon Dioxide (CO₂) Laser

The carbon dioxide laser is that which is most commonly used by the gynaecological surgeon. It is capable of producing very high power densities and its energy is totally absorbed within a depth of 90 μm. It releases its energy where the beam strikes the tissue and works by vaporising water in tissue at the speed of light. Since human tissue is 70%–90% water the absorption of the carbon dioxide in the tissue can be related to the water content of the tissue. There is very little natural scattering and this property makes the CO₂ laser particularly suitable for the removal of tissue by vaporisation (Fig. 15.4). In contrast, the energy of the Nd Yag laser beam is absorbed within a few millimetres and some of the

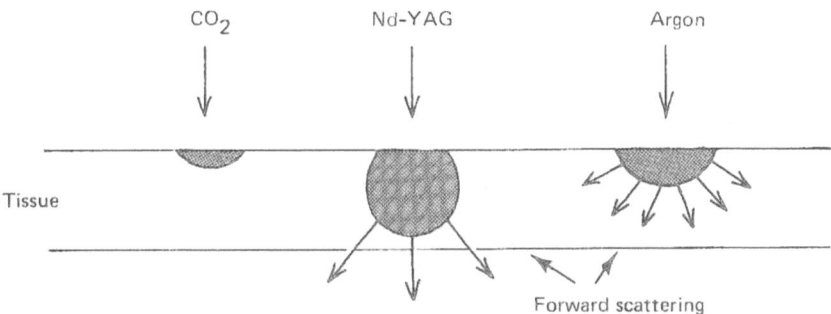

Fig. 15.4. Tissue destruction with different types of laser. There is no forward scattering with the CO₂ laser but there is a large amount of forward and lateral scattering with both the Nd-YAG and argon lasers.

energy is scattered laterally. This means that tissue is destroyed to a much greater depth than with the CO_2 laser and the amount of necrosis at the edge of the laser beam due to scattering is much greater than that of the CO_2 laser. The argon laser scatters its energy much more diffusely and approximately 100 times as much energy is scattered laterally as is directly absorbed. Haemoglobin absorbs the wavelength of the argon laser so that in vascular tissue the argon laser will be absorbed within the first few millimetres. The argon laser is therefore of particular value in coagulating tissue, for example, of the retina, but its colour-sensitive absorption and deep penetration combined with significant lateral scattering make it poorly suited to precise surgical procedures.

The CO_2 laser is particularly suited to gynaecological surgery because in most instances the surgeon wishes to destroy tissue, for example premalignant disease of the lower genital tract, warts, or division and vaporisation of adhesions. It allows a very precise vaporisation of surface epithelium with a very limited zone of injury due to heat damage (this is in contradistinction to the Nd Yag and argon lasers where the forward scattering may result in very extensive tissue injury below the surface).

The CO_2 laser beam has a wavelength of $10\cdot6\ \mu m$. Because it is in the infrared range of the electromagnetic spectrum, it is invisible and the surgeon must have some means of knowing exactly where the laser beam is focused. The CO_2 laser therefore has a small helium-neon (He-Ne) laser built into the laser system; this produces a red spot focused at the same point as the CO_2 laser beam and therefore acts as a "finder beam". The CO_2 laser beam is usually directed through a system of mirrors attached to an operating microscope, thereby allowing very great precision in its use. However, it can also be delivered through a hand-held attachment or through a laparoscope.

Treatment of Cervical Intraepithelial Neoplasia (CIN)

Removal of CIN by local destruction is gaining popularity and in approximately 1977 laser vaporisation of CIN was introduced as an alternative to cryotherapy and radical diathermy. The principle behind any destructive method is to remove abnormal epithelium and in recent years the efficacy of laser vaporisation has been confirmed in several reports (Baggish 1980; Anderson 1982; Burke 1982; Evans and Monaghan 1983; Jordan et al. 1985). Of greater importance than the technique of laser vaporisation is perhaps the criteria for patient selection. This applies to any destructive method and the prerequisites are summarised as follows:

1. The patient must be seen and assessed by a competent colposcopist.
2. The endocervical margin of the lesion and the transformation zone must be visible.
3. There must be no cytological suspicion of invasion.
4. There must be no colposcopic suspicion of invasion.
5. There must be no histological suspicion of invasion.
6. There must be no suspicion of atypical glandular cells in the cytology specimen, for this may suggest the coexistence of an underlying adenocarcinoma in situ. In this instance, an excision cone is obligatory.
7. The laser treatment should be performed by the colposcopist.
8. There must be every prospect of adequate follow-up.

These principles dictate the success or failure of the method. It is stressed that the appearance of abnormal glandular lesions is of particular concern and it is important that these lesions should be excluded before laser vaporisation is contemplated.

Technique of Laser Vaporisation

When vaporising a CIN lesion, the operator must be conscious of one thing, namely the depth of destruction. In most centres the preliminary results of laser vaporisation were disappointing but analysis showed that these failures could be explained quite simply by the fact that the operator had not destroyed tissue to an adequate depth, thereby removing not only the CIN from the surface of the cervix but the CIN which had extended into the cervical crypts. Anderson and Hartley (1980) examined histologically the depth of crypt involvement in cone biopsy specimens and concluded that in $99\cdot8\%$ of patients with CIN the lesion did not extend to the crypts for more than 4 mm. Since it is obviously impossible to measure 4 mm with any degree of accuracy, the figure of 5–7 mm depth of destruction is offered as a good guide for the clinician.

The technique of laser vaporisation is straightforward. The laser is attached to an operating microscope and a spot size between 1·6 and 1·8 mm diameter is chosen. The lesion is outlined and gradually destroyed with the actual depth of destruction usually being measured by a simple measuring stick graduated in millimetres. The power density employed will vary between machines and surgeons but is usually between 500 and 1200 W/cm². In many instances it is possible to undertake treatment without any form of analgesia being used, but if the operator finds that some form of pain relief is necessary, then he has the option of injecting local anaesthetic directly into the cervix, in which case it is best to use a dental syringe employing a fine-gauge needle, with the needle being inserted into the cervix at four points outside the lesion: if this technique is used, most surgeons include a vaso constrictor mixed with the local anaesthetic. An alternative is a paracervical block using a local anaesthetic only. In some instances a general anaesthetic will be necessary particularly if the lesion is large and the patient apprehensive. Bleeding is occasionally a problem, but with skill can usually be overcome quite simply: occasionally it may be necessary to insert a cervical suture, and very rarely the patient will require admission for the bleeding to be dealt with on an inpatient basis. Postoperative bleeding necessitating hospital review will occur in about 1·5% of patients. This can usually be controlled with the application of silver nitrate or Monsel's solution, but from time to time it will be necessary to anaesthetise the patient to control the bleeding with a cervical suture. Bleeding after the first 48 h is extremely uncommon.

Technique of Laser Excisional Conisation

Destructive methods have not replaced cone biopsy entirely. Far from it! Cone biopsy is still mandatory if the lesion extends into the endocervical canal more than about 5 mm, if there is discrepancy between cytology, colposcopy and histology (in other words if any of these modalities suggest that there may be occult invasive disease) or if the cytology suggests that there may be an abnormal glandular lesion.

Cervical conisation is not without its complications and problematical bleeding has been reported as occurring in between 5·7% (Boutselis and Ullery 1964) and 20·3% (Hollyock and Chanen 1972). Postoperative cervical stenosis is also a problem and may lead to menstrual problems. Also because it may restrict access to the squamocolumnar junction, adequate follow-up examination by colposcopy and cytology may be impossible.

In an attempt to overcome these problems the CO_2 laser has been used to perform the conisation. Dorsey and Diggs (1979) reported a significant reduction in incidence in operative and postoperative haemorrhage. A reduction in cervical stenosis with easy assess to the squamocolumnar junction has been reported by Fenton et al. (1986). The procedure is best carried out under general anaesthesia with the patient in the lithotomy position. The usual haemostatic sutures are placed through the cervix laterally at 3 and 9 o'clock and as close to each lateral fornix as possible. A vasoconstrictor is then injected into the cervical tissue using a fine-gauge needle attached to a dental syringe. The cone can be cut by using either the laser attached to the operating microscope as for laser vaporisation, or by using a hand-held attachment at the end of the articulated arm of the laser. In either event the aim is to use a small spot size (0·5 mm) which allows a very high power density to be used (up to 2500 W/cm²). In this way, the cone can be cut very rapidly. The lesion should be outlined microscopically by the use of either acetic acid or Schiller's iodine solution. The ectocervical limits of the cone are marked out rapidly, with the laser beam allowing approximately 5 mm of normal tissue between the edge of the lesion and the line of incision. The laser should then cut a volume of tissue which is more cylindrical than the traditional cone shape. When the operator has cut the cone to the desired depth, he will then use a scalpel to cut the upper end of the biopsy. The power density is then reduced by enlarging the spot size and the surgeon then vaporises the apex of the defect. Still using the larger spot size with lower power density, as in vaporisation cone, he will then laser all of the cut surface of the defect to minimise haemorrhage. Most patients having this sort of procedure can be discharged home in 24–48 h. As mentioned above the intra- and postoperative haemorrhage rate seems to be reduced. Also at the first postoperative visit it will be seen that the cervix looks totally different from the usual cold knife conisation cervix in that there is minimal distortion, there is minimal cervical stenosis and the squamocolumnar junction is usually visible or at least accessible for cytological assessment.

Combined Vaporisation and Excisional Conisation

This is a technique which combines laser vaporisation with excisional conisation and is employed in those instances where for reasons already mentioned excision of the endocervical canal is thought to be necessary, but where the ectocervical lesion is very extensive, involving large areas of the ectocervix and occasionally the upper vagina. In these cases, provided there is no suspicion of invasive carcinoma, it is possible to treat the peripheral part of the lesion by simple vaporisation followed by removal of the endocervical canal by the excisional technique already described. This combined technique has given excellent results for patients who might otherwise have been treated traditionally by total abdominal hysterectomy, occasionally with upper vaginectomy (Wright 1984).

Follow-up After Laser Treatment for CIN

The healing process occurs extremely rapidly and scanning electromicroscopic studies of the healing epithelium (Jordan and Mylotte 1982) show that new squamous cells appear on the surface of the vaporised tissue within 8–10 days: this study also confirmed that any residual abnormal epithelium, usually in the crypts, will remain on the surface of the regenerating tissue during the healing process and can usually be recognised at the first follow-up visit. Most gynaecologists using this technique feel that there is little point in seeing the patient before 4 months and at that time the majority of patients with residual disease will be detected.

Treatment of Vaginal Intraepithelial Neoplasia (VAIN)

Vaginal intraepithelial neoplasia is asymptomatic and its presence is usually suspected by cytology or colposcopy. It usually occurs in conjunction with a pre-existing CIN and, less commonly, with vulval intraepithelial neoplasia (VIN) (Wade-Evans 1976). VAIN has the same colposcopic characteristics as CIN in that it is acetowhite with a punctation or mosaic vascular pattern and Schiller positive. When found in conjunction with CIN it is easy to detect but when it is present following a hysterectomy it may not be easy to localise because usually it is found in the vaginal angles at 3 and 9 o'clock and since there are often deep "pockets" of tissue in the angles it may be difficult to assess the full extent of the lesion.

For many years the traditional treatment of VAIN was partial or total vaginectomy or irradiation.

However, colposcopy allows the lesion to be identified and located and more recently laser vaporisation has changed the approach to this condition, the treatment to a large extent depending on the colposcopic findings.

Laser Vaporisation of VAIN When the Uterus is Present

In approximately 4% of patients with CIN, the lesion will extend off the cervix onto the vagina, and the gynaecologist then has the problem of how to treat the vaginal part of the lesion. Laser vaporisation has proved equally effective in the management of this type of lesion as it has in the management of CIN alone. The principles behind the use of laser vaporisation for the treatment of VAIN in association with CIN are of course exactly the same as those for CIN and detailed above. Having established that the lesion is premalignant the operator then has the problem of knowing how deep to vaporise. It has been established that laser vaporisation of CIN should be to a depth of 5–7 mm to take account of possible extension of CIN into the cervical crypts or clefts. Such a depth of destruction is unnecessary with VAIN because the subepithelial clefts in VAIN are relatively superficial and therefore a depth of destruction of 3 mm is enough to achieve adequate destruction. The spot size and power densities are identical for the treatment of CIN alone.

The operator must at all times be aware of the proximity of the rectum, bladder and occasionally urethra. If the patient is postmenopausal then the epithelium is often atrophic, in which case it may be prudent to give a 6-week course of oral oestrogen before treatment is carried out. If the VAIN coexists with CIN, as it usually does, then the cervical lesion must be treated on its merits either by laser vaporisation alone or by a combined vaporisation and excisional conisation technique or alternatively by hysterectomy. If it is the intention to perform a hysterectomy then it is tempting to remove a vaginal cuff at the same time, but an alternative, which is particularly attractive if the vaginal extension is quite extensive, is to vaporise the vaginal lesion and then, on a subsequent occasion, perform a hysterectomy without removal of vaginal tissue.

Laser Vaporisation of VAIN Following Hysterectomy

Hysterectomy has been the standard treatment for CIN for many years, particularly in North America, and follow-up studies have shown that subsequent VAIN occurs in between 0·9% and 6·8% of cases. Progression of this lesion to invasive malignancy has also been reported (Lee and Symmonds 1976). Traditionally the treatment of this problem has been surgical excision by partial or total vaginectomy with radiotherapy reserved for patients considered to be a poor operative risk. However, the morbidity associated with these procedures has encouraged the search for conservative forms of therapy. These have included the local application of antimitotic agents such as 5-fluorouracil (Woodruff et al. 1975) and the use of the laser.

The provisional results of laser vaporisation of VAIN following hysterectomy were good and the combined results of four series (Stafl et al. 1977; Capen et al. 1982; Townsend et al. 1982; Petrilli et al. 1980) suggested that it had been successful in 60 of 67 patients treated. However, this claim was based on limited follow-up, with only seven patients being followed for 12 months or more. More recently Woodman et al. (1984) showed that laser vaporisation was often inadequate treatment for VAIN following hysterectomy and that other methods should be considered. They presented 23 patients with VAIN following hysterectomy of whom laser vaporisation was used as the initial treatment in 14. Only 6 of the 14 lasered remained free of disease after a mean follow-up of 30 months. Not only were the results disappointing but two of those patients subsequently developed invasive carcinoma. They concluded that the poor results were due to a combination of two factors. First the period of follow-up was significantly longer than in previous case reports. Second, they commented on the problem of not knowing how much vaginal tissue was above the vaginal vault suture line following hysterectomy, i.e. it was impossible to say how much VAIN was buried above the vaginal vault and it was therefore impossible for the laser surgeon to decide during treatment how deep the laser vaporisation should be.

In conclusion, laser vaporisation for VAIN in conjunction with CIN is effective and particularly suitable for the majority of patients especially those who are young, sexually active and desirous of children. In the case of VAIN following hysterectomy, it is less effective but provided the restrictions mentioned above are borne in mind it should be considered: if it is then it is particularly important to ensure that representative biopsies are taken to exclude occult invasive carcinoma and usually this will mean biopsy under general anaesthesia.

Treatment of Vulval Intraepithelial Neoplasia (VIN)

Until recently VIN was usually diagnosed by its clinical appearances. The lesions vary tremendously, being white, grey, pink, dull red or any shade of brown, and may be small and sharply localised or cover the entire vulva and spread to the perineum and perianal areas. It is uncommon and the Third National Cancer Survey in the United States estimated the incidence rate for VIN was 0·53 cases per 100 000 white women (Hensen and Tarone 1977). It tends to occur in a slightly older age-group than CIN and Freidrich et al. (1980) estimated that the average age at diagnosis was 38 years. There is also a definite association between VIN and other malignancies. Freidrich et al. (1980) showed that 30% of patients with VIN had a malignancy at some other site and 20% had CIN. They also showed that there was a correlation between VIN and sexually transmitted diseases, with a sexually transmitted disease of any type occurring in 60% of cases, and condyloma accuminata in particular in 26% of cases.

Treatment can be very difficult particularly since the lesions are frequently multicentric but as with other premalignant diseases, treatment can be subdivided into methods which require local destruction and those which rely on surgical excision. If it is decided to perform local destruction then CO_2 laser vaporisation is the method of choice (Baggish and Dorsey 1980; Ferenczy 1983; Reid 1985–6). In all cases prior colposcopic assessment is essential.

The depth of destruction is just as important in the treatment of VIN as for CIN although much greater care must be taken. Dorsey (1985) pointed out that skin appendages (sebaceous glands, apocrine glands) empty directly into the epithelium through ducts and are composed of cells which have a special function but which are able to help in the re-epithelialisation of injured surface epithelium. These skin appendages usually penetrate to 8–10 mm below the surface. In Dorsey's original series of 35 cases, about 18% had demonstrable skin appendage involvement. Theoretically then the vulval skin should be lasered to a depth of 1 cm but this is associated with an unacceptably high morbidity with delayed healing and scarring.

Unfortunately, there is no standard depth of destruction as there is for the cervix and the operator must be fully cognisant of the anatomy of the epidermis, dermis and underlying fat and should learn to recognise the various layers as laser vaporisation takes place. This technique has been described in detail by Reid (1985a, b) and Reid et al. (1985). In general, one should aim to destroy the epidermis, the superficial papillary dermis and appendage ducts while leaving the entire reticular dermis and lower or glandular portion of the skin appendage intact (Dorsey 1985). In this way, the VIN will be removed while the ability for regeneration will be preserved.

The same principle applies whether the operator is removing one or more small lesions or doing a superficial skinning laser vulvectomy removing all of the vulval skin with or without some of the perianal skin. In the latter case of course healing is much more protracted but the results of either method are good provided the surgeon has an understanding of what he is doing as described above.

Treatment of Benign Conditions

Many conditions can be treated successfully with the carbon dioxide laser such as chronic cervicitis, cervical endometriosis, cervical stenosis following cone biopsy, adenosis and symptomatic cervical ectopies.

There is also one reported case of a capillary haemangioma being treated with the laser (Bellina et al. 1980): they described a large cervical haemangioma which was unresponsive to other treatments and which was being considered for treatment by hysterectomy. The ability of the laser to coagulate blood vessels was used to remove the tumour with minimal blood loss and maintenance of the structural and physiological integrity of the cervix.

It has also been used in patients with infertility due to poor sperm penetration thought to be secondary to cervicitis. The laser in this instance has been used to remove the inflammatory tissue involving the ectocervix and the lower part of the endocervical canal. All laser surgeons have reported unexpected incidences of pregnancy following this procedure but as yet there is no report which shows that the technique gives statistically significant results.

Human Papilloma Virus (HPV Infections)

The human papilloma viruses are a diverse group of site-specific oncogenic viruses. They induce benign epithelial tumours (warts) on susceptible epidermal or mucosal surfaces. Sexually transmitted papilloma viral infections are associated with a spectrum of disease ranging from benign warty proliferation through varying degrees of intraepithelial neoplasia and occasionally to invasive malignancy (Reid 1984). This infection can affect either the cervix, the vagina or the vulva and can present either as exophytic condylomatous or papillomatous lesions or as subclinical "microwarts" which are only visible following the application of acetic acid to the infected surface. It is important to remember that without treatment of any kind many of these lesions will disappear (Woodman et al. 1986). It must also be remembered that there is a very definite link between HPV infection and squamous neoplasia in the lower genital tract (Reid et al. 1982). Those lesions which do not resolve spontaneously are often suitable for treatment with topical caustic therapy but those infections which remain unresolved may pose a very difficult problem in management particularly when the infection involves a large area of vulva, perineal and perianal tissue. The carbon dioxide laser offers some hope for such patients by allowing the surgeon to perform a "superficial laser vulvectomy", which destroys the entire area of abnormal epithelium to a shallow depth so that rapid healing will occur from the keratinocytes in the underlying pilosebaceous glands (Reid 1985; Reid et al. 1985). Before undertaking such treatment, however, the surgeon must have convinced himself there is no associated intraepithelial neoplasia and must be, by any standards, an experienced laser surgeon who can exercise precise control over the depth of tissue destruction. Also, it should be remembered that the source of infection is usually the sexual partner and he should also be assessed for the presence of overt HPV infection.

If concomitant intraepithelial neoplasia has been excluded, then whether or not to treat will depend to a large extent on the site of the HPV infection and the symptomatology associated with it. If the disease is simply cervical or vaginal, and the patient is asymptomatic, then treatment is not mandatory. If, however, the infection involves the vulva then the patient may present with overt condylomatous lesions for which she requests removal: a small number of such lesions can usually be removed by laser vaporisation under local anaesthesia, but extensive areas will need general anaesthesia. There is, however, another, though less common, form of presentation, that in which the patient complains of burning or pain at the vulva following intercourse or micturition. While the vulva may appear clinically normal colposcopic examination of the vulval tissue following the application of 5% acetic acid for

1–2 min will often show the presence of "micro-papillae" typical of subclinical HPV infection. This subclinical infection should always be considered even in the presence of overt condylomatous lesions and should also be treated, otherwise the risk of reinfection is high. When present, a subclinical lesion usually involves quite large areas of the labia and must of necessity be removed under general anaesthesia.

When removing such lesions by laser vapor-isation it is particularly important to remember that if ablation is too deep then the surgeon will produce the equivalent of a third-degree burn with sub-sequent scarring. While this may not be a problem if it involves a very small area of the vulva, it is certainly a problem where large areas are involved. Since the vulvar epidermis is only $100–200\,\mu m$ thick, it is obvious that microscopic direction of the laser beam is imperative if the surgeon is to prevent the inadvertent destruction of too much tissue.

The small areas can safely be removed by using a large spot size ($1\cdot5–2$ mm) with a relatively low power density (in the region of $500\,\text{W/cm}^2$) but using this method the surgeon must remember that a large spot size with low power density produces adjacent thermal necrosis and makes control of the depth of destruction more difficult and can lead to inadvertent scarring. For large areas this method has obvious disadvantages and ideally the laser energy should be delivered for the shortest possible time which means using very high power densities. Using this technique the margin for error is rela-tively small, but if the technique is properly applied so that only the epidermis is removed then healing is rapid and the cosmetic result is excellent. However, it must never be forgotten that the tech-nique of skinning vulvectomy should only be used by those who have detailed knowledge of laser physics and whose knowledge of the anatomy of the vulva allows them, under colposcopic direction, to remove no more tissue than that which is required.

Herpes Simplex Virus Type II

This is a cutaneously induced viral infection which may present as a vesicular or ulcerative lesion of the vulva, vagina or cervix. It is increasing in inci-dence and poses a very difficult management problem both physical and psychological! As yet, there is no treatment for this disease although the vaccination programme described by Skinner et al. (1982) has reduced the incidence of reinfection and minimised the likelihood of a non-affected partner being infected. The use of laser vaporisation has

also been described (Bellina and Bandieramonte 1984; Baggish 1982). They advocate laser ablation of the vesicular eruptions which precede the ulcer-ative stage of the disease: by destroying the DNA core of the virus, they prevent migration of the viral particles of the dendritic processes to the dorsal root ganglion. This also removes some of the pain so typical of the early stages of herpes virus infection.

The virus is inactivated at 100°C. Because the viral pathology is in the superficial layers of the epidermis, once the virus has become associated with the dendritic process, the laser is obviously ineffective. They suggest using the laser with a large spot size (2–3 mm) with a very low power density in the region of $100\,\text{W/cm}^2$. Destruction should be very superficial otherwise the heat necrosis associ-ated with a large spot size and low power density may result in scarring.

The long-term effects of this method of treatment are not yet available and extreme caution should be used in applying it to the management of herpes infection in its acute stage.

Other Conditions of the Vulva

Occasionally patients with symptomatic vulval dys-trophy resistant to other forms of treatment will have symptoms which are such that some form of treatment is indicated, that treatment usually being a simple vulvectomy. Likewise a small group of patients have persistent pruritus vulvae for which no cause can be found and they also may be con-sidered for simple vulvectomy. However, skinning laser vulvectomy as described above offers an alter-native form of management. It must be stressed however, that all other, more conservative, forms of therapy should first be tried and that skinning vulvectomy should be regarded as a last resort. Also that while the initial results are almost always invariably good, long-term results vary and it may be necessary to repeat the procedure or to remove part of the superficial vulval skin 3, 4 or 5 years later. This, however, is not a contraindication to treatment in the first instance.

Endometrial Ablation with the Nd-YAG Laser

The Nd-YAG laser works at a different wavelength to the CO_2 laser and therefore has different properties. While on the one hand the CO_2 laser exerts its destructive effect at the point of impact, the Nd-YAG laser not only destroys at the point of impact but also penetrates the tissue, thereby exerting a destructive effect below the surface.

In the case of endometrium, it can be delivered through a fibreoptic cable through a hysteroscope and used to ablate the endometrium in patients with menstrual disorders. It destroys the endometrium down to the basalis layer and the superficial part of the myometrium. It was first used for this purpose in 1979 by Goldrath in the Sinai Hospital of Detroit (Goldrath et al. 1981). Goldrath's concept was to treat patients suffering from severe menorrhagia by using the Nd-YAG laser to photocoagulate and photovaporise the endometrium.

Patients are selected as being those who have a straightforward menstrual disorder for which hysterectomy has been advised. Preoperatively the patient should have a hysteroscopy and curettage and there must be no histological suggestion of malignancy or premalignancy. The operation is preceded by 4–6 weeks of endometrial suppression using Danol 200 mg tds.

The procedure is performed under general or epidural anaesthesia. The cervix is dilated to a diameter slightly larger than the hysteroscope so allowing the irrigating fluid to fall out of the uterus into the vagina and so provide a constant flow of fluid at low pressure to remove blood and gas bubbles from the operative field. The hysteroscope is inserted through the endocervical canal into the endometrial cavity with continuous flushing of the irrigation solution. Initially Goldrath used 70% dextran but dextrose saline will do just as well. The irrigation solution is injected through the hysteroscope by an assistant using 50-ml syringes. A vaginal pouch is used to collect the fluid which comes out of the uterus and drains over the perineum so that the operator and the anaesthetist know how much fluid is being injected and how much is being collected. The reason for this is that the "raw" endometrial surface following ablation allows absorption of some of the fluid into the patient's circulation. If this absorption is excessive then a diuretic such as Lasix should be given intravenously during the procedure. The operation takes 30–40 min in a normal size uterus and most patients can be discharged home within 24 h.

The operation is not an easy one to perform and in the foreseeable future it is probable that it will be carried out in no more than a few centres. However, it has a place, and in patients selected for treatment, good results can be expected in about 93% of cases.

Management of Infertility

Those properties which make the CO_2 laser useful in the treatment of premalignant disease of the lower genital tract can be utilised in the surgical treatment of infertility. Compared with conventional techniques, the advantages of the laser in infertility surgery include greater precision of application, an unobstructed operating field, sealing of smaller vascular channels (thereby reducing bleeding), minimal damage to adjacent normal tissue, reduced postoperative sequelae, reduced operative time, faster healing time and preservation of the reproductive, anatomical and sexual integrity of the patient (Bellina and Bandieramonte 1984). Those conditions which cause and contribute to infertility, such as endometriosis, tubal occlusion and adhesions, can now be treated with the CO_2 laser; it is proving particularly useful for adhesiolysis, fimbrioplasty, salpingostomy, tubal reanastomosis and cornual reimplantation. It must be stressed, however, that this method does not replace present microsurgical techniques; it is simply an adjunct to existing techniques. Before using the laser for infertility surgery, it is imperative that the surgeon is properly trained in microsurgery and is thoroughly familiar with the biophysics of the laser.

For adhesiolysis the surgeon will use power densities ranging from 2000 to 10 000 W/cm². This high-power density will result in minimal damage to adjacent tissue, but of course the procedure must always be carried out under microscopic control and damage to adjacent tissue can easily occur unless the operator is thoroughly familiar with what he is doing. Following division of the adhesions themselves, the serosal surface is then treated with a low power density of approximately 700 W/cm² to reduce postoperative adhesion formation. If the adhesions are under a structure such as the ovary, then the laser beam can be redirected using a front-silvered surface mirror.

The operations of fimbrioplasty and salpingostomy give particularly good results with laser treatment. Any adhesions are first freed as described above. The tubal ostia are identified either directly or by transillumination but if this is not possible, an artificial opening can be created with a small spot size using a high power density. The ostium is cannulated with a glass probe and transilluminated: radial incisions are then made in the serosal surface as vascular radiations are identified. A high power density is again employed, thereby utilising the ability of the laser beam to seal microcapillaries but at the same time causing minimal thermal injury to surrounding tissue. Arterioles greater than 1 mm in diameter may require high-frequency micro-coagulation. Following the radial incisions, the serosal surface immediately adjacent to the incisions are treated at very low power densities of 100–300 W/cm^2: this produces surface heating with tissue contraction thereby causing eversion of the tubal mucosa. If necessary three to four fine sutures can be placed, serosa to serosa, to assure eversion.

Tubal reanastomosis following sterilisation is becoming more and more common in gynae-cological practice and the laser is useful here also. The serosal layer is first vaporised with a power density of approximately 800 W/cm^2, thereby exposing the muscularis layer of the tube. This is then incised with a high power density small spot and then the mucosa itself is divided using fine scissors. Closure of the defect is then accomplished by microsuturing.

Cornual reimplantation is technically difficult under any circumstances and the results, as meas-ured in numbers of pregnancies, are relatively poor. Bellina (1986) describes the technique which has given him significantly better results than tra-ditional microsurgical techniques. He infiltrates the myometrium with Pitressin (1 ml of 1 in 2000 Pitressin in 5 ml normal saline). The uterine cavity is distended with hypertonic solution to compress the endometrium and absorb the exit laser energy. A cornual neo-ostium is created using a hand-held laser with a power density of approximately 100 000 W/cm^2. A cylindrical incision is completed and the excised myometrium submitted for histo-pathology. Intrauterine fluid pressure is reduced to stop the transabdominal flow. The diameter of the neo-ostium is enlarged to accommodate the distal tubal segment. The distal tubal site is prepared by vaporising the serosal surface with a power density of 800 W/cm^2. This process exposes the muscularis layer. The terminal tubal fibrotic cap is incised with a small spot and high power density to the mucosal level and the mucosa is incised using scissors or a knife. The distal tubal segment is transfixed into the cornual neo-ostium with microsutures, thereby allowing a mucosa-mucosa, muscularis-muscle and serosal-serosal closure.

The laser can also be employed for the operation of linear salpingostomy to remove an ectopic preg-nancy. The principle of treatment is exactly as described above, namely opening the tube with a high power density small spot. The gestational sac and blood clot are removed under microscopic control and the small bleeding points obliterated by using either the laser or cauterisation. The tube is then repaired with microsutures.

Endometriosis lends itself particularly to laser treatment. Deposits of endometriosis in the pouch of Douglas or other serosal surface are vaporised with a low power density. With care, this can also be used for endometriosis which is present on the surface of bowel or over large vessels. If there is concern about an underlying structure, then infilt-ration of the tissue underneath the deposits of endo-metriosis using saline injected by a fine needle will allow the laser energy to be absorbed completely by the saline. Deposits in inaccessible areas such as underneath the ovary can be reached quite simply using a reflecting mirror. Small endometriotic cysts of the ovary are treated by decapitating the cyst with an incision around the ovarian-endometrioma junction. The removed tissue is submitted for path-ology. The cavity of the endometrioma is then washed free of debris and the laser beam using a low power density of approximately 300 W/cm^2 is used to coagulate the internal walls of the endo-metrioma. It is not necessary to close the defect. Used in this way Bellina (1986) confirms that second-look laparoscopy has revealed the defect to close spontaneously and rarely to adhere to adja-cent structures. Larger endometriomas (greater than 2 cm) are treated in the same way but the defect is approximated using microsurgical sutures. Small implants on the ovaries are vaporised in the same way as those on serosal surfaces. Since the CO_2 laser usually leaves some degree of car-bonisation this should be thoroughly washed free prior to closure of the abdomen.

Finally, the laser has been used in the treatment of uterine anomalies (Bellina 1986) such as septal defects, bicornuate uterus, removal of small fibroids, removal of polyps within the lumen of the fallopian tube, treatment of bifid fallopian tube and defective fimbrial ovarica.

The carbon dioxide laser should not be regarded as the magical cure for infertility requiring surgery, but rather as an adjunct to existing methods. It is stressed, however, that the technique is only as good as the surgeon and that it should never be embarked upon without a pre-existing expertise in microsurgical technique and a knowledge of laser physics. If, however, these prerequisites are met then those who are using it claim that it has improved their results (Klink et al. 1978; Bruhat et al. 1979; Bellina and Bandieramonte 1984; Bellina 1986).

Laser Endoscopy

It was only a matter of time before a suitable delivery system allowed the CO_2 laser to be used through an endoscope. Bruhat et al. (1979) first described the use of the CO_2 laser through a laparoscope using a single-puncture technique and, later, Tadir et al. (1981) used a double-puncture technique. Both of these authors used a focused CO_2 laser beam. Several conditions lend themselves to treatment in this way. Endometriosis is obviously the first thing which springs to mind and the preliminary reported data are encouraging. Daniell and Pittaway (1982) reported their experience with patients treated for endometriosis, 20% of whom conceived within 6 months of follow-up. Kelly and Roberts (1983) reported a conception rate of 67% for treatment of mild endometriosis and 14% for moderate endometriosis with laparoscopic CO_2 laser treatment. Keye and Dixon (1983) performed photocoagulation of peritoneal implants with an argon laser delivered via a 600-μm flexible quartz fibre and claimed that this may be more effective than a CO_2 laser because of the selective absorption of the argon laser energy by the haemoglobin of the deposits of endometriosis.

The technique of salpingostomy at laparotomy has already been described but terminal salpingostomy using CO_2 laser and a laparoscope is now possible. The occluded fimbrial end is identified by hydrotubation and a radial incision made using a small spot size with high power density (10 000–30 000 W/cm^2) followed immediately by directing the defocused beam with low power density (1000 W/cm^2) along the margin of the incision, thereby causing retraction of the serosal flap and everting the fimbria.

Dysmenorrhoea is still a difficult problem to treat at times and Feste (1984) described a technique of using the CO_2 laser to destroy the Fragenheim ganglion in the uterosacral ligament, reporting a 73% moderate to marked decrease in dysmenorrhoea following the procedure.

The incidence of ectopic pregnancy has risen significantly in the recent past (Beral 1975). It is now possible to detect tubal pregnancy more quickly than in the past and laparoscopic treatment of tubal pregnancy has been reported by several authors (Bruhat et al. 1980; DeCherney et al. 1981; Shapiro and Adler 1973). Using a laparoscope it is technically possible to perform a linear salpingostomy followed by removal of the pregnancy mass. This is obviously an extremely difficult procedure to carry out and requires skill and expertise of the highest order. Small uterine fibroids can be removed by laser vaporisation using a defocused beam and low power density. It may be argued that this is unnecessary because such small fibroids are asymptomatic. On the other hand, large fibroids begin as small fibroids and the vaporisation of small fibroids visible at the time of laparoscopy for some other procedure will, undoubtedly, in some cases, prevent major surgery in the future.

Finally it is natural to think of the laser for sterilisation but while this is technically possible (Tadir et al. 1981) recanalisation can occur and at the moment other techniques of laparoscopic sterilisation would appear to be more suitable.

The Future

It is many years since any single development had such an impact on surgery as the laser. There are several types of laser each with its own special properties: as years go by others will be developed as will the delivery systems. However, whatever developments the future holds, it is not the lasers themselves which will produce the hoped for end point, but the quality and expertise of the person operating them. To those of us trained to use traditional surgical tools, the effect of the laser beam appears almost magical, but a knowledge of the underlying biophysics of each type of laser allows us to realise that the property of each beam is predictable and so is its effect on tissues. This knowledge is essential to anyone wishing to practise laser microsurgery; without it the effects can be disastrous but with it the effects can be all that a surgeon would ask for.

The key to laser microsurgery is therefore an understanding of the laser, an understanding of the clinical properties of the laser, proper patient selection, but above all to accept the laser as being yet another surgical tool which will allow the surgeon to do the best for his patient. It does not replace current surgical techniques; it is simply an adjunct to them.

References

Anderson MC, Hartley RB (1980) Cervical crypt involvement by intraepithelial neoplasia. Obstet Gynecol 55:546–550

Anderson MC (1982) Treatment of cervical intraepithelial neoplasia with the carbon dioxide laser: report of 543 patients. Obstet Gynecol 59:720–725

Baggish MS (1980) High power density carbon dioxide laser therapy for early cervical neoplasia. Am J Obstet Gynecol 136:117–125

Baggish MS, Dorsey JH (1980) CO_2 laser for the treatment of vulval carcinoma in situ. Obstet Gynecol 57:371–375

Baggish M (1982) CO_2 laser treatment of viral venereal disease. In: Atsumi K, Nimsakul N (eds) Proceedings, IV international congress of laser surgery. Tokyo, Japan, November 1981, Inter Group Corp, 1982, pp 13/10–13/11

Bellina JH (1974) Gynecology and the laser. Cont Obstet Gynecol 4:24–74

Bellina JH, Gyner DR, Voros JI, Raviotta JJ (1980) Capillary haemangioma managed by the CO_2 laser. Obstet Gynecol 55: 129–131

Bellina JH, Bandieramonte G (eds) (1984) Principles and practice of gynecologic laser surgery. Plenum, London, p 182

Bellina JH (1986) Tubal surgery. In: Sharp F, Jordan JA (eds) Gynaecologic laser surgery. Royal College of Obstetricians and Gynaecologists, London, pp 217–236

Bennett WR, Herriott DR, Javan A (1961) Population inversion and continuous optical maser oscillation in a gas discharge containing a He-Ne mixture. Phys Rev Lett 6: 106–110

Beral V (1975) An epidemiological study of recent trends in ectopic pregnancy. Br J Obstet Gynaecol 82:775–782

Boutselis JG, Ullery JC (1964) Intraepithelial carcinoma of the cervix in pregnancy. Am J Obstet Gynecol 90:593–609

Bruhat M, Mage C, Manhes M (1979) Use of the CO_2 laser via laparoscopy. In: Kaplan I (ed) Laser surgery III. Proceedings of the third international society for laser surgery, Tel Aviv, Ot-Paz, p 275

Bruhat MA, Mage C, Pouly JL (1979) Use of the CO_2 laser in neosalpingostomy. In: Kaplan I, Ascher PW (eds) Laser surgery, vol III, Part 1. Proceedings of the third international society for laser surgery. Tel Aviv, Israel, Ot-Paz, pp 271–273

Bruhat MA, Manhes H, Mage G, Pouly JL (1980) Treatment of ectopic pregnancy by means of laparoscopy. Fertil Steril 33: 411–414

Burke L (1982) The use of the carbon dioxide laser in the therapy of CIN. Am J Obstet Gynecol 144: 337–340

Capen CV, Masterson J, Magrina Javier F, Calkins JW (1982) Laser therapy of vaginal intraepithelial neoplasia. Am J Obstet Gynecol 142: 973–976

Daniell, JF, Pittaway DE (1982) Use of the CO_2 laser in laparoscopic surgery: Initial experience with the second puncture technique. Infertility 5:15

DeCherney AH, Romero R, Naftolin F (1981) Surgical management of unruptured ectopic pregnancy. Fertil Steril 35:21–24

Dorsey JH, Diggs ES (1979) Microsurgical conization of the cervix by carbon dioxide laser. Obstet Gynecol 54:565–570

Dorsey JH (1985) Understanding CO_2 laser surgery of the vulva. Colposcopy and gynaecologic laser surgery. 1, 3, 205–213

Einstein A (1917) Zur quanten Theorie der Strahlung. Phys Zeit 68: 121–122

Evans A, Monaghan J (1983) The treatment of cervical intraepithelial neoplasia using the carbon dioxide laser. Br J Obstet Gynaecol 90: 553–556

Fenton DW, Soutter WP, Sharp F, James C (1986) "A comparison of knife and CO_2 laser excisional cone biopsies". In: Sharp F, Jordan JA (eds) "Gynecologic laser surgery." Royal College of Obstetricians and Gynaecologists, London, pp 77–84

Ferenczy A (1983) Using the laser to treat vulvar condyloma acuminata and intraepidermal neoplasia. Can Med Assoc J 128: 135–137

Feste JR (1984) CO_2 laser neurectomy for dysmenorrhoea. Laser in Surg and Med 3:327 (Abstract)

Friedrich EG, Wilkinson EJ, Fu YS (1980) Carcinoma in situ of the vulva: a continuing challenge. Am J Obstet Gynecol 136

Goldrath MH, Fuller TA, Segal S (1981) Laser photovaporisation of endometrium for the treatment of menorrhagia. Am J Obstet Gynecol 140:14–19

Hensen D, Tarone R (1977) An epidemiologic study of cancer of the cervix, vagina and vulva based on third national cancer survey in the United States. Am J Obstet Gynecol 129: 525–532

Hollyock VE, Chanen W (1972) The use of the colposcope in selection of patients for cervical cone biopsy. Am J Obstet Gynecol 114:185–189

Jordan JA, Mylotte J (1982) Treatment of CIN by destruction—laser. In: Jordan JA, Sharp F, Singer A (eds) Preclinical neoplasia of the cervix. Royal College of Obstetricians and Gynaecologists, London, pp 205–211

Jordan JA, Woodman CBJ, Mylotte M, Emens JM, Williams DR, Macalary M, Wade-Evans T (1985) The treatment of cervical intraepithelial neoplasia by laser vaporisation, Br J Obstet Gynaecol 92: 394–398

Kelly RW, Roberts DK (1983) CO_2 laser laparoscopy. A potential alternative to danazol in the treatment of stage I and II endometriosis. J Reprod Med 28:638–640

Keye WR Jr, Dixon J (1983) Photocoagulation of endometriosis by the Argon laser through the laparoscope. Obstet Gynecol 62:383–385

Klink F, Brosspietzsh R, Klonzing LV, Endell W, Husstedy W, Oberheuser F (1978) Animal in vivo studies and in vitro experiments with human tubes for end to end anastomotic operation by a CO_2 laser technique. Fertil Steril 30:100–102

Lee RA, Symmonds RE (1976) Recurrent carcinoma in situ of the vagina in patients previously treated for in situ carcinoma of the cervix. Obstet Gynecol 48: 61–64

Maiman T (1960) Stimulated optical radiation in ruby masers, Nature 187: 493–494

Patel CKN (1968) High power carbon dioxide laser. Sci Am 219: 23–24

Petrilli ES, Townsend DE, Morrow CP, Nakao CY (1980) Vaginal intraepithelial neoplasia. Biologic aspects and treatment with topical 5-fluorouracil and the carbon dioxide laser. Am J Obstet Gynecol 138: 321–327

Pulanyi TG, Bredemeier HC (1973) Experimental carbon dioxide laser surgery of the vocal cords. Eye, Ear, Nose, Throat, Monographs 52:171–172

Reid R, Stanhope CR, Herschman BR, Booth E, Phibbs GD, Smith JP (1982) Genital warts and cervical cancer, I. Evidence of an association between subclinical papillomavirus infection and cervical malignancy; Cancer 50:377–373

Reid R (1984) Papillomavirus and cervical neoplasia. Modern implications and future prospects. Colp and Gynecol Laser Surg 1: 3–34

Reid R (1985a) Superficial laser vulvectomy, I. The efficacy of extended superficial ablation for refractory and very extensive condylomas. Am J Obstet Gynecol 151:1047–1052

Reid R (1985b) Superficial laser vulvectomy, III. A new surgical technique for appendage-conserving ablation of refractory condylomas and vulvar intraepithelial neoplasia. Am J Obstet Gynecol 152:504–509

Reid R, Elfont EA, Zirkin RM, Fuller TA (1985) Superficial laser vulvectomy, II. The anatomic and biophysical principles permitting accurate control over the depth of dermal destruction with the carbon dioxide laser. Am J Obstet Gynecol 152:261–271

Schawlow AL, Townes CH (1958) Infrared and optical masers. Phys Rev 42: 1940

Shapiro HI, Adler DH (1973) Excision of an ectopic pregnancy through the laparoscope. Am J Obstet Gynecol 117:290–291

Sharp F, Jordan JA (1986) The 15th Royal College of Obstetricians and Gynaecologists Study Group 1985—Gynaecologic laser surgery, RCOG, London

Skinner GRB, Woodman CBJ, Hartley CE, Buchan A, Fuller A, Durham J, Synnott M, Clay JC, Melling J, Wiblin C, Wilkins J (1982) Preparation and immunogenicity of vaccine Ac NFU$_1$ (S) MRC towards the prevention of herpes genitalis. Br J Ven Dis 58:381–386

Stafl A, Wilkinson EJ, Mattingly RJ (1977) Laser treatment of cervical and vaginal neoplasia. Am J Obstet Gynecol 128:128–136

Tadir Y, Kaplan I, Zuckerman Z, Ovadia L (1981) Laparoscopic CO_2 laser sterilisation. In: Semm K, Mettler L (eds) Human reproduction. Excerpta Medica, Amsterdam, p 429

Townsend DE, Levine RU, Crum CP, Richart RM (1982) Treatment of vaginal carcinoma in situ with the carbon dioxide laser. Am J Obstet Gynecol 143, 565–518

Wade-Evans T (1976) The aetiology and pathology of cancer of the vagina. Clin Obstet Gynaecol 3: 229–241

Woodman C, Jordan JA, Wade-Evans T (1984) The management of vaginal intraepithelial neoplasia after hysterectomy. Br J Obstet Gynaecol 91: 707

Woodman CBJ, Byrne P, Fung SY, Wade-Evans T, Jordan JA (1986) Cervical HPV infection—a self limiting disease? Colposcopy Gynecol Laser Surg 2:9–13

Woodruff JD, Parmley TH, Julian CG (1975) Topical 5-fluorouracil in the treatment of vagical carcinoma in situ. Gynecol Oncol 3: 124–132

Wright VC (1984) Laser surgery for cervical intraepithelial neoplasia. Acta Obstet Gynecol Scand Suppl 125:17–24

Section C:

POSTOPERATIVE

16 · Intensive Care and Resuscitation: A Medical and Surgical Overview

Julian M. Leigh and Philippa Keyes-Evans

Metabolic Response

The metabolic response to trauma has been well documented in the century or so following the first description of postoperative negative nitrogen balance by Bauer (1872). In general terms, it does not appear to be a wholly favourable adaptive response and, consequently, interest has also been shown in the possibilities of blocking or reversing it.

The response itself consists of disordered carbohydrate metabolism, salt and water retention, negative nitrogen balance and increased oxygen consumption.

The triggering mechanisms are various, and include soft issue trauma, haemorrhage, other types of fluid losses, severe illness, burns, sepsis and both pain and psychological stress.

Mediation seems to be integrated in the hypothalamus and the hormonal changes are summarised in Table 16.1. Humoral mechanisms involving kallikreinins and prostaglandins are also concerned in the initiation of the response.

The metabolic phenomena can be blocked in part or wholly during surgery by combinations of epidural or spinal analgesia, barbiturates, morphine, neuroleptanalgesia and adrenergic blocking agents.

Carbohydrate Metabolism

The interaction of catecholamines, growth hormone, cortisol and glucagon together with diminished insulin secretion and increased resistance to its peripheral activity cause hyperglycaemia and inhibit both the intracellular transfer and the metabolism of glucose (Hinton et al. 1971).

Mineralocorticoid secretion and altered renal perfusion have led Flear (1970) to suggest that the primary disturbance at cell membrane level consists of inhibition of the sodium pump. This would explain the intracellular sodium retention with extracellular hyponatraemia, the simultaneous

Table 16.1. Hormonal changes and effects during the metabolic response to trauma

Organ	Hormone	Effect
Pituitary: Posterior	↑ADH	Water retention, glycogenolysis
	↑Oxytocin	Vasoconstriction
Anterior	↑ACTH	↑Cortisol, ? ↑aldosterone
	↑GH	Insulin antagonism, ↑FFAs
Adrenal: Cortex	↑Cortisol	Permissive hyperglycaemia, ↑FFAs
	↑Aldosterone	Na retention, K lost in urine
Medulla	↑Catecholamines	CVS stimulation, hyperglycaemia
Pancreas: β-cells	↓Insulin	Hyperglycaemia
α-cells	↑Glucagon	↑FFAs, ↑liver glycogenolysis, ↑ACTH, ↑insulin, ↑GH
Thyroid	↑Thyroxine	Contributes to catabolism
Kidney	↑Renin and angiotensin	↑Aldosterone, sodium retention

opposite effects on potassium, and the consequent shifts in water. The potassium losses are also related to the increased nitrogen excretion.

Support for a single "biochemical lesion" in this area of intermediary metabolism is demonstrated by its inhibition by the glucose, potassium, insulin regimes advocated, for example, by Hinton et al. (1971).

Negative Nitrogen Balance

The balance between protein synthesis and destruction in the body obviously fluctuates but on average a steady state situation produces 8–12 g nitrogen excretion/day. The dietary nitrogen required for equilibrium is represented by the same amount. Calorie requirements are based on those of nitrogen with a ratio of approximately 200–250 calories/g nitrogen. Although a nitrogen deficit may be explained in part by inadequate intake of protein, anorexia and gastrointestinal failure (ileus), this does not explain the negative balance.

Part of the explanation is that there is a reorientation of protein synthesis. There is a shift towards production of fibrinogen and the immunological plasma proteins, and diversion of amino acids for increased leucocyte activity.

However, the explanation remains incomplete. From a clinical standpoint the patient appears to be catabolising protein as amino acids are broken down to provide intermediates for the Krebs cycle. This starts to occur after about 12 h, once the body stores of glycogen are used up. A 1-g nitrogen loss is equivalent to 6·25 g protein or 25–30 g lean muscle tissue. This process can be inhibited by glucose/insulin infusions, together with the administration of amino acid solutions. Parenteral nutrition in this way may be started on the second postoperative day if a patient is expected to starve for a long period; otherwise unnecessary expense is incurred. Protein catabolism takes precedence over the healing process and reduces the ability of defence mechanisms to inhibit infection. Fat is also catabolised at this time, causing a ketosis which is non-acidotic because the intermediates are still metabolised. The ketosis also has a useful inhibiting effect on catabolism.

During the recovery phase anabolism attains dominance and continues until the pre-insult state is reachieved.

In gynaecological patients, the catabolic response to trauma in routine clinical practice does not usually become significant enough to require the initiation of parenteral nutrition. If a regime is required, the solutions should be administered via a central venous line as they are, on the whole, hypertonic. A standard feeding regime is appended (Table 16.2).

If there is no ileus, which would be rare in the context of a severe catabolic response, then patients should be fed enterally via a nasogastric tube if normal eating is not possible.

Postoperative Deficits Following Routine Surgical Procedures

Patients who have an intravenous infusion commenced either prior to "major" surgery or for prophylactic reasons, e.g. prior to Caesarean section, and who are in a normal state of nutrition, merely have a free water deficit due to lack of drinking. Their first requirement, therefore, is that this should be made up and all i.v. infusions should be commenced with 1 litre 5% glucose/water. Blood should be given if necessary if losses attain 1 litre. Subsequently, balanced salt solution (as Hartmann's solution) on a 100 ml/h basis is reasonable for an adult. This regime may be continued for 24 h or so; the only additive that may be required is KCl which should be administered according to daily assessments of serum potassium. After 48 h parenteral nutrition may be started as indicated earlier.

Admissions to Intensive Care Unit

Our own Health District has three Consultant Obstetricians and Gynaecologists serving a population of 180 000. In the last 10 years, 28 cases were transferred to the intensive care unit (ICU) out of 40 034 total obstetrical and gynaecological admissions—an incidence of 7/10 000. Of these, 17 had surgical complications, an incidence of 4·3/10 000. These patients represent only those with the most severe problems requiring advanced resuscitation techniques and, of course, do not indicate the overall rate of complications in the cohort.

The precipitating causes of admission are summarised in Table 16.3.

Differential Diagnosis in the Collapsed Obstetrical and Gynaecological Patient

There are 14 patients in whom non-specific "collapse" might have made differential diagnosis

Table 16.2. Intravenous nutrition via a central venous catheter

Requirements for normal nutrition in the female:

CALORIES	30–40 cals/kg/day $\simeq$ 2000/day
NITROGEN	0·15–0·20 g N_2/kg/day $\simeq$ 10–14 g N_2/day $\simeq$ 60 g protein
WATER	40 cm/kg/day $\simeq$ 2·5–3 litres/day

These figures are raised by up to 50% in fever and severe trauma
Insensible water loss is 10 ml/kg/day $\simeq$ 700 ml/day, which increases by 10%/°C pyrexia
Normal kidney function will sort out a moderate excess of fluid intake
Additional requirements supplied by:

Parentrovite I and II daily	i.v.
Konakion (vit K) 10 mg daily	i.m.
Folic acid 15 mg twice weekly	i.v.
Neo-Cytamen (vit B_{12}) 500 μg monthly	i.m.

After 1 month, consider vitamin and trace element preparations Vitlipid and Addamel (10-ml vials added to Intralipid and Vamin Glucose twice weekly)

A regime for intravenous feeding might reasonably be A+B with one from C, D or E, depending on requirements. Commonsense should prevail

A	20% Intralipid 500 ml [a]	given together over 6–8 h	Supplying 2650 cals with 9·4 g $N_2 \simeq$ 60 g protein in 2 litres Na 50, K 20, Ca 2·5, Mg 1·5, Cl 55 mmol, essential fatty acids and phosphates
	Vamin glucose 500 ml		
	50% glucose 500 ml + 20 units sol. insulin	given together over 6–8 h	
	Vamin glucose 500 ml		
B	Hartmann's sol. 1000 ml	in 6–8 h	Na 131, K 5, Ca 2, Cl 111, HCO₃ 29 mmol. KCl supplement should be added according to daily requirements
C	Synthamin-17 500 ml	in 6–8 h	Supplying 8·25 g $N_2 \simeq$ 54 g protein, Na 36·5, K 30, Mg 2·5, acetate 75, Cl 35, phosphate 15
D	Glucose 20% 500 ml or Glucose 50% 500 ml	in 3–4 h	400 kcals Soluble insulin should be added to prevent 1000 kcals hyperglycaemia
E	Plasma protein fraction 400 ml Freeze dried plasma 500 ml Whole blood 200–500 ml (weigh bag to determine amount and bear in mind that SAG-M blood is now the commonest product supplied)	in 3–4 h	Given only if required Fresh frozen plasma may be needed for extra clotting factors

[a] The equivalent number of calories (1000) can be supplied in 500 ml 50% glucose at approximately one-seventh the cost.
Insulin at one unit per hour given subcutaneously should be given for its anabolic effect. Glucose levels should be monitored with BM sticks and a colorimeter; this is especially important if the energy administration regime is interrupted for other fluids

difficult, i.e. excluding the three patients with ileus/obstruction. In fact, all the haemorrhage cases were due to primary bleeding to the exterior—admission to the ICU being due to its intractable nature with the onset of resistant shock.

In the event that haemorrhage had been concealed, the chances that collapse in the post-operative obstetrical and gynaecological patient is due to septicaemic shock are 62·5%, with a 25% chance of haemorrhage being the main cause.

There was a 12·5% chance that the collapse was due to a myocardial infarction, but both patients who sustained coronary thrombosis had a previous history. The chance that coronary thrombosis is the cause of postoperative collapse, without a relevant previous history, is extremely small in obstetrical and gynaecological practice, bearing in mind also that the incidence of coronary thrombosis is three times higher in males than in females.

Although patients had had pulmonary emboli on the obstetrical and gynaecological wards during this 10-year period, their history and clinical features were classical. In the minor cases, there is no collapse anyway and the patients were treated on the ward. After massive pulmonary embolism, no case survived to reach the ICU.

Table 16.3. Obstetrical and gynaecological admissions to the intensive care unit in a 10-year period

Diagnosis	History	Deaths
Planned admission (3)	Hysterectomy in an unstable epileptic	
	Pelvic exenteration	
	Repair of ruptured diaphragm in second trimester	
Anaesthetic complications (4)	Aspiration during induction (1)	
	Failure to breathe following intra-abdominal surgery (3)	
Severe eclampsia (2)	Postpartum renal failure	
	Fulminating pre-eclampsia	
Coronary thrombosis (2)	Cardiomyopathy and hysterectomy for malignancy	Death
	Severe hypertension and gross obesity. Laparotomy and sterilisation: failed to breathe postoperatively. Cardiac arrest	Death
Haemorrhagic shock (4)	Ectopic (1)	
	Lower segment Caesarian section (3)	
Septicaemic shock (10)	Posthysterectomy (5)	
	Post—lower segment Caesarian section	
	—Dilatation and curettage	
	—Spontaneous abortion and evacuation of retained products: cerebral haemorrhage and DIC	Death
	—appendicectomy and premature labour with faecal peritonitis	
	—hysterectomy with clostridial bowel infarction	Death
Ileus (1)	Electrolyte imbalance following hysterectomy	
Intestinal obstruction (2)	Posthysterectomy	

It is noteworthy that during this period the patient who died from gut infarction and septicaemic shock mentioned above was diagnosed initially as pulmonary embolism. Collapse in this patient occurred 3 days postoperatively and was, therefore, not typical of pulmonary embolism.

Another case died before reaching the ICU after normal delivery following previous Caesarean section. This patient was initially diagnosed as having supraventricular tachycardia and disseminated intravascular coagulation—she in fact had a ruptured uterus. Clearly medical causes of collapse should not be diagnosed until surgical causes have been totally excluded.

Differential Diagnosis

It would be reasonable to conclude that the differential diagnosis in the collapsed obstetrical and gynaecological patient lies between:

Septicaemia—abscess formation
           —gut leakage
Haemorrhage—slipped ligature ⟨reactionary / primary
Coronary thrombosis
Pulmonary embolism

Less common—biliary colic
           —peptic perforation
           —acute pancreatitis
           —dissecting aortic aneurysm
           —intestinal obstruction and inadequate fluid replacement
           —superior mesenteric artery thrombosis

Faced with a hypotensive shutdown and oliguric patient, how should the clinician arrive rapidly at the diagnosis? It is imperative that there should be a high index of suspicion and a willingness to accept a surgical complication as the diagnosis rather than to espouse a medical cause of collapse.

Symptoms and Signs

The type of surgery performed and the possibility of bleeding, together with significant events in previous history, such as ischaemic heart disease, form the background on which to build the pathway to diagnosis.

The timing of the collapse in relation to the surgical intervention is important. Collapse from endotoxic shock can follow within a very short time of, for example, instrumentation of the urethra, but its occurrence can be at any time in the postoperative period. A rigor may be a presenting feature in septicaemic shock and would indicate the diagnosis from the outset. Primary surgical haemorrhage usually manifests itself well within the first 12 h. In gynaecological practice, haemorrhage may present as vaginal bleeding or as steadily increasing lower abdominal distension, with a rising pulse rate and a falling blood pressure. This may initially be improved by restoration of blood volume, but again will subsequently deteriorate, unless surgical intervention occurs. If haemorrhage is concealed, the most apparent difference from other causes of collapse or shock is the waxen appearance of the lips and mucous membranes of the gums. In both myocardial infarction and pulmonary embolism, the features tend to be blue or grey. However, the pulmonary embolism patient is typically beset by agitation, while the patient with severe myocardial infarction and shock has a resigned attitude.

Pain

One of the most helpful indices, on taking a history from the patient, is the character and distribution of any pain. The pain of myocardial infarction is characteristically central and crushing or vice-like and may radiate to either arm or jaw. In pulmonary embolism, there may be no pain at all, or, if it does occur, it is lateralised and pleuritic in nature. Chest pain is invariably absent, when there is either intra-abdominal sepsis or haemorrhage and, indeed, any guarding, pain and tenderness may be elicited by abdominal, pelvic or rectal examination.

The pain of a perforated peptic ulcer has a characteristic distribution in the upper central hypochondrium. However, it is unusual for these patients to be grossly shocked.

Pain and indeed septicaemia may follow gall bladder colic and cholecystitis. The incidence of gall bladder symptoms should be sought from the patient and stones may be present on the abdominal X-ray. Pain radiating through to the back would assist in establishing the gall bladder as a source of problem, if other characteristic features of the main diagnoses are not present. Similar pain could also be caused by acute dissection of the thoracic aorta. However, this is an extremely rare event in a female. Also, theoretically, pericarditis might be a cause but the patient should also exhibit a pericardial rub on auscultation and possibly the signs of cardiac tamponade.

The pain in superior mesenteric artery thrombosis is severe and persistent and will be accompanied by physical signs in a patient with auricular fibrillation and known atherosclerosis. There is repeated vomiting, facial pallor and fall in systolic blood pressure. Abdominal rigidity is a late sign. Rebound tenderness may be present and in late stages the patient may pass blood per rectum. On X-ray gas is usually completely absent from the small bowel.

The pulse rate is rapid in haemorrhagic shock, usually rapid in septicaemic shock and may be slow, rapid or unchanged in both myocardial infarction and pulmonary embolism.

The *temperature* may be raised in septicaemic shock but this is *often* not the case. A small rise in temperature does occur also in myocardial infarction.

The *jugular venous pressure* is unequivocally lowered in haemorrhagic shock and may be raised in the other three. Characteristically, however, the patient with pulmonary embolism can lie flat, whereas in severe myocardial infarction the patient cannot lie flat. Both the latter may have a cough. In myocardial infarction the patient may cough up frothy pink sputum, whereas in pulmonary embolism the sputum will be normal in consistency but blood stained. Auscultation in cardiogenic shock may reveal crepitations at the lung bases and a third heart sound or a gallop. In pulmonary embolism, initially there will be no chest signs, though bronchial breathing may develop later if there is a pulmonary infarction. However, a right sternal edge fourth heart sound may be heard.

Haemorrhagic shock itself is not usually associated with sputum production. A patient with septicaemic shock may have greenish coloured sputum if the septicaemia originates from a lung infection.

Investigation

A chest X-ray which shows bats-wing pulmonary oedema (Fig. 16.1) would fit in with left ventricular failure associated with cardiogenic shock. A picture of widespread patchy infiltration may be consistent with the "shock lung" syndrome (Fig. 16.2), associated with septicaemic shock, or, if there is a consolidated patch with an air bronchogram, this may be consistent with a focus of lung sepsis associated with septicaemia. The chest X-ray in haemorrhagic shock will probably be normal and in pulmonary embolism may be unaffected unless a pulmonary infarction occurs later on.

An erect abdominal or lateral decubitus X-ray may show free gas (Fig. 16.3) if septicaemia is associated with gut perforation or may show pelvic collections of gas, if gas-producing anaerobic abscesses are present. Gut fluid levels with ileus may be present in all the named conditions.

The *electrocardiogram* is an important inves-

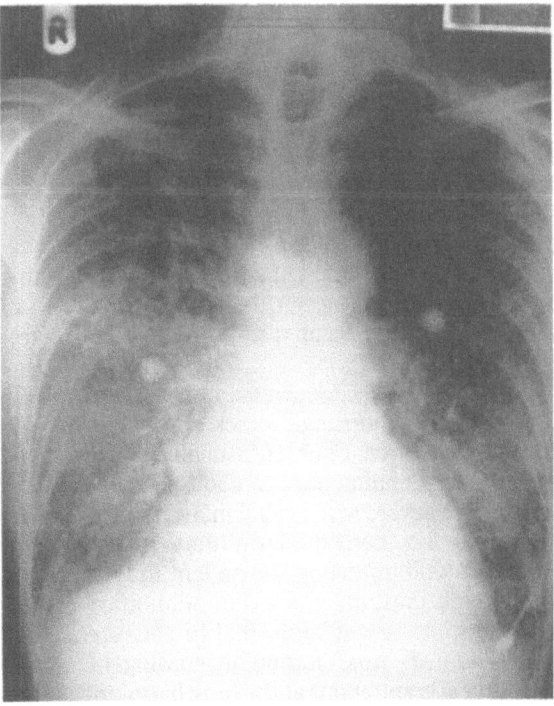

Fig. 16.1. Chest X-ray in acute left ventricular failure: bat's wing pulmonary oedema is present. The X-ray appearance is invariably asymmetrical, as shown here, and may mislead the unwary into diagnosing a unilateral pneumonia.

tigation to assist in these cases. However, it is important to recognise that generalised ischaemic ECG changes can occur when the hypotension is not in fact due to myocardial infarction but merely due to myocardial hypoxaemia. Such changes disappear completely within hours of successful treatment.

Initially in myocardial infarction ST segment changes occur with elevation in the leads which overlie the damaged areas of myocardium. If there is full-thickness myocardial infarction then Q-waves develop in the relevant leads. It is usually assumed that a pathological Q-wave must be more than 0·4 s in duration and more than 25% of the succeeding R-wave. It is important to realise that Q-waves do not appear until muscle necrosis occurs and may be delayed for some hours.

If the infarction is anterior then the most affected leads are I, AVL and the chest leads; in anteroseptal infarction the early chest leads show the maximal changes (Fig. 16.4); if the infarction is anterolateral then V4 to V6 demonstrate the main effects; and on some occasions extensive infarction may be manifest in all the anterior chest leads. In inferior infarction the main changes are in leads II, III and AVL (Fig. 16.5).

In pulmonary embolism the ECG changes are characteristic (Fig. 16.6). There is right axis deviation and, with the onset of right ventricular strain,

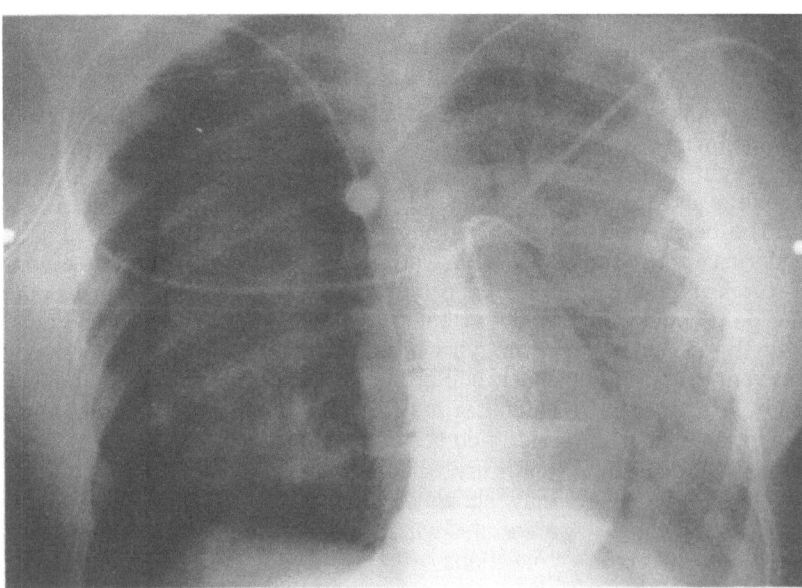

Fig. 16.2. Shock lung syndrome: chest X-ray of a teenage girl showing a pneumothorax on the right and a chest drain in place. A Swan–Ganz catheter has been passed via the right subclavian vein into the left pulmonary artery for monitoring and measurement.

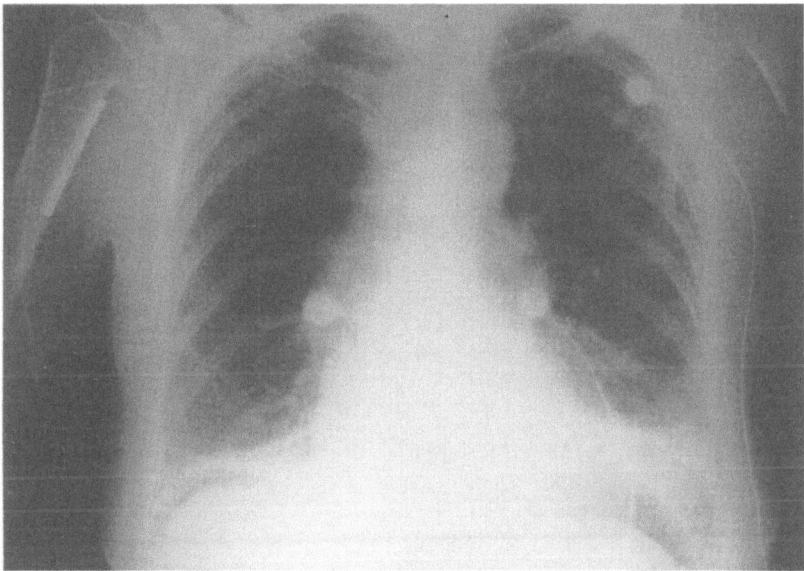

Fig. 16.3. Gas under the diaphragm: in this erect chest X-ray, the presence of free gas can be seen under both domes of the diaphragm following perforation of the duodenum.

the development of an S-wave in lead I, a Q with an inverted T in lead III, and T-wave inversion in V1 to V3. There is a pronounced atrial wave (P pulmonale) and right bundle-branch block.

Enzyme Changes

A rise in the serum creatinine phosphokinase (CPK) starts to occur 6 h after myocardial infarction and

Anterior infarction

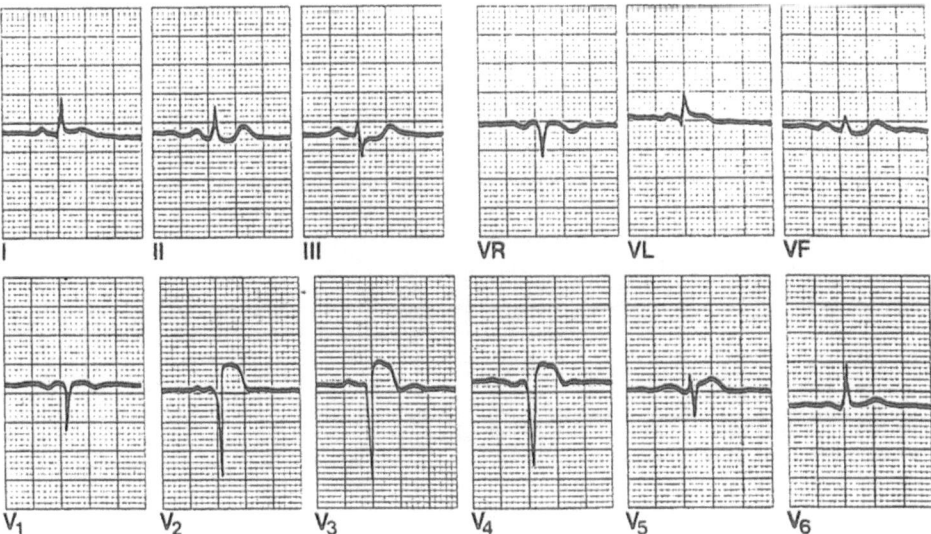

Fig. 16.4. ECG to show anterior myocardial infarction.

ACUTE MYOCARDIAL INFARCTION

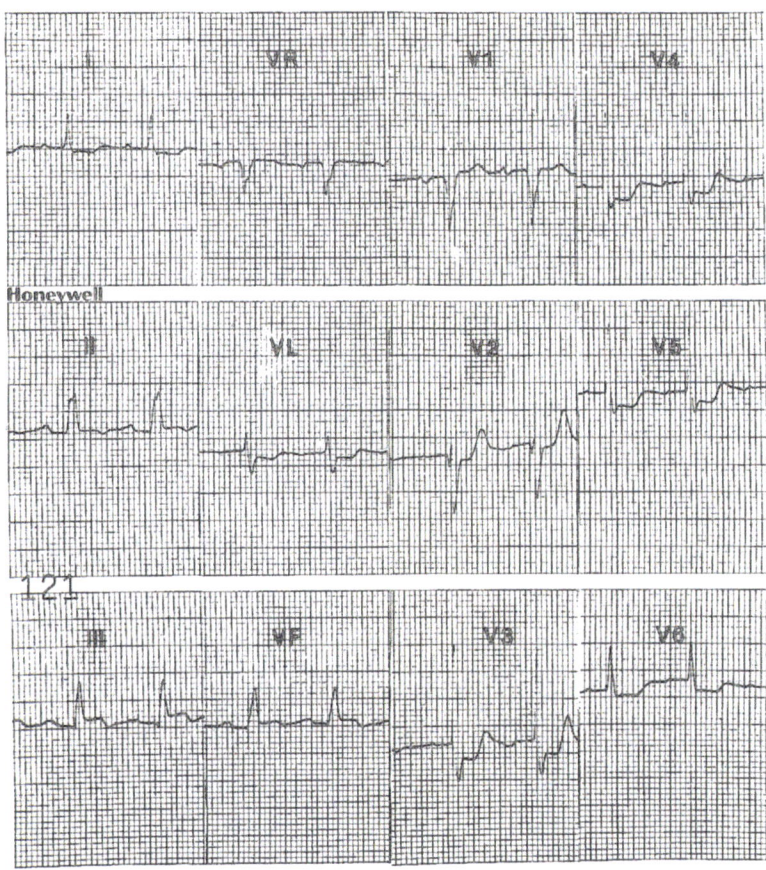

Fig. 16.5. ECG to show acute inferolateral myocardial infarction.

Pulmonary embolus

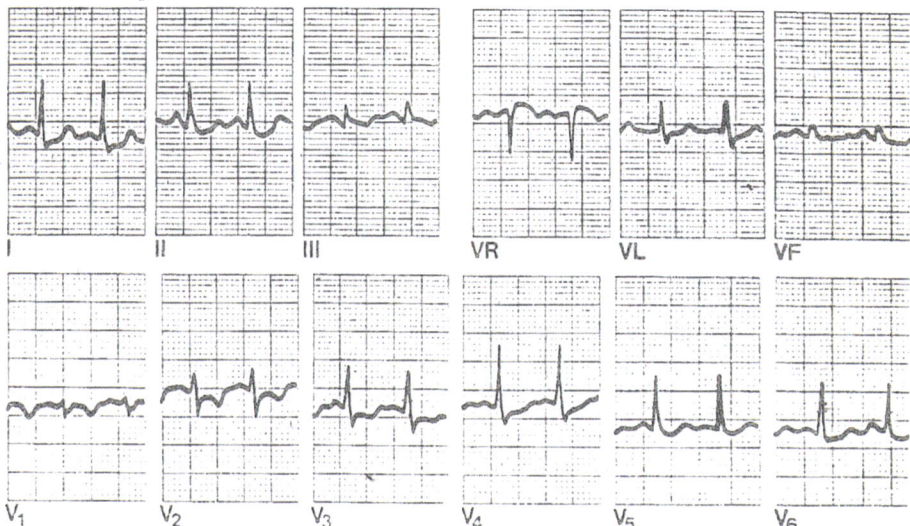

Fig. 16.6. ECG in the presence of pulmonary embolus.

reaches a peak in about 24 h, whereas in pulmonary embolism a small rise occurs. Another isoenzyme, CPK-MB, which is said to be specific for the myocardium, may prove invaluable in the future but is still not as totally specific as was hoped. SGOT (aspartic aminotransferase) rises after 12–24 h while lactic dehydrogenase (LDH) rises after 72 h. Acute pancreatitis is confirmed by a raised serum amylase level.

The *white cell count* is of little use in differential diagnosis. In septicaemic shock it may not be significantly raised over that found in other postoperative patients.

Direct Central Venous Pressure Measurements

A CVP line will be a further aid in diagnosis. The catheter is inserted via the subclavian vein, usually approached infraclavicularly and connected to a saline manometer zeroed at the level of the right atrium. This will certainly enable the accurate detection of the low CVP of haemorrhagic shock and thereafter enable monitoring of the response to transfusion. The CVP is often lowered in septicaemic shock also. By contrast, the CVP will be raised in pulmonary embolism and is usually raised in cardiogenic shock.

Treatment

Immediate

If the patient appears to have myocardial infarction then she will be taken over by the appropriate team. However, initial management should consist of pain relief with diamorphine, which is a vasodilator besides being a narcotic analgesic. In pulmonary embolism full heparinisation should be commenced immediately.

In haemorrhagic shock initial resuscitation should be by colloidal infusions, such as Haemaccel or Hespan, while awaiting cross-matched blood and at the same time organising surgical intervention.

In the event of the most likely diagnosis, i.e. endotoxic shock, management is aimed at initial definitive diagnosis, very early medical treatment and delayed surgical intervention.

Initially, two samples of blood should be drawn under sterile conditions and inoculated into culture medium and sent for incubation. Then antibiotics must be commenced immediately with metronidazole 1 g intravenously, gentamicin 120 mg and amoxycillin 1 g. This regimen will cover Gram-negative rods, staphylococci and haemolytic streptococci. Fluid therapy with Haemaccel or HPPF should be commenced in order to bring up central venous pressure and improve renal perfusion. Steroids in the form of methylprednisolone, 30 mg/kg, should be given initially and every 6 h thereafter for 24–48 h to combat the effect of endotoxin which will persist in the circulation even following bacterial destruction.

The bladder should be catheterised and if there is oliguria then dopamine should be administered in "nephrogenic" doses, i.e. 3–5 μg/kg per hour. Surgery must then be contemplated, e.g. to drain pus from the abdomen or rectify soiling from gut spillage and secure the leak(s) as appropriate. All these patients are prone to develop acute renal failure unless renal perfusion is ensured. While diuretics are appropriate in severe myocardial infarction, the use of dopamine as above as a prophylactic measure, even in the absence of oliguria, is advisable.

Supportive Measures

In the circumstances under discussion oxygen therapy will benefit all groups. If the patient is in severe pain then it is cruel to withhold analgesics, even if final diagnosis might not yet have been made. Short-acting drugs, such as diamorphine or fentanyl, can be used at this stage, given in small doses intravenously. Patients in extremis from the causes discussed pass rapidly into respiratory failure and should be intubated and undergo intermittent positive pressure ventilation. All of them should naturally be transferred to ICU.

Management of Disseminated Intravascular Coagulation

If it is considered that haemorrhage is in fact associated with disseminated intravascular coagulation (DIC), the occurrence of this syndrome should be confirmed in the laboratory by measuring levels of fibrin degradation products in the serum. Fresh frozen plasma should be given to remedy the deficit and a metronidazole/gentamicin regime commenced as bacterial infection is a main factor in triggering this response. Heparinisation has now largely been abandoned in the management of this condition.

Extreme Emergency Situations

When the situation is rapidly deteriorating and the differential diagnosis between cardiac infarction, pulmonary embolism and septicaemic shock is unclear, then the regime outlined above for the immediate treatment of septicaemic shock *must* be initiated. Such a step will not further harm the infarct or embolism patient but will produce dramatic improvement in the septicaemic patient. The longer the delay the worse the outlook in the latter condition with the onset of multiorgan microcirculatory failure and its consequences, shock lung syndrome (ARDS), acute renal failure, etc. We have been very thankful on a number of occasions that this approach had been adopted.

References

Bauer J (1872) Ueber die Zersetzungsvorgänge im Thierkörper unter dem Einflusse von Blutentziehungen. Z biol 8:567–585

Flear CTG (1970) Electrolyte and body water changes after trauma. J Clin Path [Suppl] 23 (4):16–31

Hinton P, Allison SP, Littlejohn S, Lloyd J (1971) Insulin and glucose to reduce catabolic response to injury in burned patients. Lancet i:767–769

Suggestions for Further Reading

Beal JM (1982) Critical care for surgical patients. Macmillan, New York

Tinker J, Rapin M (1983) Care of the critically ill patient. Springer, Berlin Heidelberg New York

17 · Intestinal Complications and How To Cope

Michael Knight

Normal Bowel Management Following Gynaecological Surgery

After any abdominal operation there follows a period during which bowel activity is at a minimum and bowel sounds cease. The mechanism of this intestinal inhibition is sympathetic overactivity stimulated by manipulation of the bowel during surgery. This adynamic period is transient and lasts for about 24 h after which time intestinal activity and bowel sounds return. During this period of transient ileus it is sensible to avoid feeding the patient and to restrict the oral intake of fluid. Although bowel sounds return after 24 h, the normal propulsive action of the intestine takes a little longer and it is not unusual for the passage of rectal flatus to be delayed for 2–3 days. The first stool is passed a few days later and is usually liquid or loose in consistency, probably a result of fluid accumulation in the bowel during the adynamic phase. These "milestones" are brought forward if the patient receives a rectal suppository or an enema. In the normal course of events it is not necessary to stimulate the bowel in this way but in patients known to have a sluggish colon pre-operatively, the accumulation of bowel gas in the postoperative period can cause abdominal discomfort and occasionally distress and it is in these patients that suppositories and enemas are most helpful. It should be remembered, however, that such stimulation can and does put a considerable strain on any bowel anastomosis and should be avoided in the early days after gut resection for fear of dehiscence.

Intestinal Complications Following Gynaecological Surgery

These are classified into minor and major:

Minor

Wound infection

Wound infection can occur after any abdominal operation but is particularly likely if the intestine has been opened inadvertently or electively during the procedure. Such infection usually presents as an area of erythema somewhere along the line of the incision 4–5 days after the operation. If there is no spontaneous discharge of pus and the area of erythema progresses to a swollen cellulitis, the overlying sutures should be removed and the wound gently probed to release any pus. Having established free drainage, the area of cellulitis rapidly settles without antibiotics, although it is a wise precaution to send a wound swab to the laboratory for bacteriological culture.

Haemorrhoids

It is not uncommon for patients with pre-existing haemorrhoids to develop troublesome perianal complications in the postoperative period following gynaecological operations. The more common of these include anal discharge and perianal skin irritation, prolapse and occasionally thrombosis of a haemorrhoid. The usual cause of these complications is an increase in intra-abdominal pressure during the adynamic ileus phase and straining by the patient in an attempt to defaecate. Attention should therefore be turned to treating the abdominal distension as well as the haemorrhoids, which usually regress after resolution of the ileus. In the meantime, the application of bland creams such as Anusol will give local relief. Steroid and local anaesthetic creams should be avoided as they may cause perianal skin complications. Prolapsed haemorrhoids should be treated conservatively in the first instance by gently replacing them with a gloved hand and maintaining the patient recumbent with the foot of the bed raised. Thrombosed haemorrhoids may require formal excision under general anaesthesia.

Major

Prolonged Ileus

After extensive surgery and prolonged anaesthesia, the return of intestinal activity may be delayed for several days, during which time gas and fluid accumulation in the adynamic bowel can cause not only gross abdominal distension and respiration difficulties but also salt and water depletion which can threaten the patient's life. Other factors which predispose to prolonged ileus include hypokalaemia, congested and oedematous bowel and surgical sepsis. It is therefore important to correct any electrolyte imbalance pre- and postoperatively and to be aware that any delay in the return of intestinal activity beyond 1 week usually indicates the presence of surgical sepsis or mechanical obstruction.

During the period of adynamic ileus no fluid should be taken by mouth and the stomach should be kept empty by nasogastric aspiration. Intravenous fluids and electrolytes should continue until normal bowel activity returns, when oral fluids may be resumed. Intravenous feeding will be required if the ileus is prolonged into the second postoperative week in the absence of sepsis of other surgically correctable cause.

Peritonitis

Peritonitis results from the presence of an irritant in the peritoneal cavity. The irritant may be blood, urine or any substance normally present in the gastrointestinal tract, e.g. gastric, duodenal and intestinal juice, pancreatic exocrine secretion, bile or faeces. Other causes include foreign bodies and the bacterial contamination from salpingitis or other septic foci in the pelvis. The peritoneum reacts to such irritants by exuding a fluid rich in fibrin which acts as an adhesive to adjacent loops of intestine and greater omentum. In this way the body attempts to wall off and localise the source of irritation, which, if successful, results in resolution of the peritonitis. If this defence mechanism fails, however, and pathogenic bacteria gain access to the area and multiply, an abscess will result which, untreated, may lead to a generalised peritonitis, septicaemia and death. Clinically, peritonitis presents with abdominal pain and vomiting associated with abdominal tenderness, guarding, rebound tenderness and eventually rigidity. The patient becomes ill with a tachycardia and quickly develops dehydration. As bacterial infection supervenes, the abdomen distends due to local or general ileus and the patient's general condition deteriorates with an increasing pulse rate and fever, hypotensive shock, renal failure and, in the final stages, the Hippocratic facies may be seen.

Peritonitis is essentially a clinical diagnosis, relying very little on investigations or imaging techniques. In the early days after an operation, the diagnosis may be extremely difficult because of the normal tenderness of a postoperative abdomen, but increasing tenderness and guarding associated with a rising pulse rate and dehydration should alert the surgeon to the possibility of peritonitis. Abdominal X-rays are generally unhelpful in the early postoperative period as they will reflect the normal consequences of an abdominal operation with distended gas-filled bowel, fluid levels from adynamic ileus and free air in the peritoneal cavity which has not yet been reabsorbed following open surgery. A peritoneal needle aspiration may be more helpful and is occasionally diagnostic if pus, urine or intestinal contents are discovered free in the peritoneal cavity.

The treatment of peritonitis is that of the underlying cause which in most instances is perforation of the bowel or an intra-abdominal abscess or both. The patient is resuscitated with plasma expanders, if hypovolaemic shock is a feature, and given intravenous broad-spectrum antibiotics after blood has been sent to the laboratory for culture. After rehydration and correction of any electrolyte imbalance the patient is operated upon as an emergency under general anaesthesia unless there is an absolute contraindication, e.g. a moribund patient, or if there is good evidence of localisation of the peritonitis. At operation there is usually no difficulty in identifying and dealing with the cause of the peritonitis, e.g. drainage of an abscess, closure or resection of a perforated viscus, or in the case of dehiscence of a large bowel anastomosis to bring the proximal end out as an end colostomy closing the distal end or bringing the distal end to the surface as a mucus fistula. Drains are positioned to allow any residual irritant free access to the exterior.

Intestinal Obstruction

Like peritonitis, the diagnosis of intestinal obstruction can be extremely difficult in the early postoperative period because the classical features of abdominal pain, vomiting, absolute constipation and abdominal distension so closely resemble those which naturally occur following surgery. It is essential, however, to make the diagnosis at the earliest possible moment because the mortality rises with every hour of delay. In general, increasingly severe colicky abdominal pain is not a feature of the normal postoperative period and should arouse the suspicion of intestinal obstruction, particularly if associated with high-pitched bowel sounds, abdominal tenderness localised at a distance from the wound, an increasing tachycardia and abdominal X-rays which show not the generalised gaseous distension of adynamic ileus but localised distension of the intestine above a contracted distal bowel (Fig. 17.1).

Intestinal obstruction is classified into simple obstruction, strangulated obstruction and functional obstruction and all of these can occur after gynaecological surgery. Simple obstruction without impairment of blood supply may occur early in the postoperative period from fibrinous adhesions or later by fibrous adhesions. Occasionally the obstruction results from herniation of a small bowel loop into a partially dehisced abdominal wound or through a defect in a reperitonealised pelvic floor or the lateral space following end colostomy. In all of these instances strangulation will occur if the blood supply to the obstructed bowel is occluded. Strangulation in turn leads to ischaemic necrosis of the bowel wall, perforation and peritonitis.

Functional obstruction following gynaecological surgery is usually due to paralysis of the intestine resulting from intra-abdominal abscess formation.

The treatment of postoperative intestinal obstruction depends upon the condition of the patient and

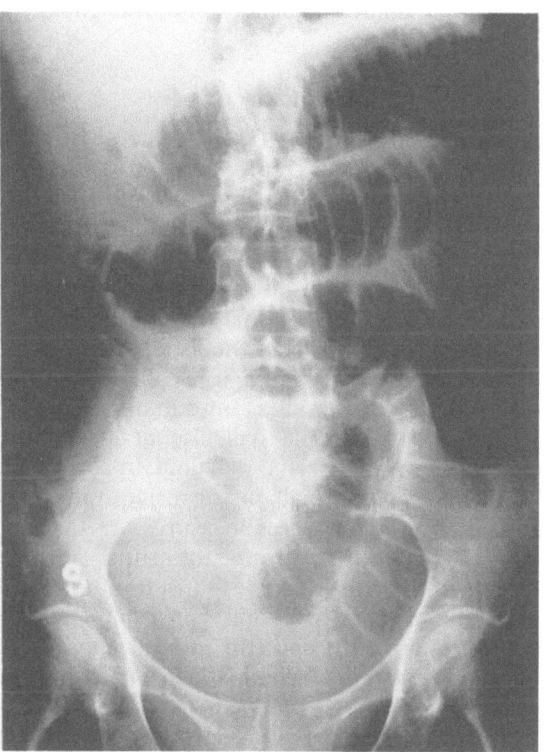

Fig.17.1. Plain supine abdominal radiograph showing loops of distended gas-filled small bowel due to obstruction.

the type of obstruction. Patients showing features of strangulation, e.g. continuous pain, tachycardia, extreme localised tenderness and guarding, should be operated upon as an emergency as soon as they have been rehydrated and their general condition allows. Patients with a simple occlusion or large bowel obstruction without signs of strangulation can be prepared for up to 12 h before the surgery necessary to relieve the obstruction. Functional obstruction is dealt with according to the underlying cause, e.g. pelvic abscess.

Fistulae

A fistula is an abnormal communication between two epithelial surfaces. An intestinal fistula may be internal, e.g. ileocolic or external in which the intestinal contents are discharged completely or incompletely onto the skin surface or into the vagina. It is a surgical maxim that a fistula will close spontaneously if there is nothing to keep it open. Conditions which keep a fistula open include distal obstruction, disease or foreign body in the fistula track and epithelialisation of the track, e.g. a colostomy.

Enterocutaneous Fistulae—Small Bowel. A small bowel fistula usually results from an undetected and unrepaired laceration inadvertently sustained during abdominal surgery. Occasionally the laceration has been repaired but for a variety of reasons has broken down and discharged bowel contents onto the skin surface. The nature of these contents will depend on the level of the fistula. A duodenal or high small bowel fistula will contain bile and pancreatic juices as well as intestinal secretion. A low small bowel fistula will discharge faeculent material as well as enzyme-rich fluid. In both cases, the fistula contents will be corrosive and cause marked excoriation unless measures are taken to protect the skin surface around the fistula. The most effective of these measures is to insert a tube drain along the fistula track and apply low-pressure suction to direct the contents into an appropriate collecting device for volume measurement and analysis.

The priorities in the management of a small bowel fistula are:

1. *Fluid* and *electrolyte replacement* using serial electrolyte estimations on the serum, urine and fistula fluid as a guide. Central venous pressure monitoring is indicated in patients with a high output fistula of the upper small intestine.

2. *Control of the fistula* using a tube drain as described above. Local applications of barrier cream to the skin around the fistula may help prevent excoriation.

3. *Identification of the fistula source* by contrast studies of the fistula itself (fistulogram) and of the small and large bowel will provide information about the size of the fistula, its site of origin and the presence or absence of distal obstruction. This information is essential in deciding whether to treat the fistula expectantly or surgically.

4. *Nutritional requirements.* A regime of fluid and electrolyte replacement must continue until the fistula closes. In addition calories must be provided either by instillation through a feeding tube positioned in the intestine distal to the fistula or intravenously through a centrally placed cannula. Approximately 3000 calories are required each day by the average adult.

A small bowel fistula will close spontaneously if there is no distal obstruction and if there is no epithelialisation, foreign body or disease such as Crohn's disease, tuberculosis or malignancy in the fistulous track. The demonstration of any of these conditions is an indication for surgery as soon as the patient's general condition allows. In the absence of these complicating factors, it is reasonable to adopt a non-operative approach and to continue fluid and nutritional support for 2–3 weeks in the justifiable hope that spontaneous closure will occur. Delay of closure beyond this time is an indication for surgery.

At operation the surgeon usually encounters adhesions and tangled bowel. Patience and careful dissection is required to isolate the segment of intestine from which the fistula arises. The diseased bowel is resected between intestinal clamps and an end-to-end anastomosis performed. In certain cases it is more appropriate to bypass the fistula if further dissection is hazardous to the patient's life.

Enterocutaneous Fistulae—Large Bowel. A large bowel fistula can result from any elective or accidental opening of the colon or rectum even though an apparently satisfactory repair was achieved at the time of the operation. A high percentage of large bowel anastomoses leak to some degree although in the majority of cases the leak is so small as to be insignificant. When the leak does assume significance and faeces appear in the abdominal wound or drain site, the situation is serious and demands urgent investigation and treatment. Signs of spreading peritonitis in association with the fistula is an urgent indication for operation to evacuate faeces from the peritoneal cavity and to exteriorise the leaking bowel usually as a Hartmann's procedure. More frequently, signs of peritonitis are absent and time allows for adequate investigation and radiological studies to determine the site and extent of the fistula and to demonstrate any distal obstruction or diseased bowel which will need resection to control the fistula.

In the absence of distal obstruction, epithelialisation of the track and pre-existing disease in the leaking segment, e.g. diverticular disease, malignancy or Crohn's disease, an expectant attitude may be adopted as the fistula is likely to close spontaneously. To encourage this development the nutritional needs of the patient are met with an elemental diet which is absorbed in the upper small bowel leaving little residual material to enter the fistulating segment of large intestine.

Enterovaginal Fistula. The discharge of intestinal contents through the vagina 7–10 days after gynaecological surgery is alarming for the patient and distressing for the surgeon. The causes, investigation and management of these fistulae are identical to those formulated for enterocutaneous fistulae except that a persistent rectovaginal fistula needs specialised repair by an experienced surgeon. A defunctioning colostomy will control the fistula until the definitive repair is attempted and this, to have any chance of success, should be delayed for at least 2 months from the time of injury to eradicate pelvic sepsis.

Suggested Reading

Dudley H, Smith R (1983) Alimentary tract and abdominal wall. In: Rob C, Smith R (eds) Operative surgery, vols 1–3, 4th edn. Butterworths, London

Maingot R (1985) Abdominal operations, 8th edn. Appleton, Century and Croft, Connecticut

18 · Urological Complications and How To Cope

Anthony R. Mundy

Classification

The close proximity of the lower urinary tract to the female genital tract makes urological complication one of the commonest types of complication after gynaecological surgery. Some of these are a direct result of urological injury at the time of surgery and are apparent either peroperatively or very early in the postoperative period. These have already been described in Chap. 12 and will be mentioned only briefly here. Other complications only become apparent with the passage of time, although some nonetheless are due to operation trauma.

It is the purpose of this chapter to describe some of the complications that become apparent after the early postoperative period has passed, usually at the time of the first follow-up outpatient appointment or thereafter. These complications may be categorised anatomically as:

1. *Ureteric complication*
   a) Obstruction
   b) Fistula
2. *Bladder complications*
   a) Functional abnormalities
   —Voiding dysfunction
   —The urge syndrome
   —The decentralised bladder
   b) Fistula
3. *Urethral complications*
   a) Sphincter weakness incontinence
   b) Erosion
   c) Fistula
   d) Obstruction

Unfortunately, although this anatomical approach to classification is a useful aide memoire its usefulness is restricted in practice because of the interdependence of the bladder and urethral function. It is therefore more satisfactory to consider complications according to the way in which they may present:

1. *Loin pain*
   a) Ureteric obstruction
   b) Vesicoureteric reflux
2. *Recurrent urinary tract infection*
   a) Ureteric obstruction
   b) Voiding dysfunction (see below)
3. *Voiding difficulty* (including retention)
   a) Outflow obstruction
   b) Reduced detrusor activity
   c) Vesicourethral decentralisation
4. *Fistula*
   a) Ureterovaginal
   b) Vesicovaginal
   c) Urethrovaginal
5. *The urge syndrome*
   a) Hypersensitivity
   b) Detrusor instability
   c) Reduced bladder capacity
   d) Reduced bladder compliance
6. *Stress incontinence*
   a) Sphincter incompetence
   b) Sphincter damage
   c) Vesicourethral decentralisation

We will now consider each of these in turn.

Loin Pain

Recurrent or persistent loin pain with or without associated urinary tract infection is strongly suggestive of ureteric obstruction, particularly if a ureteric injury was sustained at the time of operation. Loin pain that occurs on voiding is suggestive of vesicoureteric reflux, but unless the ureteric orifice was damaged peroperatively, or a ureteric reimplantation was inadequately performed, it is rare to find reflux on micturiting cystography.

The simplest screening test for loin pain is an ultrasound study of the affected side to look for a hydroureteronephrosis (Fig. 18.1) and to exclude gallstones as a cause in patients with right-sided pain. In patients who are known to have had a ureteric injury, because of the higher diagnostic yield, it is as well to proceed straight to an intravenous urogram (IVU) as this is more likely than an ultrasound study to show the site of ureteric obstruction. Otherwise the IVU is reserved for those with an abnormal ultrasound study.

The demonstration of a dilated ureter and hydronephrosis, although suggestive, does not prove a ureteric obstruction unless a preoperative IVU is available for comparison and even then it is not conclusive. Firstly, if a ureteric injury has been treated a transient hydroureteronephrosis (HUN) is to be expected and this should improve with time. Secondly, the patient may have had a pre-existing HUN due, for example, to vesicoureteric reflux or to the effects of a previous pregnancy. It is wise therefore to confirm the obstruction by means of a diuresis renogram (Fig. 18.2), which should also give an assessment of differential renal function, which is helpful when it comes to a consideration of management.

If renography confirms obstruction and there is a useful degree of residual function in the obstructed kidney (i.e. more than about 20% of total renal function) then the obstruction should be treated. If the obstruction is confirmed but there is insufficient residual renal function to warrant operative resolution of the obstruction then nephrectomy is indicated.

If surgical resolution of the obstruction is decided upon then this should be performed by a urologist (as should the preoperative assessment). The exact technique depends on the site of obstruction and the cause. Distal pelvic ureteric obstructions are due either to direct injury or indirectly to a stitch abscess or postoperative fibrosis, although some are due to

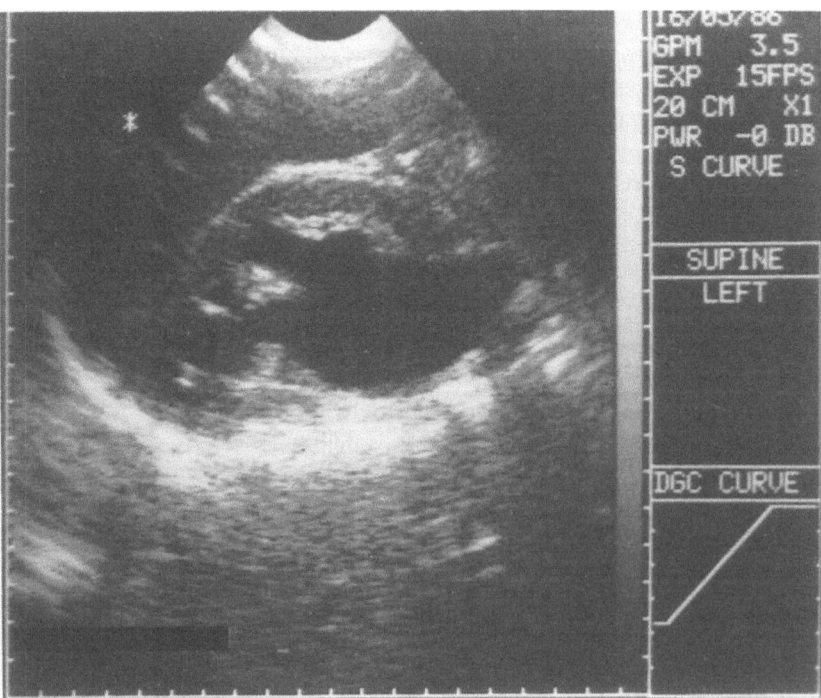

Fig. 18.1. Ultrasound scan of a kidney showing hydronephrosis.

Recurrent Urinary Tract Infection

Recurrent bacteriologically proven urinary tract infection (UTI) (as distinct from bacteriologically negative frequency and urgency, with or without scalding, due to the urge syndrome or the urethral syndrome) is suggestive of either obstruction to the upper or lower urinary tract or the presence of residual urine which may or may not be due to obstruction.

When associated with loin pain, the investigation and subsequent management should be as outlined in the last section.

If, on the other hand, the symptoms seem to localise the focus of the recurrent UTI to the lower urinary tract, the first step is to arrange a preliminary screening of bladder function with an ultrasound scan of the bladder before and after voiding with a flow study of the voiding pattern. It is obviously important that this should resemble the patient's normal voiding pattern as closely as possible, so that the first ultrasound study should take place when the patient has a full bladder and her usual desire to void, the flow study should be sitting in privacy and the postvoid ultrasound should follow immediately, before the bladder has started to fill again. This investigation studies four parameters: bladder capacity, the flow rate, the flow pattern and voided volume and the completeness or otherwise of emptying. A low flow rate, a long drawn-out or intermittent flow pattern and incomplete emptying are signs of a voiding dysfunction which may require further investigation.

An essentially normal study (good capacity, normal flow rate, normal flow pattern and complete emptying) means that further investigation is usually unnecessary. Such patients are treated according to the frequency of the infections. Three episodes a year or less should be treated as and when they occur with an appropriate antibiotic as judged by sensitivity testing. Prophylactic, long-term antibiotic treatment probably confers no benefit. It is obviously important to distinguish recurrent UTI from persistent UTI with an organism which has never been completely eradicated. Such patients have several episodes of UTI in close succession with the same organism and may well benefit from 6 weeks or so of low-dose antibiotics after the initial "curative" course (for example trimethoprim 200 mg bd for 1 week followed by 100 mg nocte for 6 weeks).

Patients who have more than three UTIs/year should have an IVU to exclude a morphological urinary tract abnormality and a cystoscopy if there is any possibility of a foreign body, such as non-

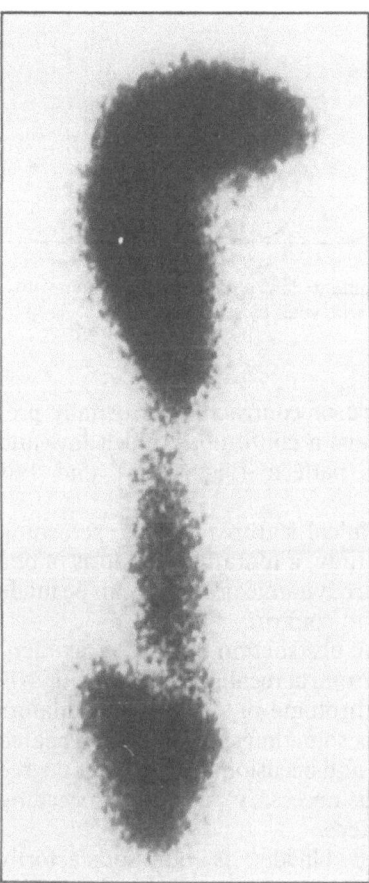

Fig. 18.2. DTPA renal scan showing distal ureteric obstruction. There is progressive accumulation and slow washout of tracer.

residual or recurrent disease, particularly in patients with cancer. More proximal obstructions, particularly at the level of the pelvic brim, are more commonly due to stitch abscesses or to the underlying disease process.

Distal injuries will usually be treated by a direct ureteric implantation as described in Chap. 12; more proximal injuries either by reimplantation into a psoas hitch (Chap. 12) or by transureteroureterostomy in which the ureter is divided just above the obstruction, mobilised, passed over the great vessels deep to the sigmoid mesocolon and the inferior mesenteric vessels and then anastomosed end-to-side to the contralateral unobstructed ureter.

It is rarely necessary to treat vesicoureteric reflux in adults but when the patient has severe symptoms, or recurrent upper tract UTI despite antibiotic prophylaxis, ureteric reimplantation is indicated if ipsilateral renal function is satisfactory.

absorbable suture, within the bladder. Any abnormality is then treated on its own merits; otherwise the frequency of infection is probably sufficient to justify long-term prophylactic treatment with a drug such as trimethoprim 100 mg nocte. This should be given for 6 months to 1 year in the first instance, at which time it is worth trying to see whether it can be discontinued.

Those patients with an abnormal ultrasound/flow study warrant further investigation with a videourodynamic (VUD) study although it is reasonable to make a tentative diagnosis of relative outflow obstruction (see below) and treat the patient with an empirical urethral recalibration to 40F with an Otis urethrotome (without the blade), reserving the VUD for those who fail to respond.

The principle role of VUD is to distinguish between a relative outflow obstruction and bladder decentralisation (often, but inaccurately, referred to as denervation), although other urodynamic abnormalities may sometimes be detected in this way. The clinical picture often helps to distinguish between obstruction and decentralisation. Decentralisation is the result of damage to the pelvic plexuses, usually during a radical type of hysterectomy, as they lie in relation to the lateral fornices of the upper third of the vagina. As a result of the neural damage, both the bladder and urethra become more or less inert giving a bladder that does not contract and a urethra that neither contracts fully to hold urine in nor relaxes fully to let urine out. On the other hand relative outflow obstruction is due to failure of the urethra to attain a normal calibre during voiding usually due to the failure of the urethral sphincter mechanism to relax properly. The term relative outflow obstruction is used to distinguish this from the more overt obstruction seen in men with a definite morphological obstruction, usually the hyperplastic prostate and sometimes seen in women after an overenthusiastic sling procedure.

Thus any patient may have a relative outflow obstruction often made worse by one of the various operations for stress incontinence in which the urethral resistance is surgically enhanced, whereas decentralisation tends to follow extensive perivaginal excision or dissection. Furthermore because decentralisation affects the urethra as well as the bladder, sphincteric incompetence causing stress incontinence is often apparent in addition to the voiding difficulty.

The ultrasound/flow study may also give some clues in this differentiation. Patients with decentralised bladder, because they are acontractile, generally void by straining, giving an intermittent flow pattern (Fig. 18.3) and a more substantial residual urine, whereas those with relative outflow obstruc-

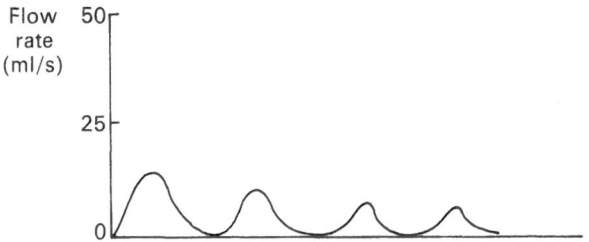

Fig. 18.3. An intermittent flow pattern in a woman with a decentralised bladder who voids by straining.

tion, because detrusor contractility is usually preserved, tend to have a continuous, albeit low and fluctuating, flow pattern (Fig. 18.4) and less residual urine.

Thus by the clinical features and the screening ultrasound/flow study, a tentative diagnosis of one or other of these urodynamic problems can be made which VUD seeks to confirm.

Relative outflow obstruction is treated, as mentioned above, by urethral recalibration to about 40F with an Otis urethrotome or using Hegar dilators up to size 14. This sometimes needs to be repeated from time to time and occasionally a greater degree of recalibration is necessary, usually proceeding upwards in 10F steps.

A decentralised bladder is not satisfactorily treated in this way as treatment of the obstructive element in this way, by reducing urethral resistance, tends to make the incontinence element worse. For this reason, if recurrent UTI is the main problem, it is safer to accept the situation and control the UTI by the use of prophylactic antibiotics. If, on the other hand, the incontinence element is a prominent factor or if the functional bladder capacity (the difference between the total capacity and the residual urine volume) is so severely restricted that the patient has marked frequency as well, then clean intermittent self-catheterisation is indicated, if the patient can perform it, to give complete emptying and to make the maximum use of the total bladder capacity.

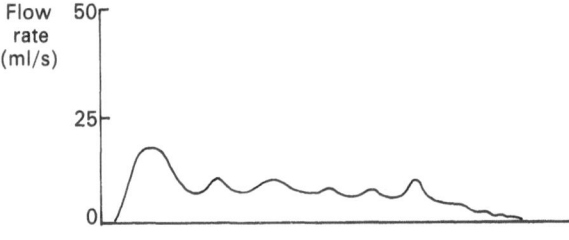

Fig. 18.4. A low, irregular, fluctuating, but continuous flow pattern in a woman with relative outflow obstruction.

The other, occasional cause of recurrent UTI is a urethral diverticulum as a result of urethral injury, which is treated by surgical excision and urethral repair.

Voiding Difficulty

Two common causes of this, relative outflow obstruction and vesicourethral decentralisation, have already been discussed. Three other postoperative complications need to be described:

1. Transient postoperative acute retention.
2. Overt outflow obstruction (which may cause either persistent retention or, when less severe, difficulty in voiding).
3. Detrusor fade.

Acute Retention

Many patients are unable to void after an operation, irrespective of the type of procedure, for a variety of reasons. Some because of pain, some because of oedema around the bladder neck and urethra induced by general pelvic dissection and some simply because they are not used to voiding into a bedpan or commode, often in an unnatural position, in a public ward. In all of these situations, spontaneous voiding can be expected to occur in a few days when pain and oedema have subsided somewhat, and particularly when the patient can go and void in a normal toilet. All that is required in the meantime is a few days of indwelling urethral catheterisation.

If in addition the patient has had an operation specifically intended to enhance outflow resistance (such as colposuspension, sling procedure or anterior repair), a temporary voiding difficulty is to be expected and for this reason a bladder catheter is left in at the end of the operation. In such a situation a suprapubic catheter is better than a urethral catheter, not only because most women find a suprapubic catheter more comfortable, but also because a suprapubic catheter can be clamped to allow a trial of voiding before removing it, whereas a urethral catheter can only be removed. Although in most patients spontaneous voiding can be re-established in 3–5 days there is an enormous variation, for no apparent reason, particularly in patients who have had sling, or similar procedures. Presumably this is related to the obstructive effect

of the sling, the patient's individual tolerance of postoperative discomfort, postoperative oedema, the contractile ability of the detrusor or a combination of these factors.

In such a situation, persistent difficulty in reestablishing spontaneous voiding tends to induce a great deal of anxiety for the patient. The author's practice therefore, after the initial trial of voiding has been unsuccessful, is to explain the situation to the patient, to reassure her that spontaneous voiding may occur, although it may take as much as 3 or 4 weeks to do so, to try again at about 10 days after the operation and if there is still no joy, to send the patient home for a week or two with an indwelling catheter on free drainage and then to readmit her at the end of that time for a further trial of voiding.

Persistent Voiding Difficulty—Overt Outflow Obstruction

If the patient is still unable to void adequately (or at all) after the first postoperative month has passed, by which time the causes of transient retention should have subsided considerably, then there is a strong possibility of outflow obstruction. It is still possible, however, that the patient has one of the other causes of voiding difficulty, particularly if the patient has not had an anti-incontinence procedure, and for this reason and because spontaneous improvement can still be expected for up to 3 months after surgery it is wise to continue with a policy of reassurance and wait-and-see.

If at the end of 3 months there is still no adequate voiding the cause should be looked for with VUD. The crucial urodynamic factor is the presence or absence of a detrusor contraction. If present then satisfactory spontaneous voiding is likely to occur with time; if not then a satisfactory result is much less likely. Other factors to look for, apart from relative outflow obstruction and bladder decentralisation (see above) and detrusor fade (see below), are bladder neck incompetence, an obstructing sling or colposuspension and evidence of urethral injury.

The normal bladder neck is closed except when the detrusor contracts; if the bladder does not contract, the bladder neck will not open. Thus if the bladder neck is urodynamically competent and the bladder is acontractile, voiding cannot occur. Hence the importance of these two factors.

The effects of an obstructive anti-incontinence procedure can only be overcome by detrusor contraction or straining or (commonly) a combination. The obvious concern is that on the one hand there is the temptation to use urethral recalibration to re-establish voiding and get rid of the increasing anxiety and on the other hand is the worry that recalibration may lead to a return of incontinence.

In all these situations so far described it is a good idea to change the patient from continuous to intermittent self-catheterisation (if the patient can cope) as this takes the heat out of the problem, gets rid of the indwelling "tube" and gives the patient the impression that progress is being made. If voiding is subsequently established then obviously the catheterisation can be stopped; if not then a urological referral for consideration of the appropriate specific treatment of the underlying problem can be arranged at leisure. This might be a urethral dilatation or relaxation of the sling or colposuspension for obstruction or a cautious (possibly staged) bladder neck incision for competent bladder neck in a patient with a bladder neck obstruction.

Patients with a urethral injury (the best example of which is a patient with stress incontinence after a radical hysterectomy and radiotherapy who has been treated by a sling procedure which has caused urethral erosion) cannot be treated in this way. Such a patient requires immediate referral to a urologist with a particular interest in such problems, for consideration for an appropriate reconstructive procedure.

Detrusor Fade

This is a comparatively uncommon cause of voiding difficulty (and hence of incomplete emptying and recurrent UTI) but nonetheless a distinct entity worth mentioning as it is sometimes confused with relative outflow obstruction. As the term implies, after an initially satisfactory start to a detrusor contraction, the contraction is inadequately sustained and the detrusor pressure "fades" away to nothing before the bladder is empty. Unlike relative outflow obstruction it does not respond to urethral recalibration, nor indeed to any other specific form of treatment. When the symptoms are particularly troublesome, intermittent self-catheterisation is sometimes helpful but the problem tends to occur in the elderly who often find the technique difficult or distasteful.

As the reader will no doubt have gathered, many of the postoperative voiding difficulties are not in fact "complications" of the surgery but pre-existing problems that have been unmasked by the operation. Some of them may be diagnosed by routine preoperative VUD evaluation and where it is possible, particularly in patients having an anti-incontinence operation, it is advisable that this should be done so that the at-risk patient can be identified and warned of possible postoperative problems. Where such facilities are not routinely available all patients should be warned of the possibility so that the unnecessary resentment that might otherwise occur from lack of preoperative discussion might be avoided or reduced.

Fistula

Of all the non-fatal complications of gynaecological surgery, fistula is the one the gynaecologists the world over seem to fear most, although ureteric injury runs a close second.

Whatever the type, the presence of a fistula is usually obvious early in the postoperative period with vaginal leakage of urine.

With ureterovaginal and vesicovaginal fistulae, the urine leak occurs from the suture line in the vaginal vault and so cannot be distinguished in this way. The first step, however, is to pass a urethral catheter in the hope that this is a vesicovaginal fistula and that an indwelling catheter will allow the defect to heal. If the patient is already catheterised and has been since the operation, a ureterovaginal fistula is more likely but it is usually easy to be sure either by instilling dilute methylene blue into the bladder to see if it escapes vaginally or with a cystogram.

If there is no evidence of a vesicovaginal leak, an IVU is the next investigation to detect a ureterovaginal fistula (Fig. 18.5). The IVU may not actually show a fistula but the upper urinary tract on the affected side will invariably be abnormal with a definite hydronephrosis. This is sufficient confirmation of the site of the fistula if a vesicovaginal fistula has been excluded.

In this way the diagnosis is made. Treatment, however, will obviously vary according to the site. Furthermore although a small vesicovaginal fistula may well heal with a few weeks of catheterisation, intubation of the ureter rarely, if ever, leads to resolution of a ureterovaginal fistula. Thus a vesicovaginal fistula can be managed expectantly, whereas a ureterovaginal fistula should be treated straight away.

Ureterovaginal Fistula

This is treated by reimplantation of the ureter into the bladder as described in Chap. 12.

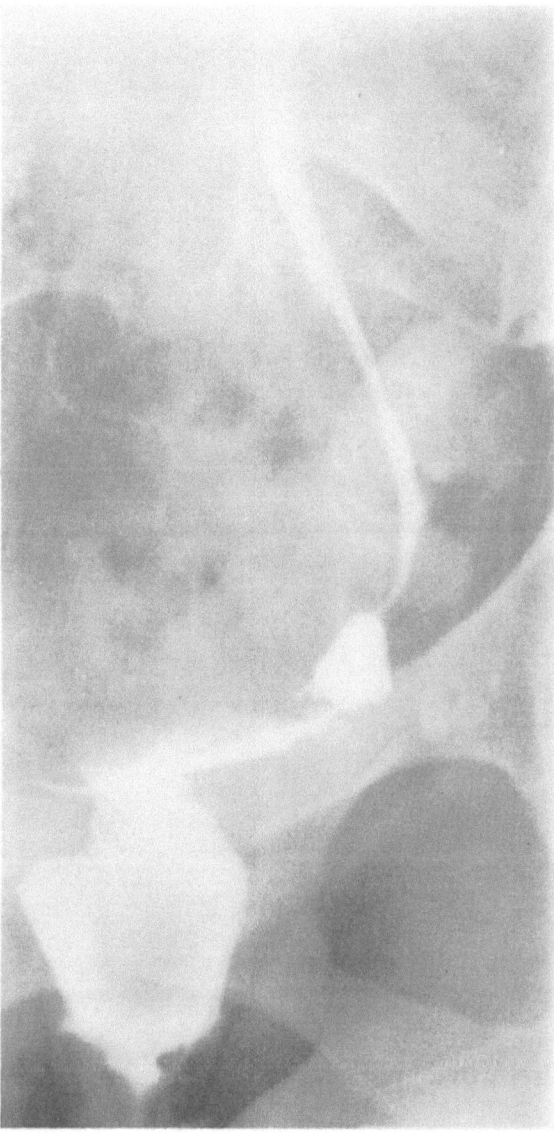

Fig. 18.5. An IVU of a woman with ureterovaginal fistula.

Vesicovaginal Fistula

It used to be said that a vesicovaginal fistula should be left for at least 3 months to allow the local tissue reaction to subside before attempting a repair, but this does not seem to be necessary. The only point in delaying is to allow the fistula to heal spontaneously and if vaginal leakage does not cease promptly with catheterisation then spontaneous healing is very unlikely. Thus if a fistula persists despite prompt catheterisation then it should be repaired as soon as the patient's general condition allows it.

The principles of fistula repair are to excise the fistula tract, to close the bladder and vaginal walls without tension and to interpose a layer of healthy tissue between—more or less the same principles, in fact, that relate to prevention of fistula formation when a peroperative bladder injury is repaired at the time of hysterectomy.

In general, gynaecologists prefer to close fistulae by means of a vaginal approach. The best approach is the one that will *guarantee* that the principles outlined in the last paragraph can be applied and, whereas this can be guaranteed with a retropubic approach, it cannot be guaranteed with a vaginal approach, particularly when the fistula is large or when the situation is complicated by extensive fibrosis or by irradiation of the tissues. A retropubic approach is therefore safer.

The first step, having exposed the bladder from above, is to open it through a vertical cystotomy incision and then to put it in a self-retaining retractor to hold the bladder open. The fistula is then identified and its relationship to the ureteric orifices determined (Fig. 18.6). If there is more than 1 cm between the edge of the fistula and the ureteric orifices then a ureteric reimplantation will probably be unnecessary. If one or other of the ureteric orifices lies any closer to the edge of the fistula, then closure of the fistula is likely to compromise that ureteric orifice and a reimplantation will probably be necessary. Whether or not a reimplantation seems likely it is a good idea to catheterise both ureters as this facilitates their identification during the rest of the procedure and also keeps the field dry by diverting most of the urine out of the bladder.

The next step is to excise the fistula and identify the plane between the bladder and the vagina. This is normally achieved by circumcising the margin of the fistula with a 0·5-cm (or thereabouts) margin of healthy bladder wall. When the plane between the bladder and the vagina is reached the bladder wall is undermined for a distance of about 2 cm in every direction, although this is easier to achieve upwards and downwards than it is from side to side because the lateral tethering by the ureters and the vascular pedicles restricts such lateral mobilisation.

If mobilisation proves difficult with the exposure as it is, the best way to improve the exposure is to split the bladder in the sagittal plane by extending the original cystotomy incision posteriorly (Fig. 18.7). This also makes identification of the plane between the bladder and the vaginal vault easier.

Having circumcised the fistula from the bladder, the vagina is then opened around the fistula tract. If the bladder wall has been mobilised from the vagina by undermining it as described above, then there should be about 2 cm of bladder wall all the way around and a similar degree of vaginal wall mobilisation on the other side.

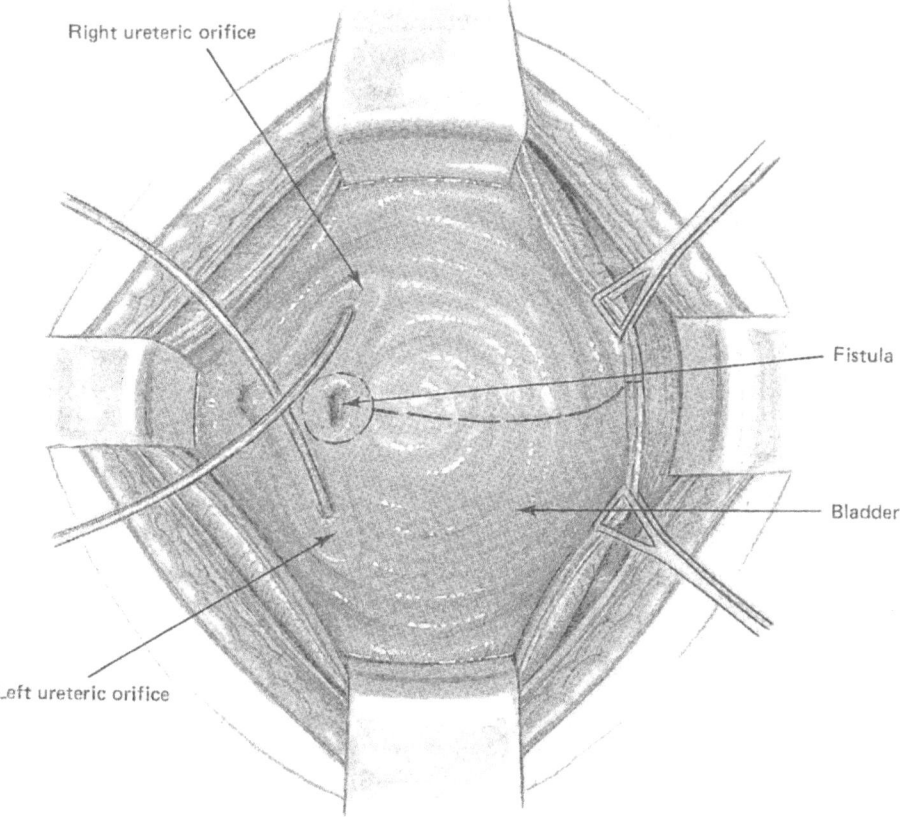

Fig. 18.6. A vesicovaginal fistula with the bladder opened and both ureters catheterised.

The vagina is then closed with 2·0 Dexon or Vicryl sutures in two layers (Fig. 18.8). The first layer closes the vagina wall and inverts it and the second layer inverts the first layer. Neither layer should be under any tension.

Before closing the bladder, a plug of omentum is pulled down between bladder and vagina, again without tension, and tacked in place with a few sutures (Fig. 18.9).

The bladder is then closed with two layers of 2·0 Dexon or Vicryl sutures in the same way as the vagina—the deeper layer bringing the muscle layer together without tension and the final, superficial layer bringing the urothelium and superficial muscle together with inverting sutures (Fig. 18.10).

To complete the procedure, the cystotomy incision is closed around a suprapubic catheter, which is left in place for 2–3 weeks to allow adequate healing before it is clamped for a 24-h trial of voiding (see Chap. 12).

Urethrovaginal Fistula

This is rare in gynaecological practice and is much more commonly seen in obstetric practice, but is occasionally seen after an anterior repair when a urethral injury lies in close approximation to the vaginal suture line. In such patients, urine is subsequently seen to leak from the suture line, but fortunately usually dries up within a few weeks of indwelling urethral catheterisation.

The Urge Syndrome

It is common for patients who have had retropubic operations, particularly around the bladder base, to

Fig. 18.7. The bladder has been bivalved to allow mobilisation
of the bladder wall around the fistula.

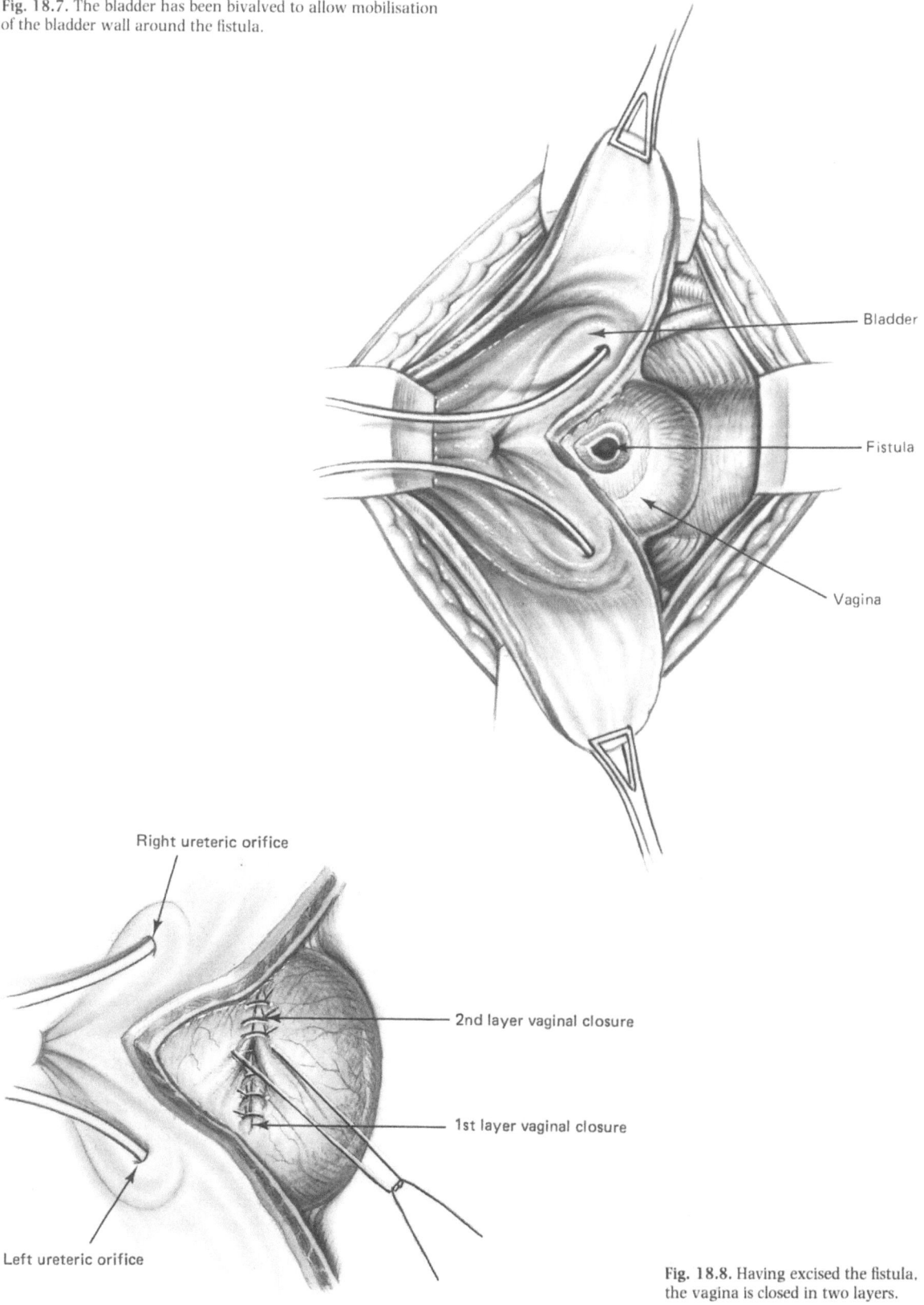

Bladder

Fistula

Vagina

Right ureteric orifice

2nd layer vaginal closure

1st layer vaginal closure

Left ureteric orifice

Fig. 18.8. Having excised the fistula,
the vagina is closed in two layers.

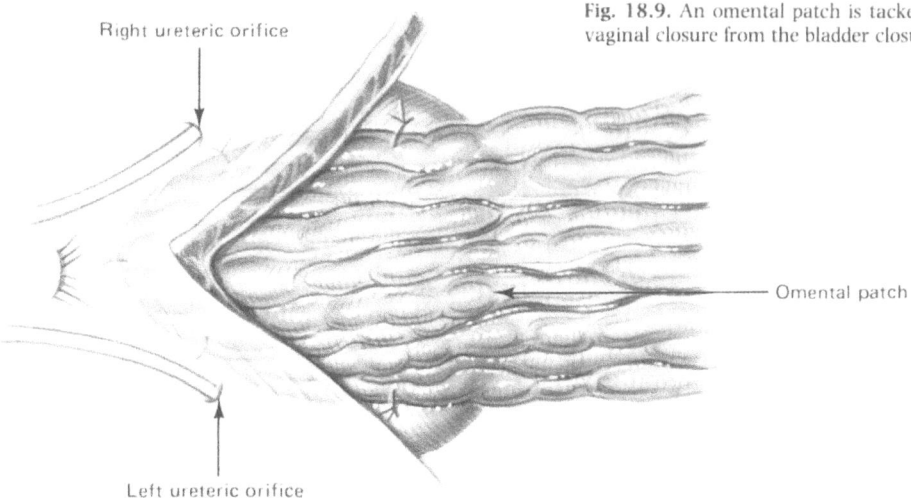

Right ureteric orifice

Fig. 18.9. An omental patch is tacked in place to separate the vaginal closure from the bladder closure.

Omental patch

Left ureteric orifice

have some frequency and urgency for the first 6–8 weeks thereafter. By 3 months this should have subsided or be obviously improving.

If frequency, urgency and nocturia persist beyond 3 months, especially if associated with urge incon-

tinence, then it should be investigated and the first investigations should be a urine culture and, if this is negative, a voided volume chart, noting the time and the volume of fluid intake and output over a 48-h period. This acts to confirm the patient's

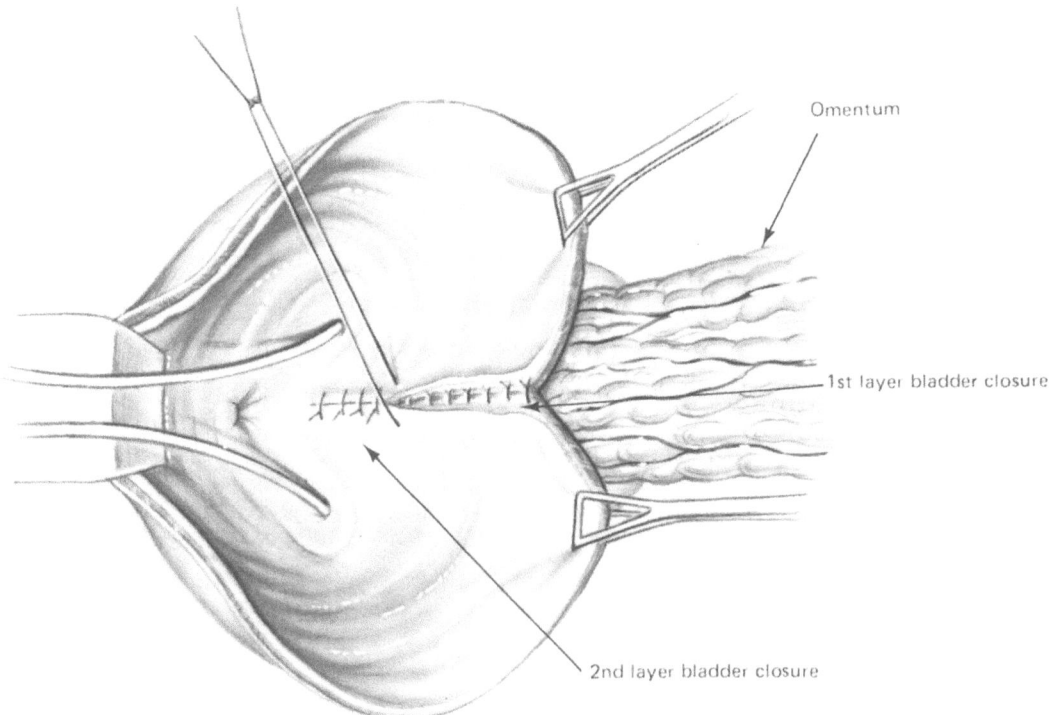

Omentum

1st layer bladder closure

2nd layer bladder closure

Fig. 18.10. The bladder is then closed in two layers.

history and to exclude a high fluid intake as the cause. In addition, the frequent passage of small but similar volumes of urine tends to suggest that hypersensitivity is the cause, whereas the passage of differing volumes at irregular intervals suggests that detrusor instability is the cause. A free urine flow rate is obtained to exclude a voiding dysfunction.

Having excluded or treated urinary infection as a cause, it is reasonable to start empirical treatment with an anticholinergic drug such as oxybutynin hydrochloride 5 mg tds or qds to see if this helps, particularly if detrusor instability seems the most likely diagnosis as judged by the voided volume chart.

If the patient does not respond to oxybutynin as anticipated then a urodynamic study is the next step to make a definite diagnosis. The commonest urodynamic abnormalities to be found in this sort of situation are:

1. Detrusor instability
2. A poorly compliant bladder
3. Bladder hypersensitivity
4. A small capacity bladder
5. Sphincter weakness incontinence
6. One of the voiding dysfunctions described above
7. A combination of any two or more of these

Multiple or severe urodynamic abnormalities are usually related to extensive pelvic surgery, particularly radical hysterectomy for cancer, and to previous pelvic radiotherapy. When both of these factors apply, the small capacity, poorly compliant decentralised bladder is a relatively common finding. A small capacity, poorly compliant bladder is otherwise an uncommon finding.

Sphincter weakness incontinence should, of course, be treated on its own merits, but when this follows an operation that was intended to deal with this (i.e. an operative failure) then the patient should be referred for further management by someone with a particular experience in this type of problem. In any case, when frequency and urgency, and particularly detrusor instability, are associated with spincter weakness, correction of the latter does not often lead to resolution of the "urge" symptoms and the patient should be warned of this.

The treatment of the other two main causes of the urge syndrome, detrusor instability and the bladder hypersensitivity, which have failed to respond to first-line treatment with bladder drill and oxybutynin, is beyond the scope of this chapter. Such patients should be assessed with a view to transvesical injection of the pelvic plexuses with phenol.

Stress Incontinence

Postoperative stress incontinence must be considered firstly as a true postoperative complication and secondly as persistence of preoperative stress incontinence despite an anti-incontinence procedure.

De Novo Stress Incontinence

In most instances this is related by the patient to a previous hysterectomy, although there is very little, if any, objective evidence to support this attribution where such a relationship has been investigated. The exception to this is the sphincter weakness incontinence associated with vesicourethral decentralisation following a radical hysterectomy. In most other patients a degree of sphincteric incompetence was almost certainly present before their operation but has become more troublesome since.

Patients in the latter category who may be said to have "simple" sphincter weakness incontinence are treated as any other new patient with a symptom of stress incontinence. Those with a history of radiotherapy and a radical hysterectomy must be viewed with caution, however, as the success rate of standard procedures, particularly of sling procedures, is very much lower because of the frequently multiple urodynamic abnormalities that they have. The complication rate is also very much higher. Such patients require detailed urodynamic evaluation and the demonstration of anything other than simple sphincter weakness is an indication for referral to a specialist unit.

Persistent Stress Incontinence

This means that either the anti-incontinence procedure was inappropriate or inexpertly performed or that there are complicating factors. An anterior repair is an inappropriate procedure and, after urodynamic confirmation of the diagnosis, a more appropriate operation such as colposuspension, Stamey-type bladder neck suspension or sling procedure should be advised. Patients who fall into either of the other two categories require full urodynamic evaluation and referral to a specialist unit.

Some of the complicating factors have already been alluded to. These include coexisting urodynamic abnormalities listed on p. 252 (the urge syndrome) and above (de novo stress incontinence). Other complicating factors include obesity, chronic respiratory tract problems and dense retropubic scarring as a result of multiple pelvic procedures. A particular complicating factor, often related to the latter, is the so-called "drainpipe" urethra in which the urethral wall is so heavily scarred that it is no longer able to function as a sphincter-active pliable conduit, but is just a rigid tube. In this situation any standard procedure is doomed to failure and implantation of an artificial sphincter is probably all that can be offered.

Conclusion

As with all complications of any type of surgery the best practice is to avoid them in the first place. With most of the more serious complications such as ureteric damage or fistula, this is almost always possible. Most of the more minor complications, however careful the surgery, will inevitably occur from time to time and this is particularly so with voiding dysfunctions and urge symptoms after anti-incontinence procedures. The important factor here is to warn the patient beforehand that they may occur, so that when something does develop, it does not come as a complete surprise. Most patients, disappointed though they may be, will appreciate that problems occur from time to time, but they are far less likely to be cooperative and understanding in such situations when they feel they have been "deceived" into believing that it was all going to be plain sailing.

Suggested Reading

Mundy AR, Stevenson TP, Wein AJ (1984) Urodynamics: principles, practice and application. Churchill Livingstone, London
Raz S (1985) Gynaecological urology. Clinics in obstetrics and gynaecology, vol 12. Saunders, London
Stanton SL, Tanagho E (1986) Surgery of female incontinence, 2nd edn. Springer, Berlin Heidelberg New York

19 · Catheters and Drains

Paul Hilton

Catheters

Introduction

Catheterisation of the bladder is one of the commonest surgical procedures; its use is apparently increasing steadily, being employed in up to 20% of all patients in hospital (Stevens et al. 1981). Whilst the use of catheterisation remains an important device in many situations in medical practice in general, and in obstetric and gynaecological practice in particular, it is well to remember that it is also associated with a significant increase in morbidity and mortality. It is the commonest cause of nosocomially acquired infection, accounting for approximately 35% of such events in the United States (National Nosocomial Infection Study 1973) and United Kingdom (Report on the National Survey of Infection in Hospital 1981). For many, catheterisation may mean considerable discomfort, significant increase in hospital stay and considerable financial implication for health services (Givens and Wenzel 1980). Despite these major implications of catheterisation, it is perhaps the very familiarity which both medical and nursing staff feel they have with catheterisation which leads them all too often to neglect the basic principles underlying bladder drainage and which may lead to unnecessary catheterisations, inappropriate timing of catheterisation and inadequate techniques of catheterisation.

Historical Perspective

The first recorded use of catheterisation appears in the hieroglyphics in the pyramid of Pharoah Khufu from the twenty-sixth century B.C., which describe the arguments of the physicians of the time over the most appropriate species of Nile reed to drain the bladder (Ingram 1978).

Developments in catheter design and materials were slow to come. It was not until the eighteenth century that Herissant suggested that rubber might be used; the first such catheters were made by a jeweller of the time, Bernard, although it is of course to Auguste Nelaton (1807–1873) that the credit for this development usually goes. The problem of retaining a catheter in the bladder was satisfactorily resolved by Foley in 1927 and urethral catheterisation as we know it today became feasible. Many further modifications to the design and materials used for urethral catheters have been introduced since but perhaps the two most important advances in bladder drainage in recent times are the description of closed suprapubic catheterisation by Hodgkinson and Hodari in 1966 and the technique of clean intermittent self-catheterisation by Lapides et al. in 1972.

Indications

The indications for catheterisation of the bladder have expanded considerably since its first use for cases of retention due to urethral stricture. The present indications are as follows:

Within gynaecology:

1. Acute urinary retention.
2. Chronic urinary retention. Catheterisation may be needed for recurrent or persistent urinary infection, evidence of upper tract deterioration or of chronic retention with "overflow" incontinence.
3. Pre- and peroperative use. Many surgeons prefer to drain the bladder prior to gynaecological operation.
4. Postoperative use. All gynaecological, urological and rectal surgery may be associated with postoperative urinary retention as a result of pain, distortion of local anatomy, clot retention, pelvic haematoma or periurethral oedema, or by virtue of bladder denervation or neuropraxia. Catheterisation may therefore be necessary following any such procedure and is perhaps best employed prophylactically in many situations. Postoperative catheterisation is positively indicated where a cystotomy incision has been made, intentionally or otherwise, to allow healing of a suture line in the bladder or urethra and to prevent development or promote healing of a urinary fistula.
5. Bladder or urethral trauma.
6. Acute vulvovaginitis.
7. Intractable urinary incontinence. Rarely, catheterisation may be required for the management of urinary incontinence which is unresponsive to alternative methods of treatment and where pads and collection devices do not render a socially acceptable level of continence.
8. Neuropathic bladder dysfunction. In patients with a neuropathic bladder, particularly those with lesions below the level of the micturition centres in the pontine reticular formation, urinary incontinence may be complicated by a dyssynergic voiding pattern and may best be managed by catheterisation.
9. For diagnostic purposes. Bladder drainage may occasionally be indicated in the investigation of a lower abdominal mass or to measure residual urine volume, although ultrasound is a more acceptable, and now widely available, technique. Catheterisation is also used during radiological assessment of the lower urinary tract, and as an integral part of urodynamic investigation.

10. To monitor urine output. Catheterisation may be required for the accurate assessment of urine output in patients with hypovolaemic or endotoxic shock, those with oliguria from other causes and those with impaired consciousness and unable to void normally.
11. In the terminally ill. If bladder management becomes a problem in the terminally ill, either because of incontinence with consequent discomfort or skin breakdown, or because micturition becomes too frequent, too painful or too difficult for the patient's comfort, catheterisation may be justified.

Within obstetrics:

1. At operative delivery. The bladder should be drained prior to assisted vaginal delivery, particularly if mid-cavity or rotational delivery is to be undertaken, in order to reduce the risks of trauma to the bladder base. Most obstetricians catheterise prior to Caesarean section. Prophylactic bladder drainage following Caesarean section is advocated where haematuria develops during the operation.
2. Epidural. Where epidural anaesthesia has been employed and is to be used for postoperative pain relief.
3. To monitor urine output (vide supra).

Methods

The bladder may be drained either continuously or intermittently through the urethra or via an artificial opening or cystostomy; the exact method used and the type of catheter employed in any individual case depends on the particular indication. The following methods will be described:

1. Urethral a) Single event
            b) Continuous indwelling
            c) Intermittent catheterisation
2. Cystotomy a) Open suprapubic cystotomy
            b) Closed suprapubic stab
            c) Vaginal cystotomy

Urethral Catheterisation

Urethral catheterisation is of course the oldest and simplest form of bladder drainage; it may be performed as a single event, as an intermittent procedure, in which case it is most usually carried out by the patients themselves, or the bladder may be drained continuously for a variable period with an indwelling catheter.

Single Event or "In-Out" Urethral Catheterisation

This is most frequently performed prior to pelvic surgery or operative delivery, where diagnostic catheterisation is used to measure the residual volume during radiological or urodynamic investigation, or where the bladder is to be filled prior to the insertion of a suprapubic catheter.

Choice of Catheter

It is a reasonable working rule in all aspects of bladder drainage always to use the narrowest and softest catheter that will serve the purpose (Blandy 1981); to this one might add that it should also be the shortest and the cheapest. The Nelaton or Jaques catheter with a tapered tip and one or more side holes is most often used; the material is of little consequence in this situation in view of the short time of contact between catheter and urethra; however, a plastic or PVC construction is most usual and a female length (20–25 cm) catheter of 8, 10 or at most 12FG is perfectly adequate.

Technique

Prior to catheterisation all materials necessary for the procedure should be to hand. The labia are separated using one hand to expose the external meatus, which is swabbed twice in an anteroposterior direction using the other hand, each swab being discarded immediately (Fig. 19.1a). The catheter is then passed into the urethra, whilst still keeping the labia separated (Fig. 19.1b): urine should start to flow into the receiver under the influence of gravity. The limiting factor on flow rate is the catheter diameter and no amount of suprapubic pressure at this stage will speed bladder

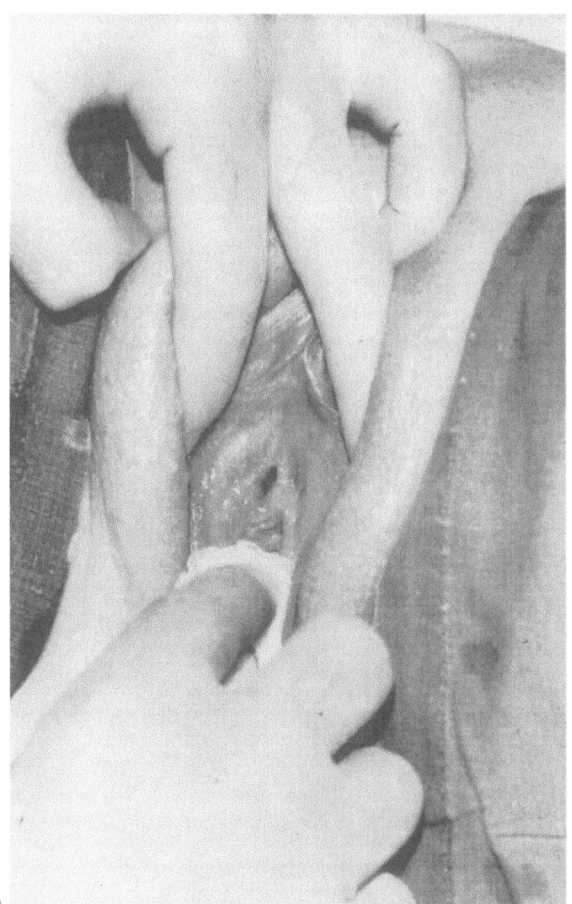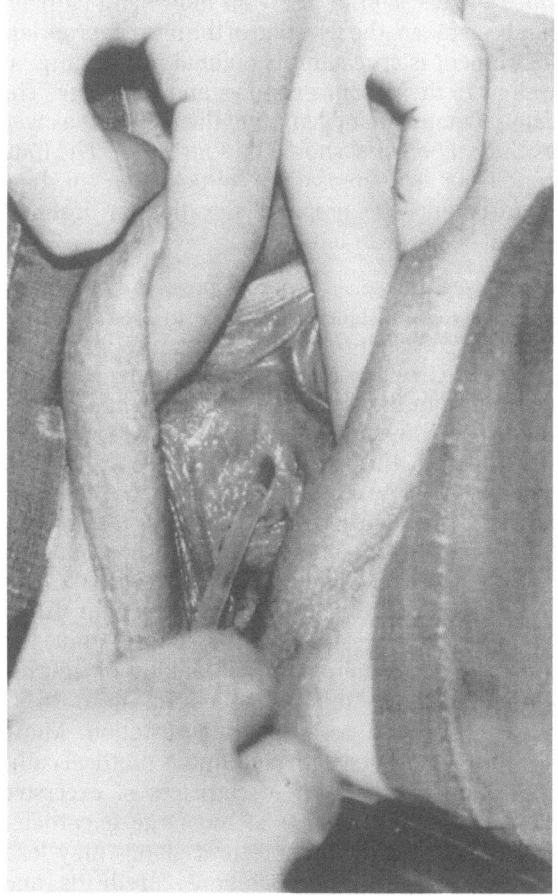

a   b

Fig. 19.1a,b. Technique of urethral catheterisation: **a** The labia are separated to expose the external meatus, which is swabbed twice in the anteroposterior direction. **b** The catheter is inserted directly into the meatus and urine drains freely by gravity. Suprapubic pressure ensures complete drainage and is continued as the catheter is withdrawn.

emptying. When urine flow slows visibly, the catheter may be advanced a little further into the urethra and only then should the labia be released. Suprapubic pressure may be applied at this stage, but, once applied, pressure should be maintained until the catheter is removed, otherwise air and potentially infection will reflux into the bladder. Under no circumstances should the catheter be passed further into the bladder after the labia have come together or infection may result.

Continuous Indwelling Catheterisation

A continuous indwelling urethral catheter may be indicated in any of the situations detailed above, although other modes of bladder drainage may be advantageous in specific situations; these are detailed where appropriate (see "Intermittent Catheterisation" and "Closed Suprapubic Stab Cystostomy" in particular).

Choice of Catheter

Once the decision to insert an indwelling catheter has been taken, the selection of the most appropriate instrument is crucial to its optimal functioning, as well as to the patient's comfort and wellbeing. The calibre, material and length of the catheter, as well as the balloon size, should be considered. The indication for catheterisation, anticipation of haematuria and the proposed duration of drainage should be borne in mind.

CATHETER CALIBRE. As noted above, the narrowest appropriate catheter should always be selected. Heavily bloodstained urine will require a catheter of 16-18 FG: otherwise a calibre 12 or at most 14 FG will suffice in the short term. The French, or Charriere, scale conventionally used for defining catheter sizes denotes the external circumference in millimetres; the flow rate obtained through a catheter, however, is proportional to its internal cross-section (at the narrowest point in its lumen). Physiological rates of bladder filling vary between 0·5 and 5·0 ml/min, so catheter sizes greater than 12 FG should rarely be necessary, assuming that the lumen is not compromised by kinking or encrustation. For longer term, a catheter of up to 16 FG may be required because of encrustation. Many problems associated with continuous urethral catheterisation are a result of catheters of excessive diameter. Long-term use of too large a catheter which occludes the paraurethral glands may lead to retention of gland secretions, urethritis and paraurethral abscess (Blandy 1981).

CATHETER MATERIAL. Until relatively recently, catheters have been made from plastic (PVC or poly-

urethane) or latex. Both have been prone to encrustation with prolonged use (Fig. 19.2); the cytotoxicity of latex in particular causes concern (Ruutu et al. 1985) and urethritis may occur in 22% of patients after 48 h use (Nacey et al. 1985). To overcome these problems, latex catheters have been coated with a variety of materials, including PTFE (Teflon) and silicone. This leads to reduction of the available internal diameter (Fig. 19.3) and flow characteristics are compromised even though encrustation may be inhibited. More recently 100% silicone catheters have become available. They have the maximum available internal diameter for a given external diameter (Fig. 19.3). In vitro studies have shown that they have better slow characteristics than coated latex catheters (Griffiths and Gallanaugh 1984) (Fig. 19.4). Where long-term drainage becomes necessary an all-silicone catheter should be considered. Some patients will require frequent changes of catheter whatever type is used,

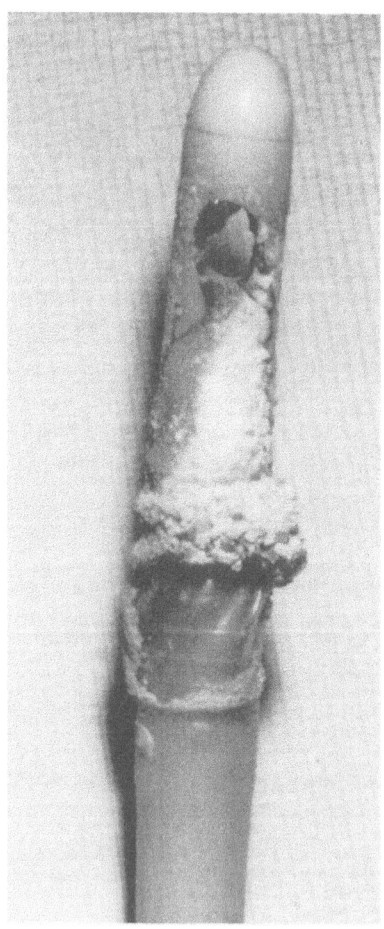

Fig. 19.2. Encrustation around the eyes and balloon of Foley catheter.

due to an increased tendency to encrustation as a result of metabolic abnormality or poor fluid intake, or repeated bypassing; for these there is certainly no advantage in silicone and coated latex or pure latex may be perfectly satisfactory if well managed (Blannin and Hobden 1980).

CATHETER LENGTH. Many hospital supply departments stock only standard "male" length catheters (40–45 cm) and many clinicians and nurses are unaware of the availability of the alternative "female" length (20–25 cm) (Fig. 19.5). The use of a "male" length catheter in a female patient has several disadvantages; firstly, it is more difficult to disguise under clothing and easier to pull accidentally; secondly, the additional length gives increased potential for kinking and blockage. Female length catheters should therefore be employed in all situations where an indwelling urethral catheter is used in a female patient.

BALLOON SIZE. Foley-type catheters are available in a number of different balloon sizes:

3–5 ml	intended for paediatric use
5–10 ml	} for routine bladder drainage
30–50 ml	
75–100 ml	for haemostatic purposes (postoperatively)

Traditionally, in the United Kingdom, 30— to 50-ml balloon catheters have been used, often inflated with less than 30 ml. Bypassing the catheter is a major problem associated with the use of large balloons. In all catheters, except the "Roberts", the drainage eyes are situated above the balloon; hence the larger the balloon, the more cranial to the bladder neck will be the eyes (Fig. 19.6) and the greater the residual urine. This will increase the likelihood of infection, and irritation of the bladder by the large balloon will encourage detrusor contractions. It is often stated that a large balloon is

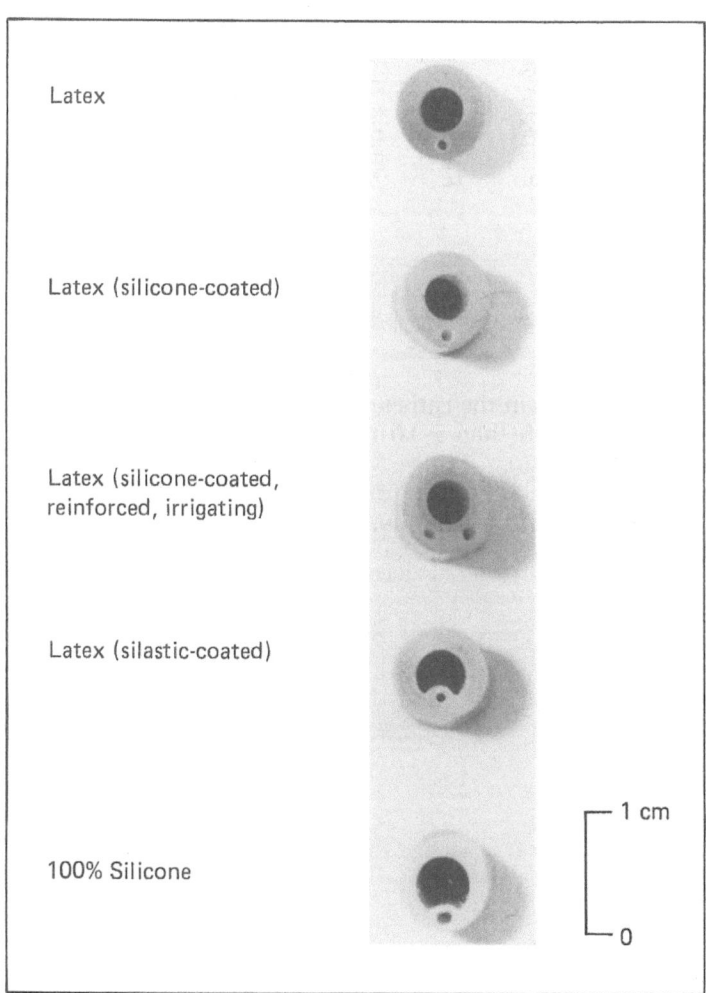

Latex

Latex (silicone-coated)

Latex (silicone-coated, reinforced, irrigating)

Latex (silastic-coated)

100% Silicone

1 cm

0

Fig. 19.3. Sections of a selection of indwelling urethral catheters (all of the same external diameter) to demonstrate variation in internal dimensions.

FLOW RATES OBTAINED THROUGH 16 FG CATHETERS

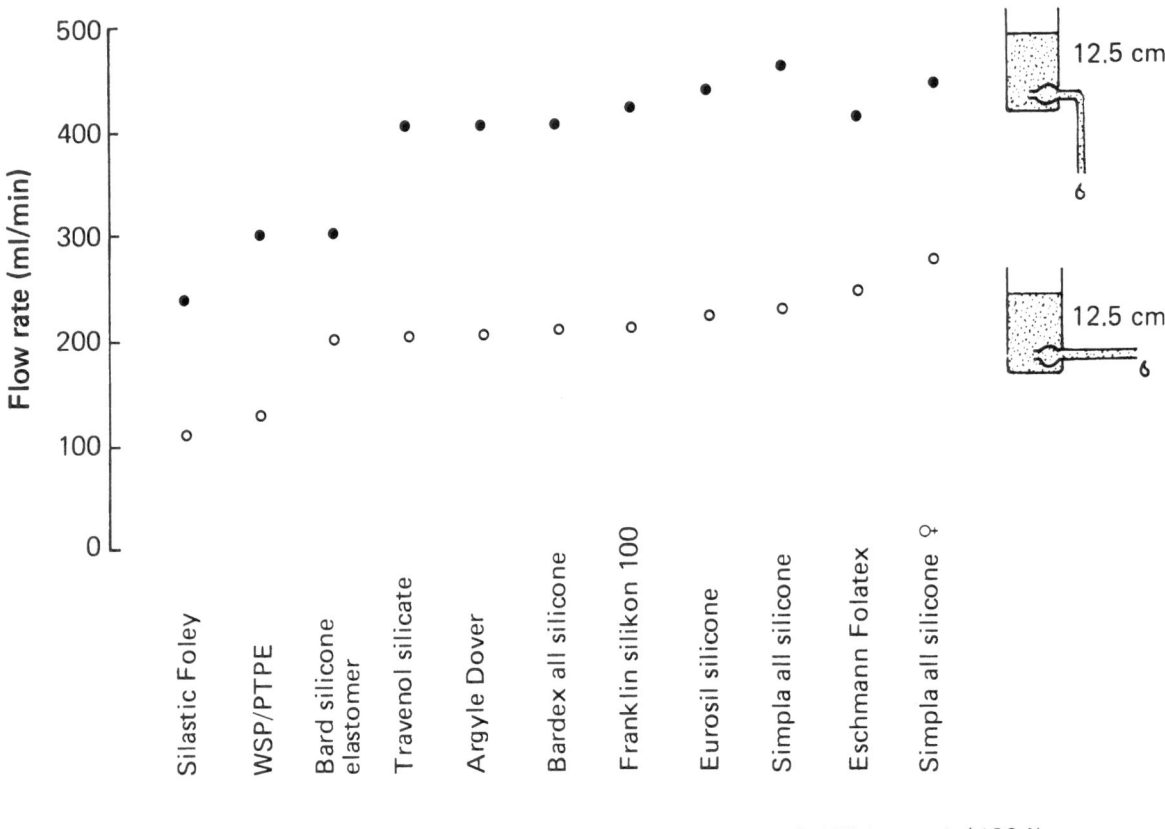

Griffiths et al (1984)

Fig. 19.4. Flow rates obtained through a selection of urethral catheters in a mechanical model. The first three are coated latex, and the remaining eight are all-silicone catheters.

required to prevent the catheter from falling or being pulled out. Bellfield et al. (1985) have shown that both large and small balloons may be rejected in patients undergoing long-term drainage. The purpose of the balloon is not to achieve continence by occluding the internal meatus, but simply to retain the catheter at the bladder neck, and rarely more than 5–10 ml is required for this purpose (Fig. 19.6).

CATHETER DESIGN. In most situations a standard "two-way" Foley catheter design will be suitable.

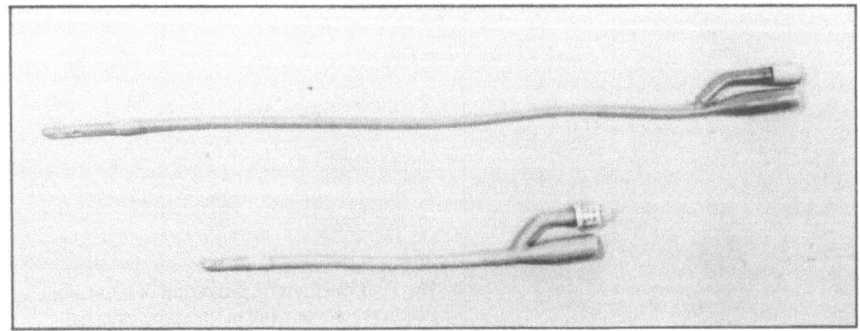

Fig. 19.5. *Top,* standard "male" length catheter (40–45) cm); *bottom,* "female" length catheter (20–25 cm).

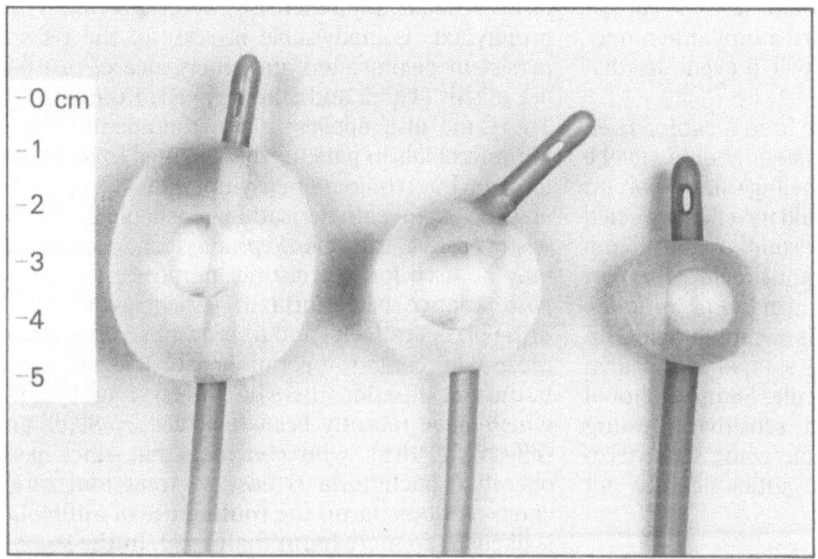

Fig. 19.6. Catheters with varying balloon size to illustrate the influence of balloon inflation on residual volume. *Left*, 30-ml balloon fully inflated—eyes 5 cm above the bladder neck; *centre*, 30-ml balloon inflated to 15 ml—eyes 4 cm above the bladder neck; *right*, 5- to 10-ml balloon fully inflated—eyes 2·8 cm above the bladder neck.

Where haematuria is likely, a wider calibre catheter is required and a three-way irrigation catheter is useful.

A double balloon catheter (Fig. 19.7) has been advocated as a means of preventing ascending infection; there is little evidence that it achieves this aim, however, and the second balloon, inflated against the external meatus, may be particularly uncomfortable. A single balloon catheter adequately secured to the thigh is preferable.

Technique

The technique of catheterisation for continuous bladder drainage is similar to that described above. Once the catheter is introduced, it should be connected to the closed drainage system whilst the operator remains gloved; the balloon is then inflated with the appropriate amount of sterile water. The practice of inflating the catheter balloon with air is not recommended; firstly, it will cause the catheter to "float" in the bladder and allow a considerable residual volume to accumulate; secondly, the air will slowly leach across the balloon wall and allow the catheter to fall out.

The catheter should then be secured to the medial aspect of the thigh to prevent dragging on the catheter and to reduce catheter movement. Several proprietary fixation devices are available which are effective but more expensive than adhesive tape. A short piece of tape placed under the catheter, with

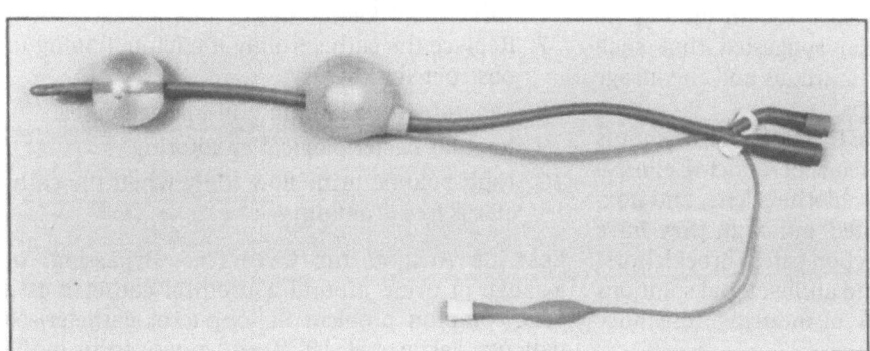

Fig. 19.7. Double balloon catheter.

a longer piece placed over the top, will discourage movement yet maintain comfort; a similar arrangement on the drainage tube will prevent its disconnection from the catheter.

When taking a urine sample from a catheterised patient the closed drainage system should not be broken; most bags have a self-sealing sample port on the drainage tubing; urine should never be collected from the bag itself. To obtain a sample a gate clamp should be applied to the tubing just below the port and left for a few minutes for urine to accumulate above the clamp. The port is cleansed with an alcohol-soaked swab and the sample withdrawn using a sterile syringe and needle. Samples should be obtained for culture and sensitivity testing every 2–3 days in patients undergoing short-term catheterisation if prophylactic antibiotics are not prescribed.

Problems of Management

The following problems may arise with any form of catheterisation; they are included here since they are much more common with continuous indwelling urethral catheters than other types.

CATHETER-ASSOCIATED INFECTION. Associated urinary infection is undoubtedly the most significant problem of catheter management and is more common with urethral than suprapubic catheters. The introduction of closed drainage systems (Kunin and McCormack 1966) has done much to eradicate ascending infection via the catheter lumen. Currently the rate of infection increases fairly consistently by 4%–5%/day of catheterisation (Hartstein et al. 1981).

Kass and Schneiderman showed in 1957 that bacteria may gain entry to the urinary tract around the catheter and, despite many changes in catheter management, this remains an important source of infection (Schaeffer and Chmiel 1983; Daifuku and Stamm 1984). Studies on the efficacy of meatal toilet regimes using povidone-iodine, non-antiseptic soap (Burke et al. 1981) and polyantibiotic ointment (Burke et al. 1983) have shown little or no benefit; indeed it has been suggested that such methods may actually be hazardous and encourage infection in high-risk groups.

The use of regular bladder irrigations or washouts has been advocated as a means of reducing clinical infection rates. Neomycin, chlorhexidene, and noxythiolin have been suggested, although they have had little influence on infection rates (Brocklehurst and Brocklehurst 1978) and antibacterial solutions at least may run the risk of inducing resistance (Warren et al. 1978).

The place of prophylactic chemotherapeutic agents remains controversial. In the case of long-term catheterisation there is general agreement that prophylaxis is inadvisable because of the risks of persistent colonisation and emergence of resistant organisms (Turck and Stamm 1981; Kunin 1979). The same also applies to the therapeutic use of antimicrobials in patients documented to have bacteriuria, but who remain asymptomatic. In the case of short-term catheterisation, particularly in the postoperative situation, prophylactic antibiotics may be used for two distinct purposes: to prevent postoperative bacteriuria in patients with sterile urine preoperatively, and to prevent septicaemia in those who come to operation with infected urine. In the first situation, there have been several studies which have recently been reviewed by Slade and Gillespie (1985), who conclude that since postoperative bacteriuria is easy to treat and rarely causes serious harm, the routine use of antibiotics is likely to do more harm than good. In the second, Hirschman and Inui (1980) conclude that the value of administering antibiotics to patients in this situation remains uncertain. It would seem therefore that antibiotic therapy should perhaps be reserved for those patients who develop signs and symptoms of urinary tract infection, or whose catheter is likely to be removed within a few days of the recognition of bacteriuria.

The prevention of nosocomial urinary tract infection was considered by Turck and Stamm (1981); their recommendations, with slight modification, are as follows:

1. Avoid catheterisation wherever possible.
2. Use a suprapubic catheter in preference to a urethral catheter.
3. Intermittent catheterisation is preferable to indwelling.
4. Use aseptic techniques for insertion.
5. Always employ a closed sterile drainage system.
6. Ensure "downhill" urine flow and antireflux valve in the bag.
7. Replace the catheter only if malfunctioning or obstructed.
8. Separate infected from non-infected cases.
9. Regular bacteriological monitoring.
10. High-volume urine flow (only when the catheter is free draining).

LEAKAGE AROUND THE CATHETER. Bypassing, or leakage of urine around a urethral catheter, is a very common problem in long-term catheterised patients (Ferrie et al. 1979) and it may occur in the short term also. The simplest reason for the problem is kinking or twisting of the catheter or drainage tubing and this should be sought immediately. If no site of occlusion is evident externally, the catheter should be gently flushed to relieve possible blockage by clot or mucosal slough. If this does not ease the problem, the catheter should be removed and examined for signs of encrustation.

If encrustation is present, then, in the long-term catheterised patient at least, it may be worth changing to an all-silicone catheter. In the absence of encrustation the most likely cause of bypassing is the occurrence of uninhibited detrusor contractions and a course of anticholinergic drugs, e.g. probanthine or oxybutinin, is often beneficial. The problem is certainly exacerbated by large balloon catheters and the temptation to increase the volume in the balloon in an effort to occlude the bladder neck must be avoided. Similarly the habit of using catheters of progressively increasing calibre is to be eschewed as it makes the urethra more and more patulous and increases the risk of urethritis and paraurethral abscess formation (vide supra).

NON-DEFLATABLE BALLOON. Traditional methods of bursting the retained Foley catheter balloon using volatile solvents such as ether and chloroform are not recommended, since they may occasionally be complicated by sloughing of the bladder mucosa as a result of spilled solvent (Clark 1985), and more commonly by calculus formation on retained balloon fragments (Chute 1962). If time is of no consequence, the balloon channel may simply be cut across and allowed to drain slowly over 24 h (Blandy 1981). Otherwise a ureteric catheter stylet may be passed along the channel to perforate the balloon (Sood and Sahota 1972). If this proves unsuccessful, the catheter may be stabilised against the bladder neck and perforated with a fine needle either percutaneously or transvaginally; this may be carried out blindly or under ultrasound control (Chin et al. 1984).

CLAMP/RELEASE REGIMES. The practice of intermittent clamping and releasing of the urethral catheter in an effort to "regain bladder tone" remains widespread, being employed by 55% of gynaecologists (though less commonly used by those with a major interest in urology) (Hilton 1986a). Although there have been reports that the technique may encourage spontaneous voiding following bladder neck surgery (Segal and Corlett 1979), it is somewhat illogical and there are potential dangers. Firstly it does not achieve its expressed aim and will actually reduce bladder tone. Secondly, on the busy ward, 4 h so easily becomes 6 h or 8 h, with consequent danger of overdistension. This will not only encourage urinary stagnation and infection, but there is evidence that bladder over-

distension actually causes impairment of contractility (Wein and Levin 1982).

MISCELLANEOUS. Several studies have shown an association between longer term catheterisation (10 years or more) and squamous cell carcinoma of the bladder (Locke et al. 1985). Collection of mucous and cellular debris will lead to catheter blockage and can be reduced by taking ascorbic acid 1 g tds.

Intermittent Catheterisation

The concept of intermittent catheterisation was introduced by Guttmann and Frankel in 1966 as the most suitable method of bladder drainage in the spinal cord injured patient. With a controlled programme of intermittent catheterisation, a much lower incidence of infection and calculus formation results and a greater proportion of patients subsequently become catheter-free (Pearman 1976). The concept of intermittent catheterisation has been taken a step further with the development of clean self-catheterisation performed by the patient—clean intermittent self-catheterisation (CISC). This technique was introduced by Lapides et al. in 1972 in patients with outflow obstruction, but it now has found a definite place in the management of children with spinal dysraphism (Lyon et al. 1975), adults with neuropathic bladders (Hunt et al. 1984) and women with chronic voiding dysfunctions (Murray et al. 1984). Early objections to the technique were based on misplaced fears of an increased risk of infection. Slade and Gillespie (1985) have shown that the major risk of infection comes after the catheter has been introduced. In fact CISC has been shown to be associated with a reduced rate of infection compared with the acceptance of a large residual urine volume or with indwelling catheterisation.

Choice of Catheter

Many different catheter types may be employed for CISC. In the author's experience patients are most easily taught self-catheterisation using a soft plastic catheter of 12 FG (Fig. 19.8), over which they perhaps have less initial reservations than metal instruments; once adept at the technique, however, many find a straight metal catheter more comfortable. The recent development of a "low friction" catheter ("LoFric", Astra-Meditec Ltd.) may also be used to advantage in some patients. This is a PVC Nelaton type catheter prepared with a hydrophilic coating of polyvinylpyrrolidone; if soaked in saline for 30 s prior to use its surface becomes extremely slippery. For patients who have difficulties catheterising without access to a mirror, the Bruijnen-

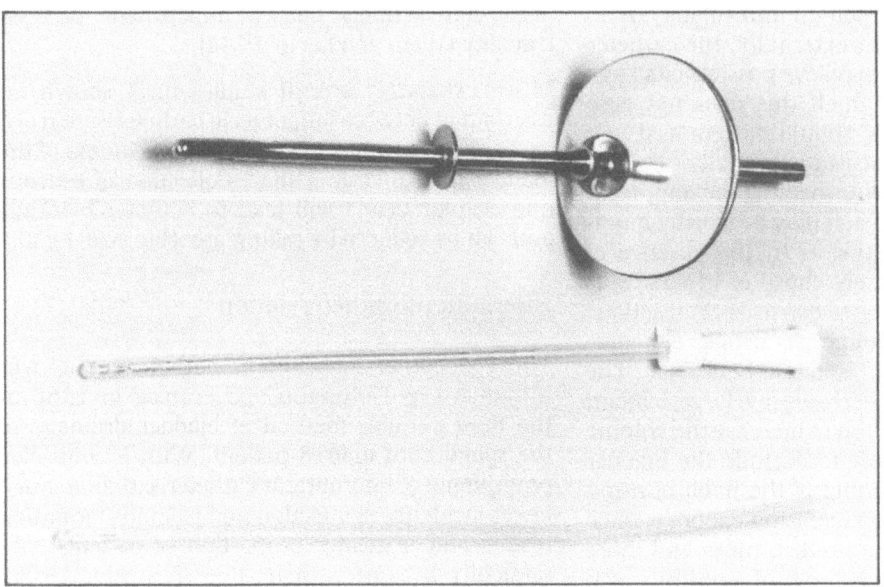

Fig. 19.8. Selection of instruments for female self-catheterisation; all 12 FG. *upper*, Bruijnen-Boer catheter; *middle*, "low friction" catheter; *lower*, PVC catheter.

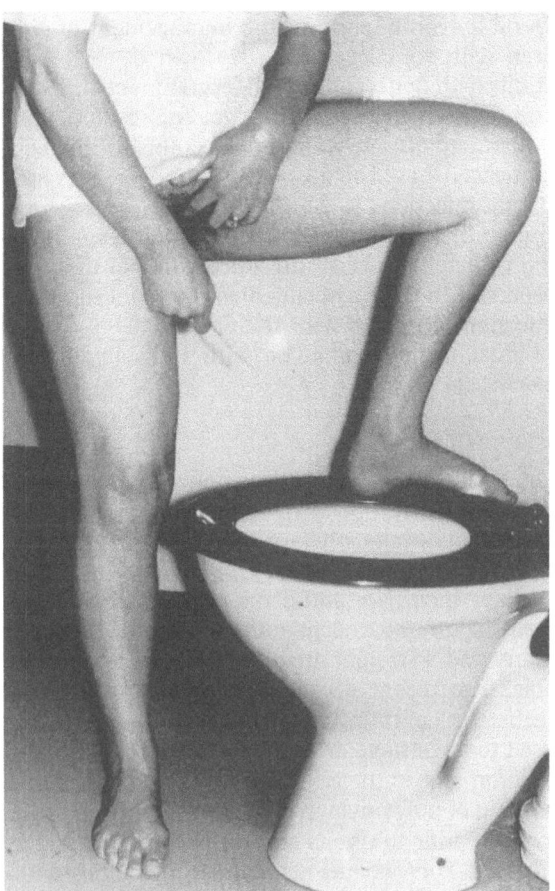

Fig. 19.9. Clean intermittent self-catheterisation.

Boer catheter can sometimes be used (Fig. 19.8) (Bruijnen and Boer 1981).

Technique

For CISC to be successful the patient should have some manual dexterity; good eyesight is also desirable, although not a prerequisite. It may be appropriate to admit neurological patients for inpatient training in self-catheterisation; however, the majority of gynaecological patients can be instructed in one or two outpatient visits. The patient should be shown the location of the external urethral meatus, first with the aid of drawings and then with the aid of a mirror placed between her legs as she lies supported on a couch; she should be encouraged to self-inspect and examine and should observe herself being catheterised in the mirror before attempting the procedure. The patient should wash and dry her hands before passing the catheter and then either lie on a couch or stand looking directly into a wall mirror or kneel on the floor over a portable mirror. Some find it easier to sit on the edge of a stool or on the toilet using a special mirror attached to the front of the seat or use the Bruijnen-Boer self-catheter. Alternatively, some stand with one leg supported on the toilet seat (Fig. 19.9). The patient should be warned that a full bladder may take several minutes to drain completely via a small calibre catheter.

Correct frequency of catheterisation is determined by the particular neurological or urological pathology, the patient's symptoms, whether she passes urine normally or is incontinent, her general state of health and finally on the amount of urine removed; an amount greater than 500 ml indicates a need to catheterise more frequently and, conversely, an amount less than 150 ml indicates less frequent catheterisation, provided that bladder capacity is normal. Most patients will catheterise two to six times a day. Once a patient is adept at this technique, it is useful for a relative, preferably spouse, to be taught the method also, so they can help in the "emergency" situation when the patient herself has difficulty or is otherwise temporarily incapacitated. Long-term antimicrobial prophylaxis is neither necessary nor helpful and bacteriuria in the absence of symptoms does not call for treatment. Regular urine culture therefore is not necessary; if the patient becomes pyrexial, however, or feels unwell and suspects infection, a catheter specimen should be taken prior to instituting antibiotic therapy. A short course of therapy may be sufficient. Recurrent proven urinary tract infection may be treated by long-term low-dose chemotherapy, i.e. one tablet trimethoprim daily.

Cystostomy

Cystostomy, the creation of an artificial opening into the bladder, is most often performed suprapubically, either by open operation or by a closed stab procedure. Vaginal cystostomy is included for the sake of completeness, but has little place in current practice.

Closed Suprapubic Stab Cystostomy

Closed suprapubic catheterisation may be employed in any of the indications outlined above, but has particular advantages over the urethral route (Hilton and Stanton 1980). Following pelvic surgery, particularly for the treatment of urinary incontinence, the patient's ability to void can be tested without removing the catheter. This appreciably reduces patient discomfort, nursing time, and urinary infection, since repeated catheterisations are unnecessary (Bonanno et al. 1970). It has also been shown to speed the return of spontaneous voiding following incontinence surgery, pre-

sumably by allowing the more rapid resolution of periurethral oedema (Andersen et al. 1982).

Following urethral trauma, urethral or bladder-neck surgery, or the repair of vesical or urethral fistulae, the presence of a catheter in the urethra, or of a catheter balloon in close proximity to the bladder neck is undesirable since it may encourage local oedema and delay healing.

Contraindications

These include:

1. Inability to distend the bladder—ideally the bladder should be distended to 400 ml, although with experience 300 ml may be adequate; at lower volumes the danger of bowel perforation makes the closed procedure unjustified.
2. Gross haematuria or clot retention—the fine calibre of most catheters designed for closed suprapubic insertion (6–16 FG) makes them unsuitable for use in the presence of gross haematuria; a larger bore catheter (e.g. 22 FG) inserted at open operation is more appropriate.
3. Recent cystotomy—an open technique at the time of operation— is preferable to closed catheterisation, as this may disrupt the vesical suture line.
4. Known or suspected bladder carcinoma—the risk of implanting malignant cells into the fistulous track makes even suspected carcinoma an absolute contraindication.

Choice of Catheter

A Foley or Malecot catheter may be inserted suprapubically either by cutting down onto a sound (Turner-Warwick 1968) or by means of the Robertson cystotrocar (Robertson 1973). Both methods are simple and straightforward, although they are presently used by only 1% of gynaecologists in the British Isles (Hilton 1986a). More usually one of the several catheter types specifically designed for closed suprapubic insertion is used. The following are among those currently in use:

BONANNO CATHETER (BECTON-DICKINSON LTD) (FIGS. 19.10A, 19.11). This is a very fine catheter (6 FG) with an inner insertion trocar which therefore has the advantage of a minimal insertion force; it is, however, for the same reason, not suitable for situations where urine is heavily blood stained. The distal end of the catheter has a preformed pigtail memory curve which prevents its passage through the urethra. Drainage is via an end hole and side holes placed around the inside of the curve, to avoid occlusion by the bladder mucosa. The original catheter (Bonanno et al. 1970) was secured to the skin with two small plastic tabs; these devices functioned

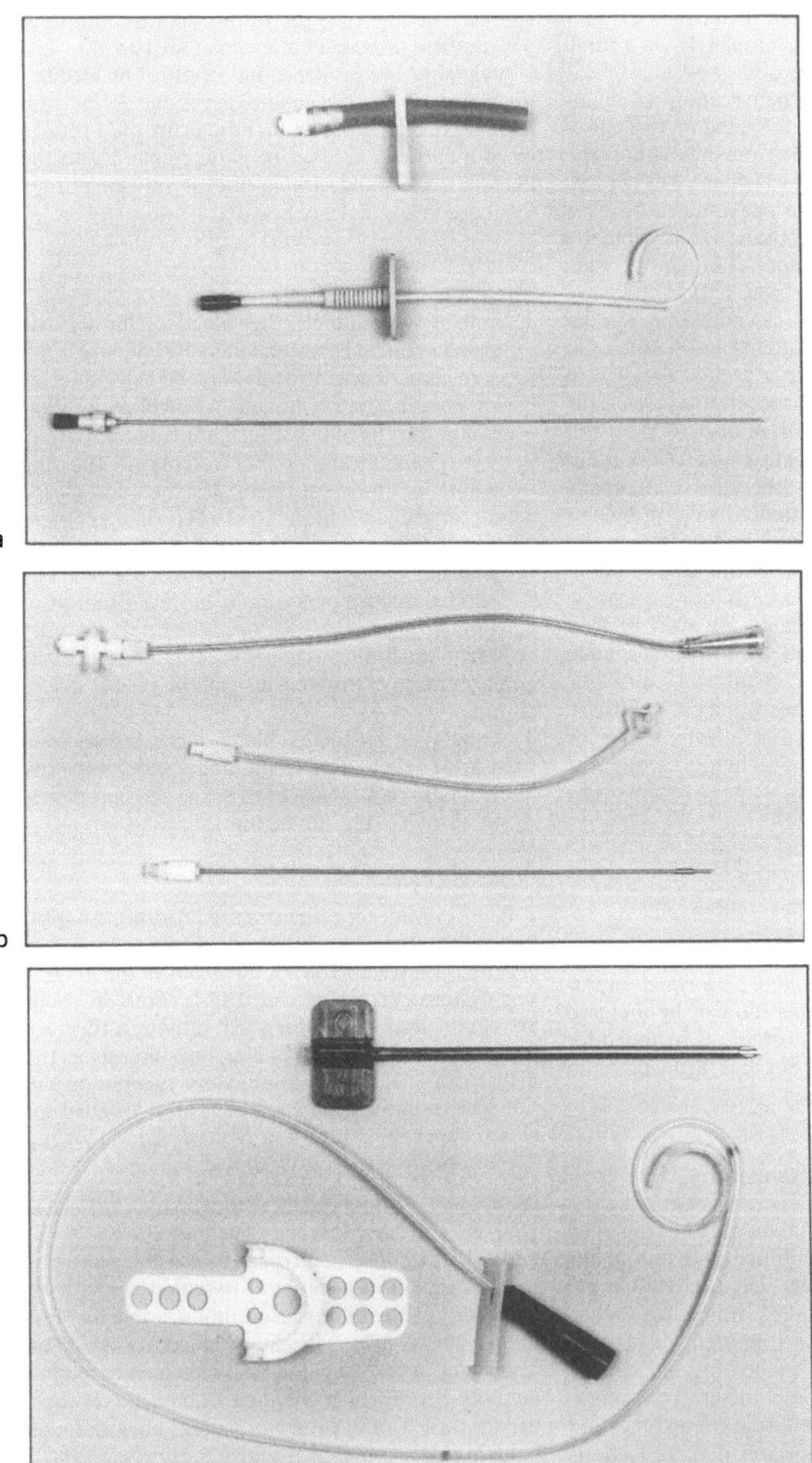

Fig. 19.10a-f. Selection of suprapubic catheters: **a** Bonanno; **b** Stamey; **c** Cystofix; **d** Cystocath; **e** Simplastic; **f** Ingram.

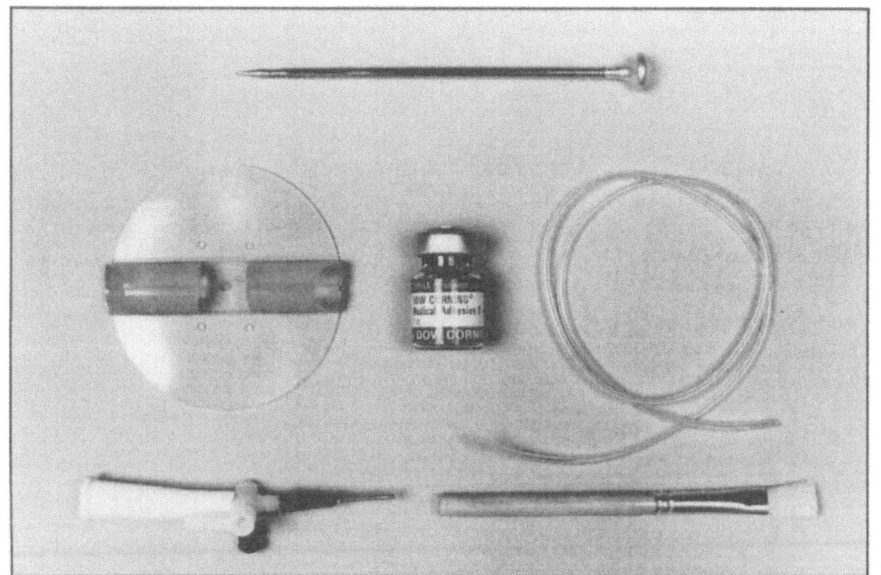

d

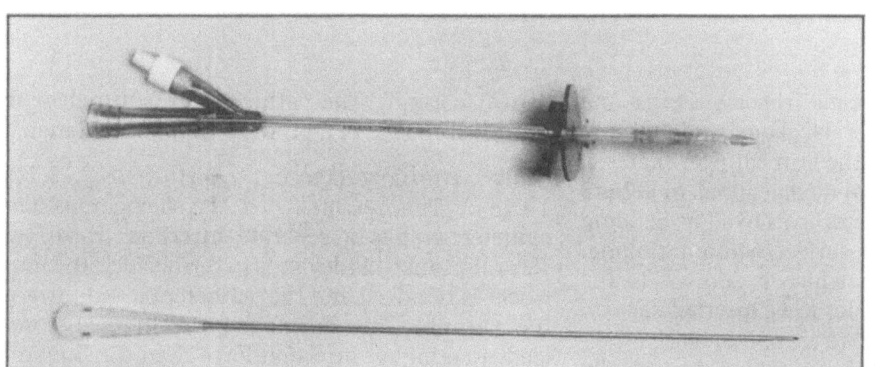

e

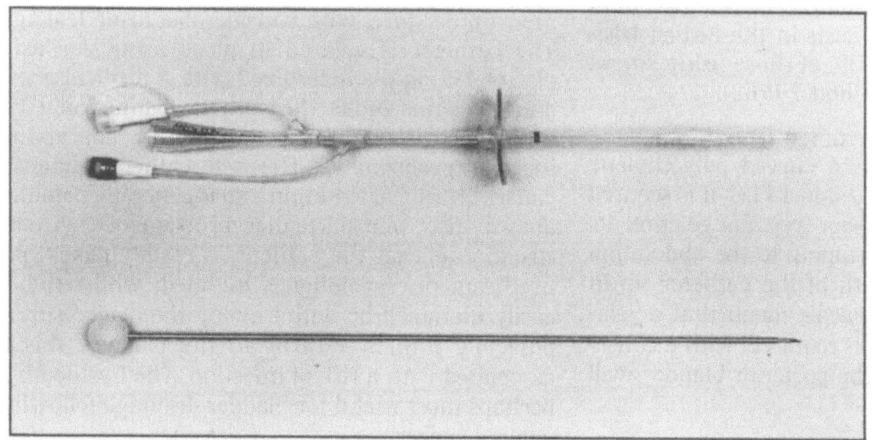

f

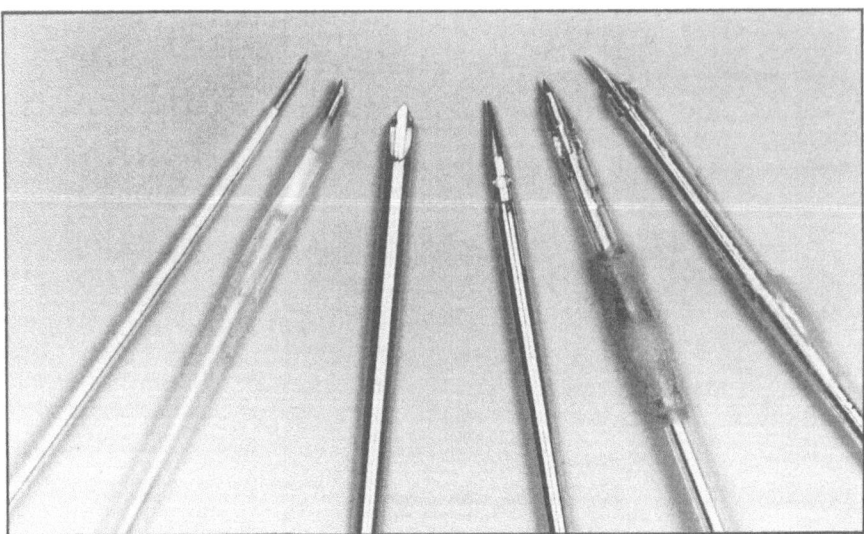

Fig. 19.11. Suprapubic catheter (or trocar) tips. *Left to right:* Bonanno, Stamey, Cystofix, Cystocath, Simplastic, Ingram.

well in general, but sporadic reports (Drutz and Khosid 1984) of catheter blockage and fracture resulting from kinking of the firm catheter material (Teflon) have led to several modifications in design. These include a concertina support to allow bending of the catheter at the skin surface without kinking, and a small ovoid flange which is sutured to the skin; this allows the catheter to be inserted close to a suprapubic incision, and to remain in place for 3–4 weeks. The present catheter is therefore ideally suited to postoperative use and is presently the most popular among gynaecologists in the British Isles, being preferred by over 70% of those using suprapubic bladder drainage (Hilton 1986a).

STAMEY PERCUTANEOUS CATHETER (COOK INC.) (FIGS. 19.10B, 19.11). This is a curved polyethylene catheter available in 10, 12 and 14 FG. It is secured in the bladder by a Malecot-type flange, and its curved shape allows easy taping to the abdominal wall. The shape and width of the catheter tip in relation to the insertion needle mean that a relatively high insertion force is required, with a consequent risk of damage to the posterior bladder wall (Floyd et al. 1983).

CYSTOFIX (B. BRAUN LTD.) (FIGS. 19.10c, 19.11). This is a polyurethene catheter of 10 or 15 FG; it has a memory curve like the Bonanno catheter, but is passed through the inside of its trocar, in contrast to most other catheters described; the trocars themselves are of 12 and 17 FG respectively, and whilst their shape ensures insertion with minimal force, they do risk a considerable degree of

tissue "coring". The catheters are sutured to the skin with the aid of a grooved supporting flange.

CYSTOCATH (DOW CORNING CORP.) (FIGS. 19.10D, 19.11). This is a soft, 8 or 12 FG silicone elastomer catheter. It has a separate insertion trocar and cannula; once this device is in the bladder, the inner trocar is removed and the catheter passed through the cannula. The conical shape of the 8 FG trocar leads to a higher insertion force than the Bonanno and the "two-stage" insertion leads to a rather messy procedure, with considerable urine leakage. The catheter is secured in place using a silastic disc of 7·5 cm diameter fixed with a medical grade adhesive; this limits the catheter's functional life and makes attachment close to a suprapubic incision problematic. The soft catheter material causes little local irritation and is generally comfortable in use; one particular problem of this construction is that the catheter is readily passed per urethram once voiding is initiated; whilst this is easily managed by withdrawing the device suprapubically until it returns to the bladder, this is associated with a risk of infection. The Cystocath is perhaps most useful for bladder drainage following vaginal surgery.

SIMPLASTIC (FRANKLIN MEDICAL) (FIGS. 19.10E, 19.11). This PVC constructed catheter is available in 10, 12 and 16 FG, and is inserted using an inner insertion trocar. It is retained in the bladder by a balloon on the shaft, and a locking flange on the skin surface. The balloon on this and the Argyle catheter may cause difficulties in insertion unless a generous skin and sheath incision is made. The rigid construction means that suction can be applied without collapse, and the negative electrostatic charge associated with the plastic is said to resist encrustation and adhesion of clot.

ARGYLE INGRAM TROCAR CATHETER (SHERWOOD MEDICAL INDUSTRIES) (FIGS. 19.10F, AND 19.11). Similar in many respects to the Simplastic catheter the Ingram is also of plastic construction, available in 12 and 16 FG, and retained by a balloon and moveable surface flange. Being similar in tip shape to the Stamey catheter (Fig. 19.11), it too suffers from the problem of requiring a high insertion force, with the risks noted above. It is generally of a more solid construction than other catheters, and is unique in having a separate irrigation channel; it may therefore be useful in patients with infected urine or with heavy haematuria, although it tends to be uncomfortable for mobile patients.

Technique

For postoperative bladder drainage the catheter will be inserted under general or regional anaesthesia; otherwise local infiltration is perfectly satisfactory. Insertion techniques vary considerably with different catheter designs, and the manufacturer's instructions should be studied beforehand by the operator and nursing staff.

The bladder is filled using a standard aseptic technique. A urethral catheter is passed and 400–

500 ml saline or irrigation fluid instilled. The suprapubic area is cleansed. The point of insertion is in the midline approximately 3 cm above the symphysis; in obese patients the catheter is most easily inserted in the suprapubic crease. When local anaesthesia is used the point of insertion should be infiltrated down to the bladder with 1%–2% lignocaine; urine may be aspirated into the syringe to confirm correct angulation of puncture. A small stab incision made through the skin with a No. 11 scalpel blade facilitates catheter introduction; in catheters requiring a relatively high insertion force (e.g. Stamey, Argyle and Simplastic) it is advisable to incise the rectus sheath also. The catheter/trocar, assembled according to the manufacturer's instructions, is introduced through the incision with a firm thrust in a slightly caudal direction. Resistance should be minimal once the bladder is entered, and correct siting is confirmed by the free flow of urine when the catheter is aspirated, or the trocar disengaged. The catheter is advanced over the trocar until its flange is flat against the skin and then the trocar is removed. In catheters without a fixed flange or balloon (e.g. Cystocath and Cystofix), or those with drainage holes proximal to their fixation (e.g. Stamey), it is important to ensure that all drainage holes, and not simply the trocar tip, are advanced well into the bladder. Otherwise, as the bladder empties, the catheter may come to lie in the retropubic space (Fig. 19.12a,b) and although initial drainage may appear satisfactory, failure may be recognised on return to the ward. The cath-

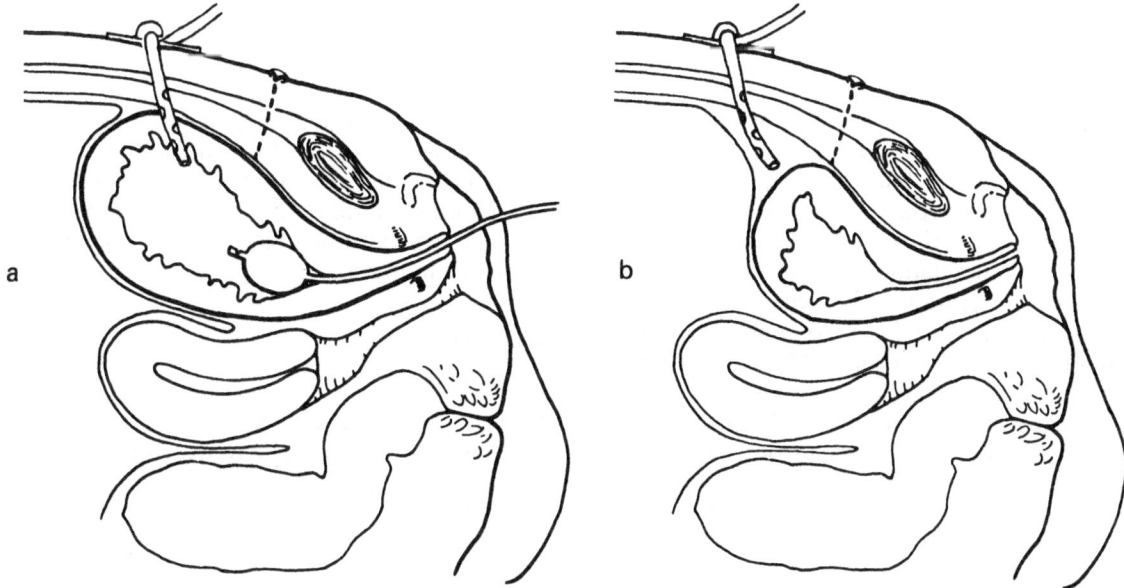

a   b

Fig. 19.12a, b. Illustration of the effects of inadequate advancement of the catheter.

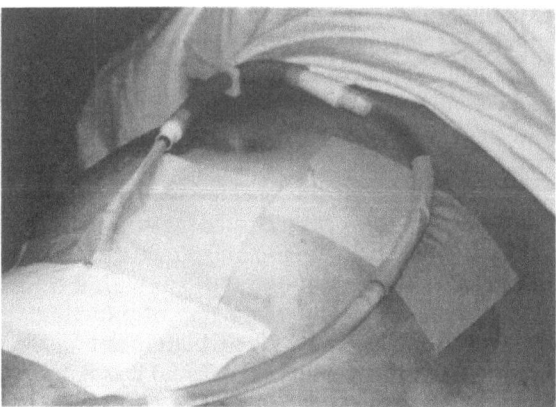

Fig. 19.13. Adequate taping of the catheter and drainage bag is essential for continuing satisfactory function.

eter is secured by suture, adhesive, balloon inflation or tape as appropriate and is connected to the drainage bag which should also be secured to the skin to prevent dragging (Fig. 19.13). The bladder is drained, and the urethral catheter removed.

Subsequent Management

The catheter should be left on continuous drainage into a closed collection system until the patient is to attempt to void. Timing will depend on the indication for catheterisation, but in the situation of postoperative drainage following incontinence surgery the author's preference is for 3 days free drainage. The adaptor or drainage connection should be clamped, or the connecting three-way tap closed first thing in the morning; on no account should the catheter itself be clamped as this will encourage fracture. If the patient is unable to void, or becomes distressed, the clamp should be released to avoid overdistension of the bladder. If she achieves normal voiding the residual volume should be checked after 8 h. The habit of checking a residual after each void is not recommended as this may give a false impression of the efficiency of micturition by masking an accumulating residual. The residual is checked by emptying the drainage bag, allowing the patient to void at her next desire, and then unclamping the catheter for 5–15 min (depending on catheter calibre). Although a high fluid intake may be encouraged whilst the catheter is on free drainage, this is to be avoided once the patient begins to attempt voiding. It will complicate the measurement of residual volumes (since the drainage will consist of the residual plus newly excreted urine), but more importantly will compromise detrusor contraction if muscle fibres are persistently overstretched by the high output. An intake of

2–2·5 litres is adequate. Practices vary considerably as to what constitutes an acceptable residual volume, but it is the author's practice to leave the catheter on free drainage overnight until the patient achieves an evening residual of less than 100 ml and is voiding volumes of over 200 ml. At this stage the catheter is clamped overnight and the residual checked after voiding in the morning. If this, too, is less than 100 ml, the catheter is then left clamped for a full 24 h, and a further residual checked the following morning; if this is less than 100 ml the catheter is removed.

If prophylactic chemotherapy is not employed, and it is not the author's practice to do so, urine samples should be obtained every 48 h for culture and sensitivity testing.

In the context of postoperative bladder drainage, where voiding difficulties are persistent, many regimes for encouraging voiding have been advocated. These include alpha-adrenoreceptor blocking drugs (e.g. Prazosin), which theoretically may reduce urethral tone, and cholinergic agents (e.g. carbachol and bethanechol), anticholinesterase preparations (e.g. distigmine bromide) and intravesical prostaglandins, which may enhance detrusor contractility. The results with all of these regimes have been inconsistent, however, and in one study the use of a benzodiazepine as night sedation was found to be the most effective pharmacotherapy to speed the return of normal voiding following incontinence surgery (Stanton et al. 1979). Undoubtedly, anxiety is a significant factor in postoperative retention, and the author's preference is to recommend discharge with a suprapubic catheter in situ for patients in whom voiding is delayed for more than 7–10 days. Whilst some patients are reluctant to take the responsibility for catheter management, the majority feel that the relief of tension which results from using their own familiar toilet facilities rather than shared hospital amenities and the removal of the sense that they have a test to pass each time a residual volume is checked and a deadline to meet for discharge allows a much more rapid return to normal voiding.

Complications

These include:

1. Failure to enter the bladder is rarely a problem if the bladder is adequately distended beforehand. If free flow of urine is not observed when the catheter and stylet are disengaged, the catheter should be aspirated with a syringe; if urine is not obtained, the whole assembly should be removed and resited after further filling. On no account must an inner trocar be advanced back

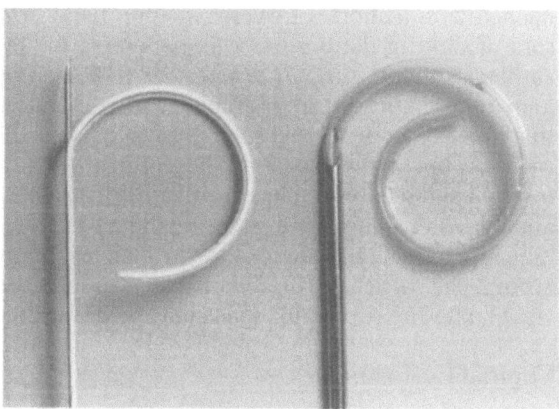

Fig. 19.14. The disastrous effects of advancing an internal trocar back through its catheter (*left*); the same may result with other catheter designs from withdrawal of a catheter through its external trocar(*right*).

into its catheter nor should an external trocar catheter be withdrawn through its trocar; in either case perforation or fracture of the catheter may result (Fig. 19.14).

2. Bowel perforation is also most usually an indication of inadequate bladder filling. The catheter should be removed and resited, and antibiotic therapy instituted with metronidazole and a cephalosporin. With small calibre catheters (6–8 FG) this is usually all that is necessary, although close observation of vital signs should be kept, and evidence of peritonism sought; with larger instruments laparotomy and bowel repair should be considered mandatory (Herbert and Mitchell 1983).

3. Haematuria may occur on the 1st day after insertion, as a result of trauma caused by catheterisation, or at a later stage, due to cystitis or mucosal irritation. A catheter specimen should be cultured, but in the absence of infection, haematuria usually settles spontaneously.

4. Detachment from the skin is rarely a problem within the usual time scale of postoperative bladder drainage; it can be managed by resuturing or taping.

5. Failure of drainage may occur at any stage and usually reflects obstruction or kinking of the catheter or drainage system; dressings and taping should be checked and adjusted as necessary, and the catheter should be gently flushed with sterile saline, to exclude encrustation or obstruction by clot. If no drainage results, it is possible that the catheter has been extruded into the retropubic space and replacement is required (Fig. 19.12).

6. Leakage around the catheter is much less of a problem with suprapubic than with urethral catheters, but it may arise for similar reasons to drainage failure. Alternatively, leakage around the catheter may result from uninhibited bladder contractions, and can be treated with anticholinergic drugs. It should be borne in mind, however, that this is much less likely with a suprapubic than urethral catheter, and the possibility of fracture of the catheter should be considered. This is more likely with the more rigid catheters, and in particular has been reported with the original version of the Bonanno catheter (Drutz and Khosid 1984); if this problem is suspected, the catheter should be removed and a replacement introduced. All catheters should be checked on removal; if doubt over completeness exists, X-ray the patient and retrieve at cystoscopy.

Open Suprapubic Cystostomy

Open suprapubic cystostomy is seldom required as a separate procedure in gynaecological practice, although many surgeons may prefer to insert a catheter by this procedure when a suprapubic incision has been made. Otherwise open cystostomy is to be preferred when there is difficulty in distending the bladder, where there is extensive scarring in the suprapubic area, or where permanent suprapubic drainage is to be instituted, as in the management of intractable urinary incontinence (Feneley 1983).

Choice of Catheter

Any of the catheters described above for closed suprapubic catheterisation may be inserted by open cystostomy, although if an incision is made into the bladder, it is as well to use a large calibre drain. A Foley or Malecot catheter is preferred of 16–22 FG with a 5- to 10-ml balloon, and of coated latex or silicone construction depending on the proposed duration of drainage.

Technique

The bladder should initially be filled and the pubic area shaved if necessary and cleansed. Under general or local anaesthesia a transverse suprapubic incision is made 2–3 cm above the upper border of the symphysis and is extended down onto the rectus sheath. The latter is incised transversely and dissected from the underlying rectus and pyramidalis muscles, which are separated in the midline. The peritoneum is pushed up off the bladder, and stay sutures are inserted above and below the proposed site of puncture. The bladder is

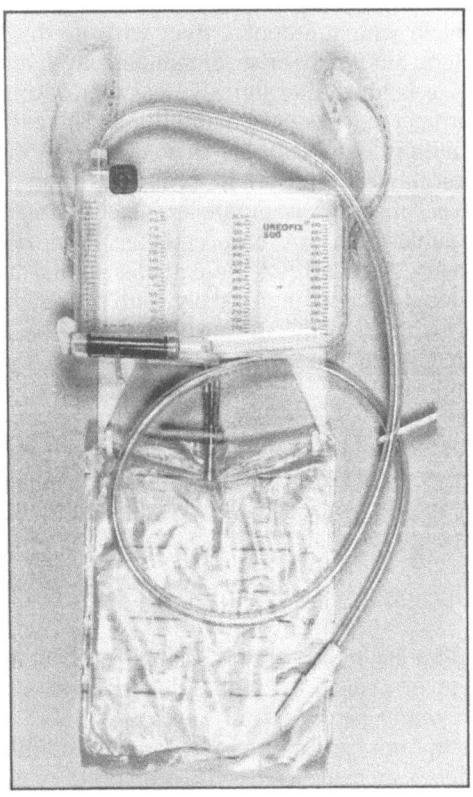

a

opened with a short transverse incision using scissors or cutting diathermy. It is preferable for the catheter to exit through a separate stab incision above the main wound; if a Foley catheter is used this must be done at this stage, before placing the catheter tip in the bladder. The catheter is then inserted and secured in place by inflating its balloon, and inserting a purse-string suture; the stay sutures may also be tied together to close the bladder snugly around the catheter. The sheath and skin are then closed, and the retropubic space may be drained.

Vaginal Cystostomy

Vaginal cystostomy has largely been superseded by the suprapubic approach.

Drainage Bags

When any catheter has been inserted with the intention of continuous drainage, it should immediately be connected to a suitable closed drainage system. Several systems are available, and the selection should be based on individual requirements

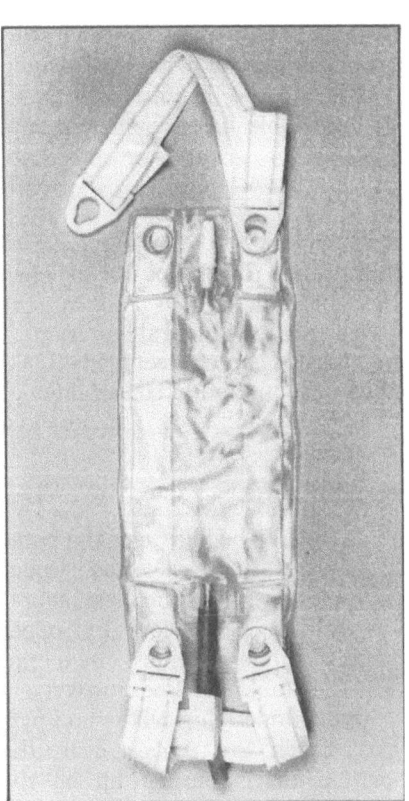

b

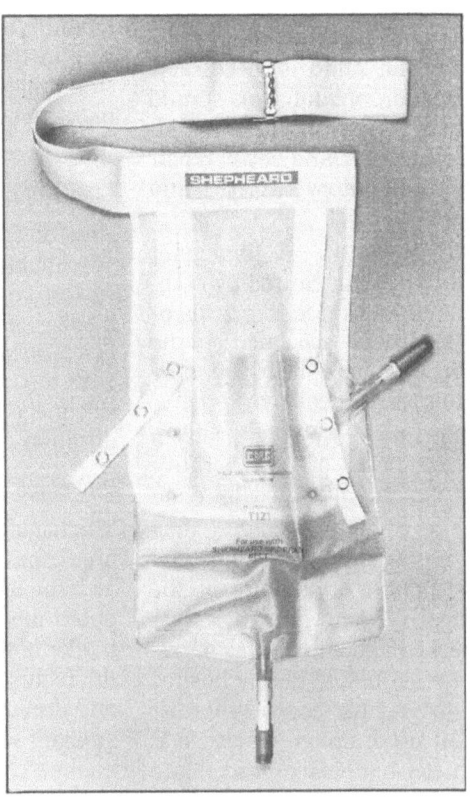

c

Fig. 19.15a–c. Drainage bags: **a** Burette system; **b** Leg bag; **c** "Sporran"-type of drainage system.

(Kennedy et al. 1983). All should be fitted with a non-return valve to prevent urinary reflux.

Two-Litre Bags

Patients who are bed bound or undergoing continuous bladder irrigation will require a large capacity drainage system. The same may be appropriate for short-term catheterisation and for overnight drainage in ambulant patients undergoing long-term catheterisation.

Burette Systems

Although most drainage bags have graduated markings, if catheterisation is undertaken for the accurate measurement of urine output several burette systems are available with capacities up to 2 litres (Fig. 19.15a).

Leg Bags

For daytime use in ambulant patients a large bag is inappropriate, and often an embarrassment. Several leg drainage systems are available with capacities of 350, 500 or 750 ml and are secured to the leg. Perhaps the best is a 350-ml bag with an elasticated fabric strap with a rubber thread woven in to increase friction without increasing tension (Fig. 19.15b).

Other Body-Worn Bags

As an alternative to the leg bag, the catheter bag may be suspended from a waist belt (Fig. 19.15c); such bags may hold up to 1000 ml and, yet, since they distribute the weight of the contained urine more effectively, may be well supported and unobtrusive under the clothing. Many alternative modifications to clothing are possible to allow the long-term catheterised patient increased freedom (Norton 1986).

Current Practices

In a recent survey of practices relating to bladder management carried out among qualified gynaecologists in the British Isles (Hilton 1986a), questionnaires were returned to 1229 individuals (43·3% response rate), of whom 960 were currently active in the speciality.

The use of routine catheterisation prior to, during and after various obstetrics and gynaecological procedures is shown in Table 19.1. Where surgery involves the bladder neck, 55·5% drain continuously postoperatively for 1–12 days (mean 3·4 days).

Gynaecologists were asked to specify a preference for urethral or suprapubic catheterisation for postoperative bladder drainage. Overall 51·5% preferred the urethral route, 38·7% the suprapubic route and 9·8% had no preference.

Table 19.1. Use of catheters by gynaecologists in the British Isles. Figures are the percentages of surgeons routinely employing pre-, per-, and postoperative catheterisation; the final column gives the mean duration of free bladder drainage postoperatively (Hilton 1986a)

	Preop.	Perop.	Postop.	Mean duration (days)
Caesarean (general anaesthetic) (n = 959)	85·1	43·8	8·4	1·1
Caesarean (epidural) (n = 955)	83·9	55·9	27·1	1·2
Abdominal hysterectomy (n = 959)	93·2	14·1	7·1	2·0
Radical hysterectomy (n = 890)	76·9	45·9	53·1	5·7
Other laparotomy (n = 959)	87·3	9·3	5·7	2·4
Vaginal hysterectomy (n = 959)	61·6	9·7	34·9	2·8
Anterior colporrhaphy (n = 959)	54·3	13·8	69·9	3·2
Posterior colporrhaphy (n = 959)	25·7	4·4	17·3	2·8
Suprapubic incontinence procedure (n = 920)	51·8	35·5	61·7	4·3

Drains

Historical Perspective

"When in doubt, drain."   Lawson Tait (1887)

The first use of drainage in surgical practice is attributed to Hippocrates (460–377 BC), who used hollow pencils to treat empyema (Moss 1981). The credit for the invention of rubber drainage tubes is given to Chassaignac in 1859. The first suction drain was introduced by Heaton in 1898, who described an open syphon drain similar to the more recent sump drains. Closed suction was employed by Raffl in 1952 and the use of the portable closed wound suction unit, which is almost synonymous with wound drainage in current surgical practice, was introduced by Redon and Jost in 1954 (Moss 1981).

Indications

It was originally stated by Halstead (1898) and repeated since (Cruse and Foord 1973) that drains must not be considered a substitute for haemostasis or a replacement for meticulous surgical technique. The place of and most appropriate techniques for drainage in surgical practice have always been the source of contention. Many of the areas of controversy remain unresolved, although in general terms surgical drainage may be indicated for therapeutic or prophylactic purposes, the former being perhaps better understood and less controversial than the latter. Drains are used therapeutically in the presence of purulent material, necrotic debris or a fistula, or to prevent premature closure of a wound. The prophylactic use of drains is intended to prevent the accumulation of blood, lymph, urine, pus, intestinal contents, bile or pancreatic secretions, and occasionally to permit the early detection of surgical complications. It is in this last context that the use of drains is perhaps most controversial of all.

Prophylactic Indications

1. Closure of certain soft tissue parietal wounds, for example the retropubic space following suprapubic incontinence surgery, and the subcutaneous tissues of obese or previously operated patients.
2. Situations of potential leakage, notably from lymphatics following pelvic node dissection in association with radical hysterectomy or vulvectomy.
3. Insecure closure of perforations, particularly of the bladder.
4. Following anastomosis where an organ lacks a strong serosal coat or is extraperitoneal, for example following ureteric anastomosis or re-implantation.

Therapeutic Indications

5. Abscess cavities.
6. Following trauma or intraperitoneal haemorrhage, where debridement or peritoneal toilet may be incomplete, for instance following ruptured ectopic pregnancy.

Types of Wound Drain

Passive Drains

Drains may be either passive or active. Passive drains are dependent on natural pressure differentials and function primarily by overflow, although they may be assisted by gravity. An element of capillary action may also be contributed by the drain itself, or an absorbant dressing, although this is insufficient to be considered active. Such drains should therefore always be placed "downhill" of the area being drained for maximum efficiency. Passive drainage is often considered as "open" if drainage occurs directly into a surgical dressing; several types of drain are currently employed in this situation (Fig. 19.16); the Lowden and Yeates drains in particular are designed to encourage capillary effects, and to prevent kinking and obstruction. The term "closed" passive drainage may be applied when a collection device is used (Robinson and Brown 1980) (Fig. 19.17).

Active Drains

Active drainage occurs when an external source of negative pressure is applied to a tube drain, creating suction in the wound. "Open wound suction" or sump drainage (Waterman et al. 1968) uses a dual-lumen tube; air enters the narrower lumen to maintain patency of the wider one through which drainage therefore occurs at minimal vacuum pressure. A sump drain provides more efficient drainage than a purely passive drain in terms of its ability to remove fluid from the peritoneal cavity (Broome et al. 1983). One of the main concerns with sump

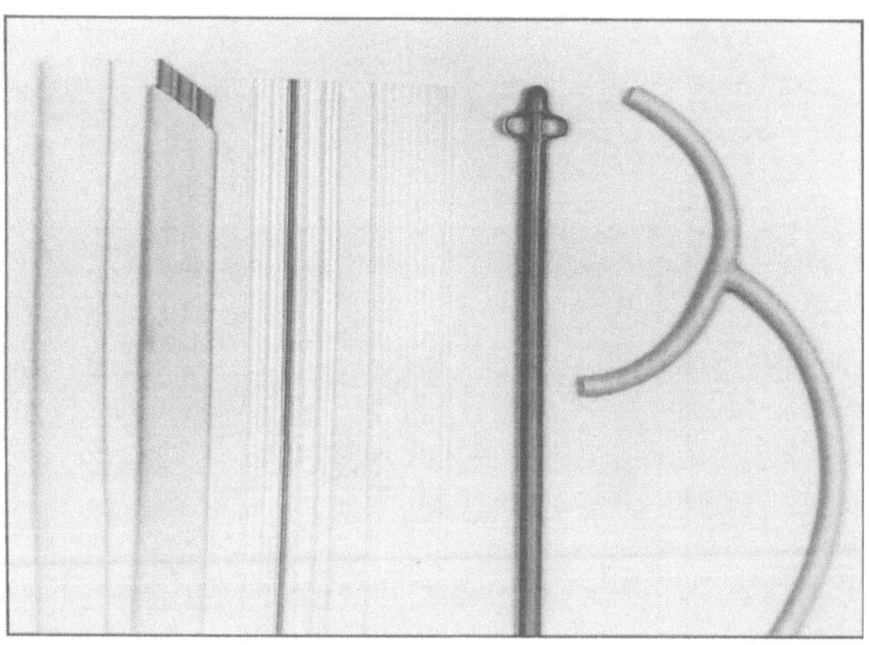

Fig. 19.16. Selection of passive open drains; *from left to right:* Penrose, Lowden, Corrugated, Yeates (capillary tube), Malecot, T-tube.

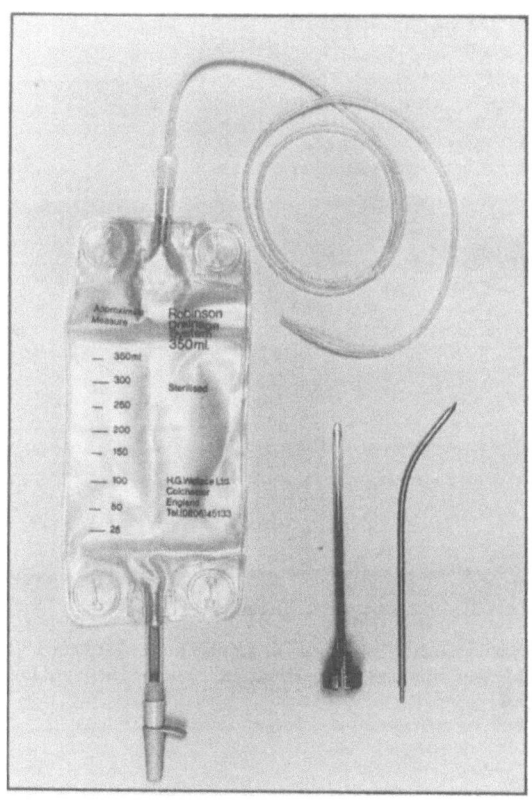

Fig. 19.17. Robinson passive close drainage (siphonage) system.

drains is the liability of airborne bacteria to be aspirated into the air vent with a consequent increase in wound and peritoneal infection. Suction levels of 80–120 mmHg are advocated to minimise this risk (Baker and Borchardt 1974), and the addition of a filter to the air inlet vent may also be beneficial.

An active drainage system which has no continuity with the atmosphere is termed "closed wound suction" and is exemplified by the original re-usable "Redivac" system (Fig. 19.18a). Many other disposable portable suction systems are now available with high or low vacuum. High vacuum pressure (300–500 mmHg) similar to that provided by the original "Redivac" system (OEC Orthopaedic Ltd) is also offered by the "Sterimed" drain (Sterimed Ltd.) (Fig. 19.18b) and the "System 600 and 150" units (Summit Medical Ltd.) (Fig. 19.18c) among others. These, aside from being disposable, are safer from breakage, and are pre-evacuated. Low-pressure (100–150 mmHg) systems are generally rechargeable by means of a bellows or bulb, and include the "Portovac" (Howmedica International Ltd.) (Fig. 19.18d), "Red-o-Pack" (Vygon U.K. Ltd.) (Fig. 19.18e) and the "Exudrain" (Astra-Meditec Ltd.) (Fig. 19.18f). The question of optimum suction pressure was investigated by Britton et al. (1979); they found that low-pressure drains drained more fluid, and were required to stay

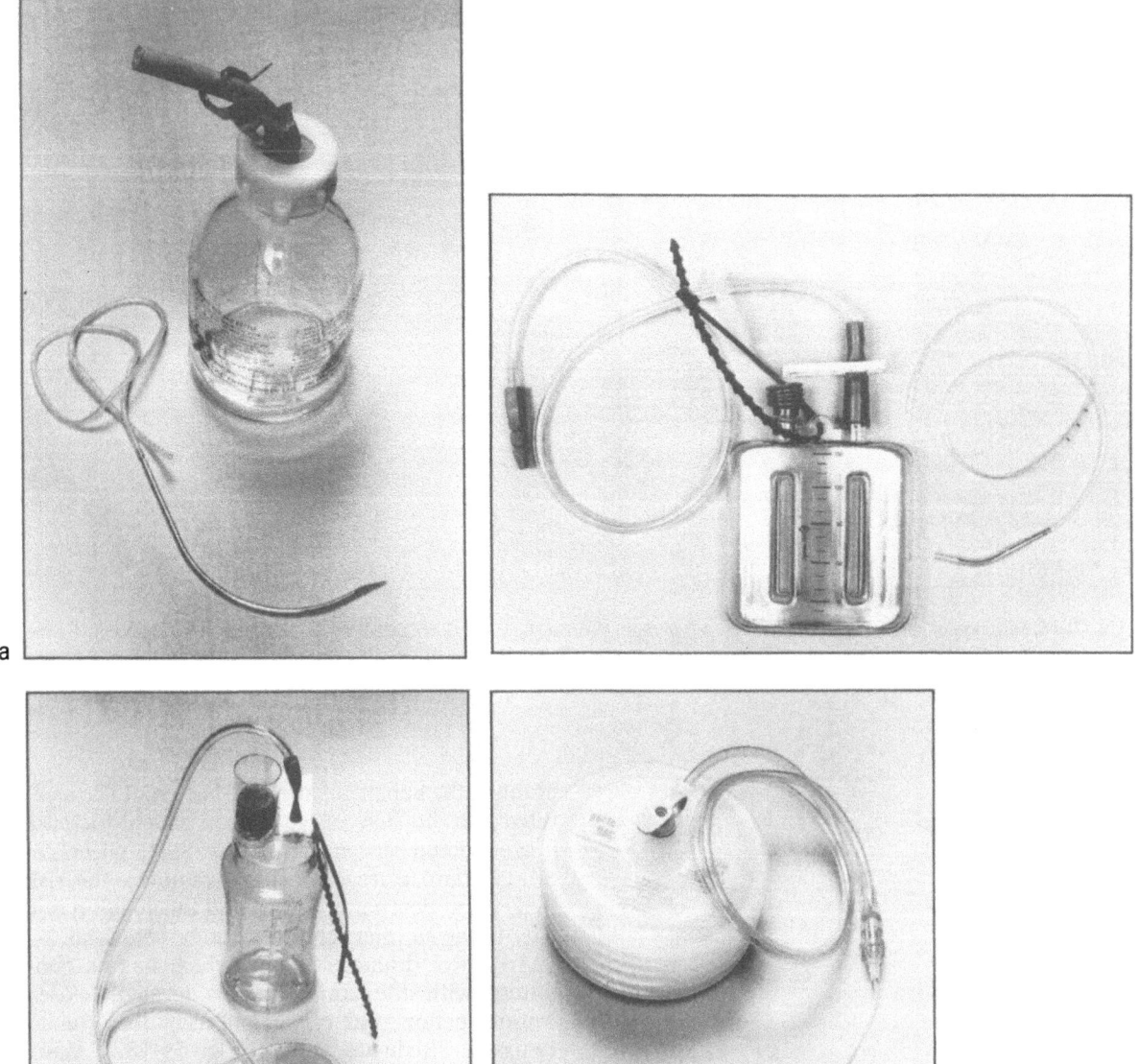

Fig. 19.18a-f. Selection of closed wound suction units: **a** Reusable "Redivac" system; **b** "Sterimed" disposable unit; **c** "System 150" drain. These are high-pressure units. **d** "Portavac" drain; **e** "Red-o-Pack" twin drain system; **f** "Exudrain" system. These are low-pressure rechargeable units.

Fig. 19.18 (*continued*)

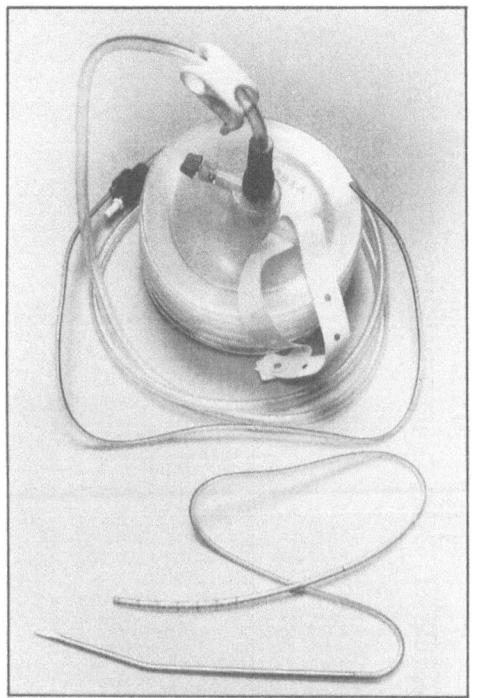

e

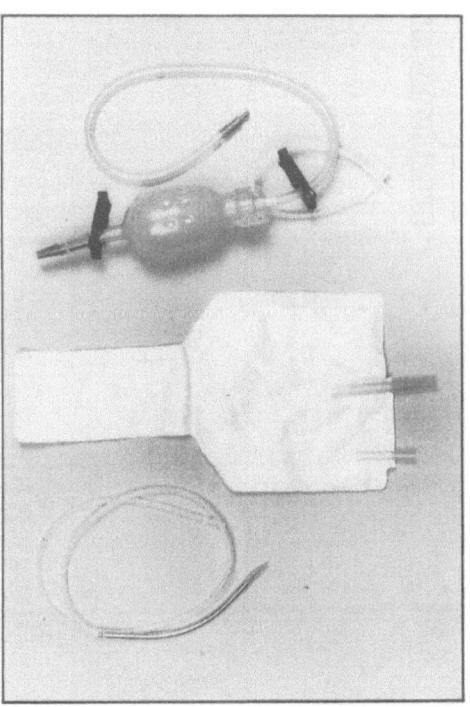

f

in place longer than high-pressure systems, and also required frequent recharging. A disadvantage of high-pressure systems, however, is that tissue encroachment into the tubing holes may impair drainage and cause tissue damage.

Complications of the Use of Drains

Infection

It has been shown that bacteria can migrate along drain tracks to contaminate deep wounds (Nora et al. 1972). The actual presence of the drain may impair tissue defences and invite infection (Magee et al. 1976), and it has been suggested that deficiency of opsonic proteins and phagocytic activity in tissue fluids within wounds may be a relevant factor (Alexander et al. 1976). Clinical studies have shown that open drainage is associated with an increased wound infection rate (Cruse and Foord 1973). Infection appears to be less of a problem when active drains are employed, and several studies have demonstrated reduced wound infection rates and reduced hospital stay with closed wound suction as compared with passive drainage (Leissner 1976). The question of infection and sump drains has been considered above; infection may, however, also spread retrogradely via low-pressure closed suction systems particularly at the time of recharging (Lumley et al. 1974); this complication may be obviated to some extent by the inclusion of a non-return valve as in the "Exudrain" or "Drevac" systems (Seely et al. 1979). High-pressure closed suction systems require little or no recharging and are therefore relatively free of this complication. The use of closed suction at hysterectomy has been shown to reduce the incidence of febrile morbidities from 25% to 11% and from 32% to 8% at abdominal and vaginal operations respectively, a similar order of benefit to that accruing from prophylactic antibiotics (Schwartz and Tanaree 1975, 1976).

Visceral Trauma

Despite the soft nature of Penrose and modern silicone drains, erosion into the bladder and intestine may occur with resultant fistula development (Hubbard et al. 1979). The use of closed suction drains within the peritoneal cavity has also been associated with bowel trauma, and Benjamin (1980) reported a case in which the perforated drain of a high-pressure device had sucked 14 full-thickness holes in the adjacent small bowel with

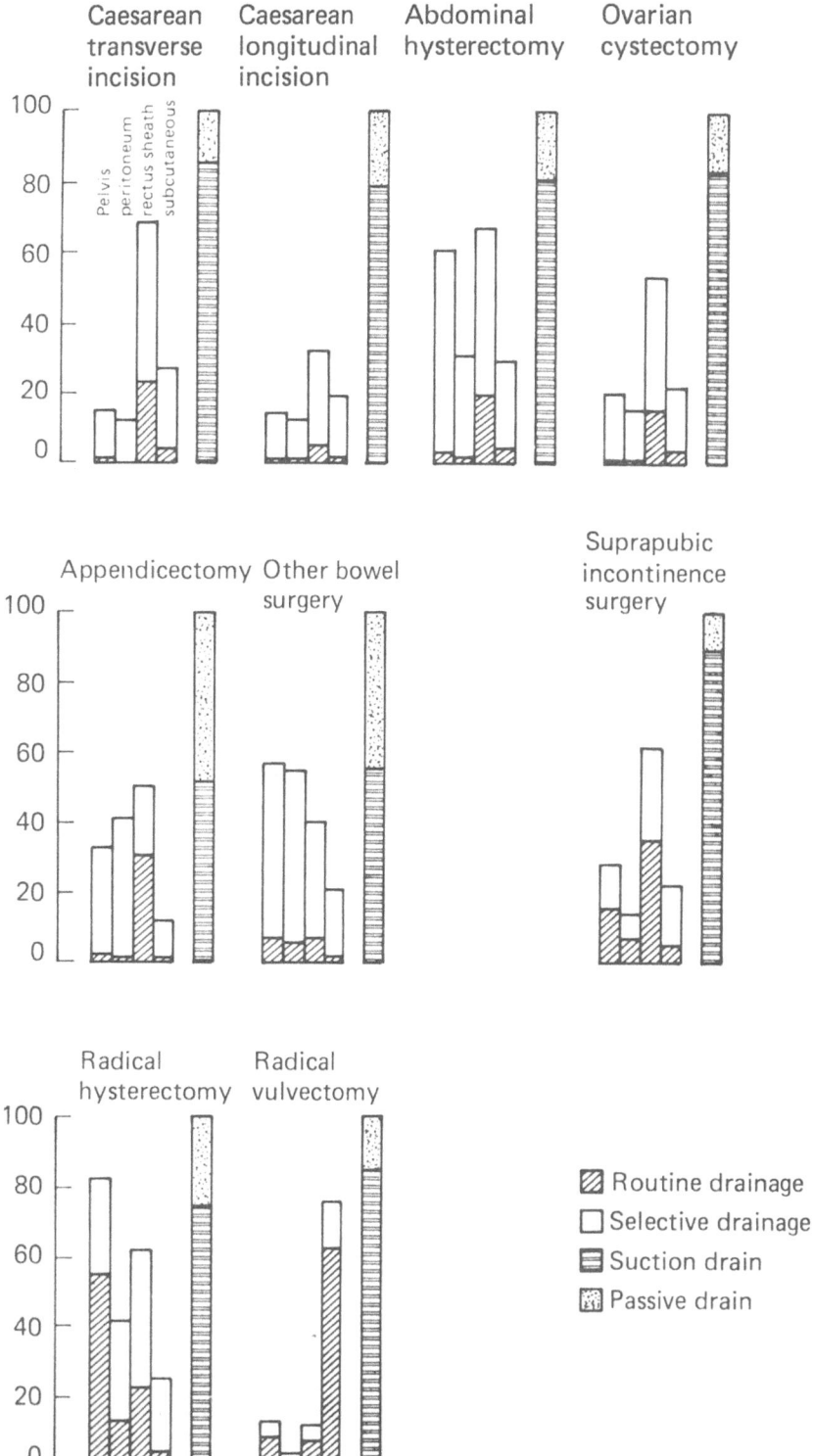

Fig. 19.19. The use of drains by British gynaecologists (Hilton 1986b). For each operation the percentage of gynaecologists using drains routinely or in selected cases, in the pelvis, peritoneal cavity, rectus sheath and subcutaneous tissues is shown by the first four columns in each case. The right-hand column shows the percentage using passive and active drainage systems.

resultant fatal faecal peritonitis. Internal hernia formation (Fulham and Pritchard 1985) and evisceration through the drain site (Shoukris and Kiff 1984) have also been documented.

Dislodgement

The commonest complication of the use of drains is dislodgement, and possible internal migration, due to insecure fixation (Smith and Gilmore 1985). The problem is usually avoided by suture fixation, although the passage of a suture through a soft drain may cause it to tear, and result in a retained fragment. The use of a safety pin through the drain is advised, and all drain materials should have a radiopaque marker.

Recommendations

In abdominal and gynaecological surgery there is no evidence to support the routine use of peritoneal drains; where drains are used, however, a "closed" passive system such as the Robinson drain (Fig. 19.17) or an "open" active drain (sump drain) with a bacterial air inlet filter should be employed. Silicone is the preferred material since it generates the least tissue reaction.

For drainage of the parietes, closed wound suction drainage using high vacuum pressure is the most effective in obliterating "dead space" and reducing the risks of infection.

Therapeutic drainage of haematomata, frankly contaminated wounds, or abscess cavities is perhaps the only place in which an "open" passive drain may be shown to be beneficial, but even here an "open" active drain (sump drain) with an air inlet filter, or low pressure "closed suction drain" may again be used to advantage. High-pressure active drains are not recommended since they may obstruct more rapidly with purulent material or clot.

Where drains are left in proximity to blood vessels, nerves, bowel or bladder they should be of a soft material. If suction is to be applied it should be either vented "open" or of low pressure, and tubing holes should be small.

Drains, whether active or passive, should never exit through the operative incision, if infection, dehiscence and hernia formation are to be minimised.

Drains should be removed as soon as significant drainage ceases. For prophylactic drains this will usually be within 24–48 h of operation, although may be much longer following lymphadenectomy.

Drains placed prophylactically can be removed straight away; those used therapeutically should be advanced by 3–5 cm/day once drainage has ceased.

Current Practices

In a recent survey of practices with regard to wound drainage (Hilton 1986b), 947 replies were obtained from qualified gynaecologists currently active in the specialty in the British Isles. Amongst other things they were asked to state whether they would routinely, selectively or never drain the pelvis, peritoneum, rectus sheath or subcutaneous tissues at each of several obstetric and gynaecological procedures. Their responses are summarised in Fig. 19.19.

References

Alexander JW, Korelitz J, Alexander NS (1976) Prevention of wound infections. A case for closed suction drainage to remove wound fluids deficient in opsonic proteins. Am J Surg 132:59–63

Andersen J, Fischer-Rasmussen W, Molsted Pedersen L, Nielsen N (1982) Suprapubic bladder drainage reduces rates of urinary infection and impaired voiding after colposuspension/vaginal repair. Proceedings of the XIIth annual meeting of the International Continence Society. Leiden pp 96–98

Baker BH, Borchardt KA (1974) Sump drains and airborne bacteria as a cause of wound infection. J Surg Res 17:407

Bellfield PW, Young JB, Mulley GP (1985) The rejection of catheters. Br Med J 291:108–109

Benjamin PJ (1980) Faeculent peritonitis: a complication of vacuum drainage. Br J Surg 67:453–454

Blandy J (1981) How to catheterise the bladder. Br J Hosp Med 26:58–60

Blannin JP, Hobden J (1980) The choice of catheter. Nursing Times 76,48:2092–2093

Bonanno PJ, Landers DE, Rock DE (1970) Bladder drainage with the suprapubic catheter needle. Obstet Gynecol 35:807–813

Britton BJ, Gilmore OJA, Lumley JPS, Castleden WM (1979) A comparison between disposable and non-disposable suction drainage units: a report of a controlled trial. Br J Surg 66:279–280

Brocklehurst JC, Brocklehurst S (1978) The management of indwelling catheters. Br J Urol 50:102–105

Broome AE, Hansson LC, Tyger JF (1983) Efficiency of various types of drainage of the peritoneal cavity—an experimental study in man. Acta Chir Scand 149:53–55

Bruijnen CLAH, Boer PW (1981) Intermittent self catheterisation: a new instrument. Br J Urol 53:198

Burke JP, Garibaldi RA, Britt MR, Jacobson JA, Conti M, Alling DW (1981) Prevention of catheter-associated urinary tract infections. Efficacy of daily meatal care regimens. Am J Med 70:655–658

Burke JP, Jacobsen JA, Garibaldi RA, Conti M, Alling DW (1983)

Evaluation of daily meatal care with poly-antibiotic ointment in prevention of urinary catheter-associated bacteriuria. J Urol 129:331–334

Chin PL, Singh RK, Athey G (1984) Removal of retained urinary catheters. Br J Urol 56:185–187

Chute R (1962) Bladder calculi formed around retained or ruptured Foley catheter balloons. J Urol 87:355–358

Clark P (1985) Operations in urology. Churchill-Livingstone, London

Cruse PJE, Foord R (1973) A five-year prospective study of 23,649 surgical wounds. Arch Surg 107:206–210

Daifuku R, Stamm WE (1984) Association of rectal and urethral colonisation with urinary tract infection in patients within dwelling catheters. JAMA 252:2028–2030

Drutz HP, Khosid HI (1984) Complications with Bonanno suprapubic catheters. Am J Obs Gyn 149:685–686

Feneley RLC (1983) The management of female incontinence by suprapubic catheterisation, with or without urethral closure. Br J Urol 55:203–207

Ferrie BG, Glen ES, Hunter B (1979) Long-term urethral catheter drainage. Br Med J 2:1046–1047

Floyd TJ, Murray K, Feneley RCL, Adams RD, Smith BJ (1983) Tissue penetration characteristics versus shape of trocar/catheters for suprapubic use. Proceedings of the XIIIth annual meeting of the International Continence Society, Aachen

Foley FEB (1937) A self retaining bag-catheter. J Urol 38:140

Fulham SB, Pritchard GA (1985) Internal hernia following T-tube drainage. Br J Surg 72:519

Givens CD, Wenzel RP (1980) Catheter-associated urinary tract infections in surgical patients: a controlled study on the excess morbidity and costs. J Urol 124:646–648

Griffiths C, Gallanaugh A (1984) Personal communication

Guttmann L, Frankel H (1966) The value of intermittent catheterisation in the early management of traumatic paraplegia and tetraplegia. Paraplegia 4:63–83

Halstead WS (1898) Concerning drainage and drainage tubes. Trans Am Surg Assoc 16:103

Hartstein AI, Garbor SB, Ward TT, Jones SR, Morthland VH (1981) Nosocomial urinary tract infection: a prospective evaluation of 108 catheterised patients. Infect Control 2:380–386

Heaton G (1898) Notes on the drainage of large cavities after surgical exploration. Br Med J 1:207

Herbert DB, Mitchell GW (1983) Perforation of the ileum as a complication of suprapubic catheterisation. Obstet Gynecol 62:662–664

Hilton P (1986a) Bladder drainage in gynaecology: a survey of practices among gynaecologists in the British Isles (in preparation)

Hilton P (1986b) Surgical drains in gynaecology: a survey of practices among gynaecologists in the British Isles (in preparation)

Hilton P, Stanton SL (1980) Suprapubic catheterisation. Br Med J 281:1261–1263

Hirschman JV, Inui TS (1980) Anti-microbial prophylaxis: a critique of recent trials. Rev Infect Dis 2:1–23

Hodgkinson CP, Hodari AA (1966) Trochar suprapubic cystotomy for post-operative bladder drainage in the female. Am J Obs Gyn 96:773–783

Hubbard JG, Amin M, Polk HCJ (1979) Bladder perforations secondary to surgical drains. J Urol 121:521

Hunt G, Whitaker RH, Doyle PD (1984) Intermittent self catheterisation in adults. Br Med J 289:467–468

Ingram JM (1978) Post-operative bladder drainage. In: Buchsbaum HJ, Schmidt JD (eds) Gynecologic and obstetric urology. Saunders, Philadelphia

Kass EH, Schneiderman LJ (1957) Entry of bacteria into the urinary tracts of patients with inlying catheters. N Engl J Med 256:556–557

Kennedy AP, Brocklehurst JC, Faragher B (1983) Comparison of 10 urinary drainage bags. Nursing Times 56–60

Kunin CM (1979) Detection, prevention and management of urinary tract infection, 3rd edn. Lea and Febiger, Philadelphia

Kunin CM, McCormack RC (1966) Prevention of catheter-induced urinary tract infection by sterile closed drainage. N Engl J Med 274:1155–1161

Lapides J, Diokno AC, Silber SJ, Lowe BS (1972) Clean intermittent self-catheterisation in the treatment of urinary tract disease. J Urol 107:458–461

Leissner KH (1976) Post-operative wound infections—32,000 clean operations. Acta Chir Scand 142:433

Locke J, Hill D, Walzer Y (1985) Incidence of squamous cell carcinoma in patients with long-term catheter drainage. J Urol 133:1034–1035

Lumley JSP, Britton BJ, Chattopadhyay B (1974) The physical and bacteriological properties of disposable and non-disposable suction drainage units in the laboratory. Br J Surg 61:832–837

Lyon RP, Scott MP, Marshall S (1975) Intermittent catheterisation rather than urinary diversion in children with meningomyelocoele J Urol 113:409–417

Magee C, Rodeheaver GT, Golden GT, Fox J, Edgerton MT, Edlich RF (1976) Potentiation of wound infection by surgical drains. Am J Surg 131:547–549

Moss JP (1981) Historical and current perspectives on surgical drainage. Surg Gynecol Obs 152:517–527

Murray K, Lewis P, Blannin J, Shepherd A (1984) Clean intermittent self-catheterisation in the management of adult lower urinary tract dysfunction. Br J Urol 56:379–380

Nacey JN, Tolloch AGS, Fergusson AF (1985) Catheter-induced urethritis: a comparison between latex and silicone catheters in a prospective clinical trial. Br J Urol 57:325–328

National Nosocomial Infections Study, Quarterly Report—third quarter of 1971 (1973) Atlanta, Georgia. United States Department of Health Education and Welfare, Public Health Service, Centers for Disease Control, vol 5

Nora PF, Vanecko RM, Bransfield JJ (1972) Prophylactic abdominal drains. Arch Surg 105:173–176

Norton C (1986) Nursing for continence. Beaconsfield, Beaconsfield, England

Pearman JW (1976) Urological follow-up of 99 spinal cord injury patients initially managed by intermittent catheterisation. Br J Urol 48:297–310

Report on the National Survey of Infection in Hospitals, 1980 (1981) J Hosp Infect 2 [Suppl]

Robertson JR (1973) Suprapubic cystotomy with endoscopy. Obstet Gynecol 41:624–627

Robinson JO, Brown AA (1980) A new closed drainage system. Br J Surg 67:299–300

Ruutu M, Alfthan O, Talja M, Andersen LC (1985) Cytotoxicity of latex urinary catheters. Br J Urol 57:82–87

Schaeffer AJ, Chmiel J (1983) Urethral meatal colonisation in the pathogenesis of catheter-associated bacteriuria. J Urol 130:1096–1099

Schwartz WH, Tanaree P (1975) Suction drainage as an alternative to prophylactic antibiotics in hysterectomy. Obstet Gynecol 45:305

Schwartz WH, Tanaree P (1976) T-tube suction drainage and/or prophylactic antibiotics, a randomised study of 451 hysterectomies. Surg Gynecol Obstet 47: 665

Seely MF, Hyde WA, Irving M (1979) A safe and effective disposable low pressure suction drain. Br J Surg 66:657–659

Segal A, Corlett RC (1979) Post-operative bladder training. Am J Obstet Gynecol 133:366–370

Shoukris M, Kiff ES (1984) Withdrawal of the appendix with an abdominal tube drain. Br J Surg 71:401–402

Slade N, Gillespie WA (1985) The urinary tract and the catheter—infection and other problems. Wiley, Chichester, England

Smith SRG, Gilmore OJA (1985) Surgical drainage. Br J Hosp Med 33:308–315

Sood CS, Sahota H (1972) Removing obstructed balloon catheters. Br Med J 4:735

Stanton SL, Cardozo LD, Kerr-Wilson R (1979) Treatment of delayed onset of spontaneous voiding after surgery for incontinence. Urology 8:494–496

Stevens GP, Jacobson JA, Burke JP (1981) Changing patterns of hospital infections and antibiotic use. Prevalence surveys in a community hospital. Arch Intern Med 141:587

Turck M, Stamm W (1981) Nosocomial infection of the urinary tract. Am J Med 70:651–654

Turner-Warwick R (1968) The repair of urethral strictures in the region of the membranous urethra. J Urol 100:303–314

Warren JW, Platt R, Thomas KJ, et al. (1978) Antibiotic irrigation and catheter-associated urinary tract infections. N Engl J Med 299:570:573

Waterman NG, Walsky R, Kasdan MN (1968) The treatment of acute haemorrhagic pancreatitis by sump drainage. Surg Obstet Gynecol 126:963

Wein AJ, Levin RM (1982) Effects of overdistension, anoxia and ischemia on bladder function. Proceedings of the XIIth annual meeting of the International Continence Society, Leiden

20 · Psychiatric Sequelae of Pelvic Surgery and Their Management

Dennis Gath and Susan Iles

In the management of the psychiatric sequelae of pelvic surgery, some issues apply to surgery in general, whilst others are specific to pelvic surgery. Accordingly, this chapter is in two parts. The first part deals with surgery in general, and the second with pelvic surgery.

Psychiatric Aspects of Surgery in General

In discussing the psychiatric sequelae of surgery, it is important to consider not only the psychiatric problems that may be detected in the surgical ward, but also those that may be detected in the outpatient clinic before the decision to operate is made. The reason for this is that the patient's psychiatric state before surgery may influence both the surgeon's decision to operate and the timing of surgery, and therefore the possible sequelae of surgery.

Several studies in the United Kingdom and elsewhere have shown that 15%–25% of patients admitted to medical or surgical wards have current psychiatric disorders, mostly in the form of emotional disorders. These studies have used standardised psychiatric measures of proven reliability and validity (e.g. Maguire et al. 1974). These high levels of psychiatric morbidity are striking, but it is also remarkable that about half of the cases of psychiatric disorder go unrecognised by the medical and nursing staff. Not surprisingly, those patients who are recognised as having psychiatric disorder tend to show outward signs such as weeping, agitation or disturbed behaviour; whilst those who are not recognised tend to be quiet or withdrawn.

Careful research has also shown that levels of psychiatric morbidity are high amongst patients referred to medical and surgical outpatient clinics, including gynaecological clinics. The evidence for this will be reviewed later.

Is it important that psychiatric disorder is common amongst surgical inpatients and outpatients? Does it matter whether these conditions are detected or not? These are important issues for several reasons. The first reason is that pre-existing psychiatric disorder may have led a patient to exaggerate or misrepresent her symptoms, and this may have led to inappropriate selection for surgery. Secondly, if untreated, preoperative psychiatric disorder may adversely affect postoperative course and rehabilitation; if the disorder is treated, these effects may be lessened. Thirdly, it is important to know whether a patient has been taking psychotropic medication, since psychiatric problems may flare up if drugs are discontinued unwittingly (and of course psychotropic drugs may interact with anaesthetic drugs). Finally, psychiatric disorder may cause the patient distress that could be relieved. Thus, in patients with mild psychiatric disorders, relatively simple measures may give considerable relief from distress; whilst for patients with more severe disorders, more specific treatments may be strongly indicated, and the risk of self-harm will need to be assessed.

These points will be taken up in more detail later in the chapter. At this stage, it is important to draw the reader's attention to some of the psychiatric conditions that may be met in surgical practice. The main syndromes and their clinical features are listed in Table 20.1. No attempt will be made to review these syndromes comprehensively here. Instead, a practical account will be given of the two groups of syndromes most commonly met in surgical practice: the organic mental states and the emotional disorders. For details of the other syndromes in Table 20.1, the reader is referred to a standard textbook of psychiatry (e.g. Gelder et al. 1983).

Organic Mental States

Organic mental states arise either from demonstrable structural brain disease (for example, brain tumours, injuries or degenerations) or from brain dysfunction due to disease outside the brain (for example, myxoedema or heart failure). Organic mental states may be acute or chronic. The acute syndromes are sometimes known as delirium or confusional states, whilst the chronic syndromes are known as dementia. For a detailed account of these syndromes, the reader is referred to the textbook on organic psychiatry by Lishman (1978).

Acute Organic Mental States

As shown in Table 20.1, the main features of these syndromes are impaired consciousness, disorientation, fearful mood and perceptual disturbances.

Acute organic mental states are important for three reasons. First, they are common in surgical practice. In one survey, the acute syndromes were found in 5%–15% of patients in surgical wards, and in 20%–30% of patients in surgical intensive care units (Lipowski 1980). Secondly, they can cause considerable distress to patients and their relatives. Third, they can present difficult management problems in surgical wards.

An acute organic mental state is not difficult to diagnose if typical features are evident, such as clouding of consciousness or disorientation. However, the condition may easily be missed in the early stages, when the only features may be some drowsiness, mild bewilderment and a tendency to make silly mistakes.

Once an acute organic syndrome is diagnosed, it is not enough simply to sedate the patient and leave it at that. The essential treatment of an acute organic mental state is the treatment of the underlying physical cause. Every effort should be made to detect the underlying cause, and to correct it. In postoperative patients, the commonest causes fall into three groups: (1) metabolic, endocrine or nutritional disturbances, including electrolyte imbalance and anoxia; (2) intoxication by drugs, particularly anaesthetics and analgesics; and (3) withdrawal from drugs, including alcohol, "street drugs" or any psychotropic medication including benzodiazepines. Apart from these more common causes, other possibilities to be considered include structural brain damage due to infection, trauma or neoplasm. The patient should undergo a full clinical examination. Blood tests should include at least haemoglobin, differential cell count, ESR, urea and electrolytes. Urine should be checked for bacteria, blood and protein. Chest and skull X-rays should be obtained. Clinical judgement should be used to assess the indications for tests such as blood gases, lumbar puncture, EEG or CT scan.

Whilst the underlying cause is being sought it is important to treat the patient's mental state, and in particular to alleviate her anxieties. Ideally, the patient should be nursed in a quiet side room which is well lit at night. Changes of nursing staff should be kept to a minimum, and staff should identify themselves regularly to the patient. They should remind the patient of her whereabouts, and give explanations of any procedures to be carried out. Acute organic mental states tend to fluctuate, and during the patient's lucid intervals the opportunity should be taken to explain what is happening to her. Visiting relatives are likely to be puzzled and frightened by the patient's state, and should therefore be given a careful explanation of what is happening.

It is often necessary to use medication to reduce anxiety and disturbed behaviour. Drug dosages should be kept to a minimum, and it is easier to achieve this goal if attention is paid to the general measures already described. It is especially important to avoid giving drugs that will reduce an impaired level of consciousness even further. By day, the patient needs to be calm but not necessarily to sleep. For this purpose, drugs such as haloperidol and chlorpromazine may be used, and may be given intramuscularly if necessary. Haloperidol is less likely than chlorpromazine to cause cardiac side effects or hypotension, a point of particular importance in treating the elderly. At night, the patient may be helped to sleep with a sedative anxiolytic drug such as a benzodiazepine; as always, such drugs should be prescribed with particular caution in the elderly.

It is recommended that a psychiatrist be asked to advise on the diagnosis and management of most cases of the acute brain syndrome, although transfer to a psychiatric ward is seldom required.

Table 20.1. Some common psychiatric syndromes and their clinical features

Psychiatric disorder	Main presenting features
Emotional disorders	
Depressive disorder	Mood sad, also often anxious and irritable. Reduction in energy, interest, self-confidence, decisiveness. Concentration impaired. Thoughts gloomy. In severe cases, biological symptoms: weight loss, appetite reduction, constipation, sleep disturbance (early morning waking), reduced sexual desire. Suicidal inclinations, expressed or concealed. Recovery from surgery may be delayed
Anxiety disorder	Fearfulness out of proportion to circumstances. Tension, irritability, sleep disturbance (difficulty getting to sleep). Autonomic symptoms, e.g. palpitations, tremor, diarrhoea, urinary frequency. Sometimes panic attacks (acute fear with autonomic symptoms). Recovery from surgery may be delayed
Mania	Behaviour typically overactive, energetic, distractable and sometimes aggressive. Mood sometimes elated, but not always, sometimes distressed, irritable. Commonly grandiose ideas, extravagant overspending, and increased sexual interest. This disinhibited behaviour may cause disturbance in the ward, and interfere with treatment
Organic disorders	
Acute organic disorders	Impairment of consciousness, with impaired concentration, thinking, memory. Disorientation common. Mood fearful. Behaviour may be restless, overactive, noisy, irritable; or slow, inactive, quiet. Visual hallucinations or illusions common. Condition often worse at night
Dementia	Slowly progressive intellectual decline, with memory impairment, poor judgement, loss of abstract thinking. Mood may be euphoric, depressed, anxious or fluctuating. Behaviour often impaired, with poor self-care and lack of consideration for others. Condition often shown by vague and inconsistent history-giving; acute emotional distress doing simple mental tasks; onset of confusion and disorientation in unfamiliar surroundings, e.g. hospital
Schizophrenia	Widespread disorder of many psychological functions, and of the connections between them. Disorder of thought including vagueness, lack of connection, and delusions (false, unshakable beliefs) which may be bizarre. Hallucinatory voices characteristic. Mood may be depressed, anxious, frightened, elated or flattened. Behaviour may be withdrawn, uncommunicative, suspicious, perplexed, aggressive or sometimes normal
Paranoid states	Delusions of persecution, often with anxious and distressed mood, and suspicious and uncooperative attitude. Patient may believe that medical and nursing staff are acting against her best interests (e.g. poisoning her with injections)
Neuroses	
Obsessive-compulsive neurosis	Obsessions are recurrent thoughts which patient resists and struggles against, but cannot exclude, e.g. thoughts about cancer or death, harming other people, contamination by dirt or germs, or religious themes. Often combined with extreme indecisiveness. Compulsions are ritualized patterns of behaviour, e.g. repeated hand washing. Depressed mood and anxiety often accompany
Hysterical neurosis	Impairment of bodily function which is not caused by physical disease. Numerous symptoms and signs, such as loss of sensation, limb paralysis, constricted visual field; these often correspond to patient's conception of the disorder but not to anatomy or physiology. Hysterical symptoms often occur with actual organic disorder. Psychiatric symptoms include memory loss and visual hallucinations, often with a mood of depression or anxiety, although patient sometimes shows *la belle indifférence*. Hysterical symptoms lead to a lowering of anxiety (the "primary gain") by avoiding contact with the stressor. They may also confer other advantages (the "secondary gains")
Personality disorder	Lifelong abnormalities of behaviour which cause suffering to the patient or other people. Patients may be demanding, manipulative and attention-seeking; shy, aloof and solitary; prone to frequent mood swings between elation and depression; aggressive, irresponsible and antisocial, etc. Patient often has a lifelong history of difficult relationships with other people and a poor work record
Alcohol and drug dependency	Most likely presentation in surgery is onset of withdrawal syndrome within 48 h of admission. Features include tremor, anxiety, and features of acute organic syndrome described above (*delirium tremens*). Dependency often not admitted, but suggested by job (e.g. publican), related physical disorders (e.g. liver disease), or demands for analgesics. Dependency often damages family and social relationships, work, finances and physical health

Reproduced by kind permission of Butterworths from: Gath D and Rose N (1985) Psychological problems and gynaecological surgery. In: Priest R G (ed) Psychological disorders in obstetrics and gynaecology. Butterworths, London, pp 31–48.

Chronic Organic Mental States

The main features of these syndromes are summarised in Table 20.1. Essentially there is chronic, progressive deterioration of intellectual capacity, affecting mainly memory, but also judgement, intellectual grasp and reasoning. It was features such as these that led to the original name of dementia. Personality and behaviour are also affected.

The surgeon is likely to meet demented patients in two main sets of circumstances. First, a patient may be known to be suffering from dementia at the time of referral. It is worth remembering that sometimes a relative initiates referral in the hope that the help provided will be general and not limited to the presenting complaint. Second, a patient in the early stages of dementia may show conspicuous features for the first time when admitted to hospital, and so removed from familiar surroundings and routine.

Demented patients may present a number of management problems in the ward. Although there is no clouding of consciousness, the patient may show disorientation in time, place and person despite frequent reminders from the staff. Such disorientation is secondary to severe deficits of short-term memory. The patient may find it difficult to cooperate with practical procedures, because of both memory difficulties and limited ability to understand explanations. Moreover, a demented patient may develop an acute organic syndrome (as described in the preceding section) in response to physical complications of surgery such as infection or electrolyte imbalance. These problems have implications for management. For example, bearing in mind that hospital admission may lead to worsening of memory loss and disorientation, and consequent agitation, it may be necessary to consider whether surgery should be replaced by a less upsetting procedure. If hospital admission is essential, it is helpful to warn the ward staff beforehand about the patient's mental state. Once in the ward, the patient should be frequently reminded where she is and why. Every effort should be made to avoid confrontations with the patient over failures to conform with ward routines. If the patient is already on medication to reduce restlessness or disturbed behaviour, careful thought will be needed about the risks of discontinuing it, or the possible advantages of increasing it. In assessing the needs for changes in medication, it may be helpful to consult the patient's general practitioner or a psychiatrist.

If an apparent chronic organic syndrome presents for the first time during a surgical admission, it is useful to inform the general practitioner and a psychiatrist so that assessments can be made, the diagnosis confirmed and treatment planned.

Emotional Disorders

The psychiatric disorders most likely to be met in surgical practice are anxiety disorders and depressive disorders. The main clinical features of these conditions are listed in Table 20.1. For a more detailed account of symptoms and signs, the reader is referred to a standard textbook of psychiatry (e.g. Gelder et al. 1983).

It should be remembered that anxiety and depression often occur together, especially in the less severe disorders often seen in general practice and general hospital practice. (The disorders seen by psychiatrists tend to be predominantly severe anxiety disorders or depressive disorders in "pure culture".)

Assuming that Table 20.1 will provide the surgeon with an adequate basic knowledge of the clinical features, this chapter will focus on methods of detecting and assessing emotional disorders, and of treating them when appropriate.

Detection of Emotional Disorders

Surgeons may feel wary of exploring their patients' emotional state for two reasons. First, and very understandably, they may feel they lack the time or the expertise to do so. Second, again understandably, they may be apprehensive about distressing the patients or making them feel worse.

On the first point, it is not suggested that the surgeon should routinely take a full psychiatric history. Such a history may take 30–40 min or more, and would clearly be impracticable. However, in the course of a normal surgical consultation, valuable information can be gained from relatively brief enquiry into emotional symptoms.

On the second point, if enquiries are carried out tactfully and sympathetically, the patient is unlikely to be made worse. On the contrary, many patients are relieved to have a chance to report their symptoms. If a patient does weep or show other signs of distress in response to questioning, the reason is likely to be a pre-existing emotional disorder rather than resentment at being asked.

Some patients with emotional disorder show obvious signs of it, whilst others do not. Patients with obvious signs may appear tearful, sad, worried, frightened, irritable or touchy. In such cases, it should not be difficult for the surgeon to enquire about the clinical features of anxiety and depressive disorders, as listed in Table 20.1. If the patient has psychological or biological symptoms, it should be possible to elicit them in a fairly short time.

If the patient does not show obvious emotional signs, then it is good practice in each case to ask a few simple screening questions concerning low mood, worries, loss of energy, sleep disturbance, poor appetite, loss of interest and so forth. If the answers suggest possible emotional problems, confirmatory evidence of an emotional disorder can be sought by a further enquiry, concerning, for example, depressive thought content and biological features of depression, or panic attacks and bodily symptoms typical of anxiety disorders. It is of course possible that some patients with emotional disorders will not give positive answers to the screening questions, but it is nevertheless very worthwhile to provide the opportunity to do so.

If the surgeon prefers not to ask routine screening questions about emotional symptoms, then self-report questionnaires can be used to detect such symptoms. There are several self-report questionnaires which can be remarkably successful in the detection and assessment of emotional disorders. The patient is required to indicate on a simple scale how far certain adjectives or descriptive phrases apply to her emotional health in recent days or weeks. These questionnaires are quick and easy to answer and can be readily completed by a patient waiting in the outpatient clinic. Most patients find these questionnaires fully acceptable. The scoring and interpretation of the questionnaire is easy, requiring no psychiatric expertise.

An example of such a questionnaire is the General Health Questionnaire, or GHQ (Goldberg 1972), which has been widely used. If the total score on this questionnaire exceeds a certain cut-off point, it is highly likely that the patient has a psychological disturbance requiring further investigation. The questionnaire is reliable and useful in clinical practice. Its potential value in a surgical clinic was shown when it was administered to 97 women attending gynaecologists in Australia (Worsley et al. 1977). Half the women scored above the cut-off point for psychological disturbance—a much higher proportion than would be expected amongst women in the general population. The authors suggested that the use of the GHQ in this way "would be of great assistance to the gynaecologist, who would then decide whether the patient should be referred to a psychiatrist ... and/or be treated by gynaecological means". It is interesting that, in emphasising the importance of such psychiatric screening, the authors pointed out that the non-recognition of emotional and social problems could lead to the inappropriate use of surgery.

Assessment of Emotional Disorders

If the methods of detection just described suggest that a patient is suffering from an emotional disorder, it is often important (time permitting) to seek further information from a relative or close friend, or from a general practitioner or psychiatrist who may have treated the patient in the past. Seeking information in this way may be very helpful because patients with emotional disorders may give an inaccurate account of their symptoms. Such inaccuracy may result from concealment, or lack of insight, or distorted self-report due to the emotional disorder itself.

As a result of such inquiries, it should be possible for the surgeon to diagnose the syndromes of anxiety or depression with reasonable confidence. If these two syndromes seem to coexist, it is important to establish which came first, and which is the more prominent, as these factors may influence the choice of treatment (see p. 291).

Certain conditions are important in the differential diagnosis of anxiety and depressive syndromes. For example, some anxiety symptoms may occur with thyrotoxicosis, and it is often important to exclude the characteristic symptoms and signs of thyrotoxicosis (such as intolerance of heat, exophthalmos and lid lag) and to check for biochemical abnormalities. Similarly, depressive syndromes may be accompanied by lack of concentration and forgetfulness, which may lead to a mistaken diagnosis of dementia (which, as explained earlier, is a primary deterioration of intellectual function). On the other hand, dementia is often accompanied by low mood, which may lead to a mistaken diagnosis of depressive disorder.

It should also be remembered that an anxious mood or a low mood can occur in patients with other psychiatric disorders, such as schizophrenia.

Once an emotional disorder has been diagnosed as a depressive or anxiety syndrome, the next step is to assess its severity, because this will provide an additional guideline to the indications for treatment. Mood disorders can range in severity from mild or near normal to extremely severe. For example, after a bereavement, grief may range from mild despondency to severe and disabling depressive illness. Skill in gauging the severity of an emotional disorder comes mainly from experience, but certain simple guidelines can be applied in general medical and surgical practice. Thus, for both anxiety and depressive disorders, a sensitive clinician should be able to judge the intensity of distress experienced by the patient, and the extent to which emotional symptoms have reduced the patient's capacity to function effectively at home, or at work, in social life, and so forth. The duration of an emotional disorder should also be taken into account, although mild disorders can be lasting, and severe disorders brief. In depressive disorders, the presence of biological features (see Table 20.1) is very important, as it points to a moderate or severe disorder. If delusions or hallucinations are present, the depressive disorder is invariably severe.

It should be borne in mind that moderate or severe depressive disorders may carry a risk of suicidal behaviour. The clinician should be alert to any hints of suicidal ideas given by the patient, and should be prepared if appropriate to enquire tactfully about any suicidal inclinations.

Assessment of emotional disorders is not complete until aetiology has been assessed. Again such assessment is important because it may have implications for treatment. Indeed it may indicate whether the patient needs surgical treatment or psychiatric treatment, or both. Thus, in a woman with an apparent surgical condition, a depressive disorder may be an understandable reaction to her physical state (such reactions, as explained later, are very common). On the other hand, a patient with a primary depressive disorder may complain of physical symptoms but not of psychological symptoms, and such complaints may lead to unnecessary physical treatments, including surgery. This point is particularly relevant to gynaecological complaints such as menstrual disorders, and will be taken up more than once in the later sections of this chapter.

Aetiological factors can be classified as predisposing, precipitating and maintaining. Predisposing factors are those which determine a patient's vulnerability to becoming mentally ill under certain circumstances; they include both hereditary factors and lasting personality characteristics such as an inability to cope with minor day-to-day stresses. Precipitating factors are events (such as bereave-

ments, broken engagements, loss of job, etc.) which occur shortly before the onset of a mental disorder and appear to have played a part in inducing it. Maintaining factors are circumstances that prolong the course of an established mental disorder, once it has started.

These three sets of factors will be reviewed in turn, starting with precipitating factors, which are usually elicited first in interviewing a patient.

Precipitating Factors.   Precipitating factors in surgical practice can be subdivided into four groups, as shown in Fig. 20.1.

GROUP (A).   Numerous physical factors can act directly on the brain to cause emotional disorders. Examples are brain diseases (for example, vascular, degenerative or neoplastic diseases); endocrine diseases (e.g. Cushing's syndrome); and various metabolic diseases (e.g. deficiency of B12 or folate). In addition, drugs used in the management of physical illnesses can directly induce emotional symptoms, such as the depression or occasional euphoria induced by steroids. When emotional symptoms are presented by patients in surgical practice, it is obviously highly important that physical causes should be excluded by careful history taking, physical examination and if appropriate by investigations.

GROUP (B).   In some surgical patients, an anxiety disorder or depressive disorder may be precipitated by the physical symptoms that led to the original surgical consultation.

GROUP (C).   In other patients, emotional disorders can be precipitated by psychological/social factors related to the surgical condition. For example, the patient may be anxious about arrangements at home while she is in hospital and convalescing afterwards; the possibility of losing her job; or financial problems resulting from admission to hospital.

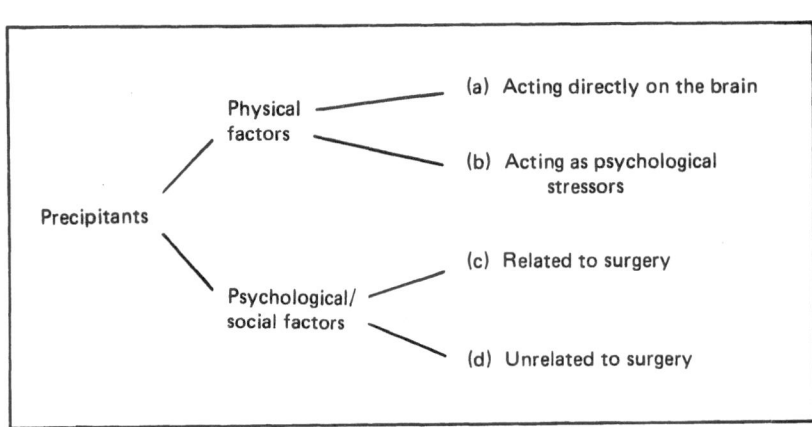

Fig. 20.1. Precipitating factors for emotional disorders.

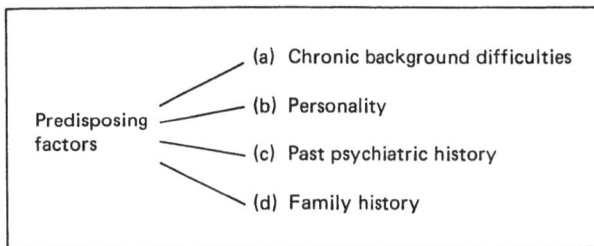

Fig. 20.2. Predisposing factors for emotional disorders.

GROUP (D). It is important to bear in mind that emotional disorders may have been precipitated by psychological/social factors totally unrelated to the surgical condition. As before, such factors may include problems in the family, at work or elsewhere. Such environmental factors are probably common in gynaecological patients—a point to be taken up in the second part of this chapter.

Predisposing Factors. Certain factors make patients more or less likely to break down emotionally when confronted by the stress of surgery. As shown in Fig. 20.2, these factors can be divided into four groups.

GROUP (A). Chronic background difficulties are environmental stressors that last for several years (and therefore differ from precipitating factors which are short-term events). For women, examples of such factors are lack of money, poor housing, lack of a confiding relationship, responsibility for small children at home and lack of employment outside the home. Research has clearly shown that such factors make some women, especially those of low socioeconomic status, vulnerable to the precipitation of emotional disorders by stressful life-events of many kinds.

GROUP (B). Certain personality characteristics make patients more likely to break down emotionally under new stresses, such as physical illnesses or the prospect of surgery. For example, patients with chronically anxious personalities react to every difficulty in life with inappropriate fear, and are likely to be made exceedingly anxious when faced with surgery. Highly obsessional patients may be unable to alter their rigid routines to cope with the new regime of a hospital ward. Several research studies have shown that highly neurotic women [for example, those scoring highly on the Eysenck Personality Inventory or EPI (Eysenck and Eysenck 1963)] are likely to have adverse emotional reactions to surgery of various kinds.

In commonsense terms, patients who have coped well in the past with stresses such as previous physical illnesses are most likely to cope well with a current illness. It is therefore useful to ascertain how well a patient has coped with such problems in the past.

GROUP (C). A previous history of psychiatric illness is a good indicator of a high risk of emotional breakdown in response to surgery. It should be stressed that such a history does not mean that an adverse emotional response is inevitable; it merely points to an increased statistical risk. It is therefore useful to find out whether or not the patient has been treated for psychiatric or "nervous" problems by a GP or psychiatrist in the past. Obtaining such information may be useful for another reason—it may indicate the type of psychiatric symptoms that could develop in response to hospital admission or surgery, since the pattern of breakdown tends to resemble that of past episodes.

GROUP (D). A family history of psychiatric disorder is statistically related to the risk of psychiatric breakdown in response to surgery, but probably has little predictive value in practice.

Maintaining Factors. If an emotional disorder is induced by a precipitating factor, such as a surgical operation, it may be maintained by other factors (such as adverse social factors). The persistence of the psychiatric disorder may in turn delay recovery from surgery.

Treatment of Emotional Disorders

For emotional disorders, as for all psychiatric disorders, there are three main approaches to treatment: psychological, physical (drugs or electroconvulsive therapy) and social. Details of these treatments can be found in a standard textbook of psychiatry. In this chapter, certain psychological measures will be discussed in some detail, and medication will be mentioned briefly.

Psychological Management. Many of the emotional disorders encountered in surgical patients can be considerably helped by explanation and reassurance.

Careful research has shown that about 90% of patients in surgical wards want to be given explanations about their illness, and about 60% believe that they have been given explanations that were not adequate. Examples of the types of information required are: how long are they likely to stay in hospital; what will be done in the operating theatre; what the postoperative treatment will be (infusions, drains, stitches, pain relief); and how soon normal activities can be resumed, including work, social life and sexual activity.

There are several reasons why many patients may not be given the information they would like. Understandably, busy surgeons may have little time to provide such explanations, whether in the clinic or on the ward. Patients are often scared of asking doctors questions. For their part, doctors often use the patients' diffidence to keep them at a distance, thus avoiding potential overinvolvement. Some doctors assume that patients will be unable to grasp the details of an explanation even if given.

In practice, it is often possible to overcome some of these barriers to communication. For example, if technical language is avoided and simple diagrams are used, most patients can be given an idea of what will happen to them and why. In providing explanations, it is important to take cues from the patient's questions as to how much she wants to know. Some patients like to have detailed explanations, whilst others are content with a broad outline.

In clinical practice, it may seem that attempts at explanation are a waste of time because patients do not remember what they have been told. Research has indeed shown that, in stressful circumstances such as an outpatient clinic or a hospital ward, new information is poorly registered and so cannot be recalled in detail. Studies by psychologists have shown that information is most likely to be remembered if presented in writing, so that the patient can read and reread it at her leisure, and possibly discuss the contents with her family or fellow patients. For this reason, there is an increasing trend to provide explanatory leaflets in hospitals and clinics. When such leaflets are provided, the surgeon's initial explanation can be quite brief. The patient can be encouraged to record any questions arising from the leaflet, and to raise them with a member of staff on admission.

Patients should be made aware (perhaps in a leaflet) that doctors and nurses on the ward can deal with many of their queries, especially those concerning the practicalities of postoperative recovery. Consultations in response to such queries are best carried out in private, rather than on a ward round when the patient is surrounded by a surgical team. The patient may still hesitate to ask certain questions, particularly about future sexual functioning. It can therefore help if the surgeon provides the opportunity by tactfully raising the question himself.

It is well within the skills of most surgeons to provide simple psychological treatment (in the form of explanation) for most of their patients who have emotional disorders. A small proportion of patients will need to be referred to a psychiatrist. The main indications for psychiatric referral are: (1) if there is uncertainty about the psychiatric diagnosis, or about the extent to which an identified psychiatric disorder is affecting complaints of physical problems; (2) if the emotional disorder fails to respond to information and reassurance; (3) if the disorder is particularly severe or if there seems to be a risk of suicide; and (4) if the patient's behaviour is disruptive in spite of reasonable explanation or simple sedation.

How far is it advisable for the surgeon to prescribe psychotropic drugs to patients with emotional problems? In the case of anxiety disorders of moderate severity, it may be appropriate to prescribe anxiolytic drugs (such as benzodiazepines), but this should only be done after explanation and reassurance have failed. Because such drugs can be harmful if prescribed long-term, they should be used only as a temporary measure. The patient should be told that the drugs are intended to tide her over a crisis, and that they will be discontinued within 3 weeks at the most.

If it appears that a patient has a depressive disorder severe enough to require antidepressant medication, it is probably advisable to refer her to a psychiatrist for advice on choice of drug and dosage. Such referral might not be necessary if the surgeon had considerable knowledge of antidepressant drugs and experience in prescribing them.

Other Aspects of the Management of Psychiatric Disorders in Surgical Practice

Three further aspects of psychiatric management are important in surgical practice—selection for surgery, timing of surgery and the management of the patient already on psychotropic medication. All these factors have particular relevance to gynaecological surgery.

Selection for Surgery

It is again stressed that physical complaints, very often gynaecological, are frequent manifestations of emotional distress. In selecting patients for any elective surgical procedures, it is important to detect any evidence of emotional disorder, and then to decide which is primary, the emotional disorder or the physical complaints. This decision is important, because in some cases psychiatric treatment could be more beneficial than surgery, a point discussed in greater detail in the second part of the chapter. At this point, it is worth noting the cautionary words of a gynaecologist, "a great deal of gynaecological surgery is elective, done to improve the quality of life and only occasionally to sustain life. Decisions to perform elective gynaecological surgery need never be taken at haste" (Smith 1979).

Timing of Surgery

It may be difficult to decide on the best time for elective surgery in a patient who is currently psychiatrically ill. If a patient is currently suffering from a major mental illness, such as schizophrenia or manic depressive psychosis, surgery may well lead to psychiatric deterioration, especially if the patient has delusions or hallucinations. Apart from this risk, patients with major mental illnesses may be difficult to manage on the surgical ward. Many major mental illnesses have a fluctuating course, and it may therefore be best to postpone surgery until the patient is in remission. By contrast, if the patient is suffering from an emotional disorder secondary to a distressing physical condition such as severe and prolonged menorrhagia, it may be desirable to proceed to surgery without delay, since psychiatric recovery is only likely to occur when the menstrual disorder has been relieved.

In planning the timing of elective surgery for a patient with psychiatric disorder, it is probably best to consult the patient's general practitioner or a psychiatrist and of course the patient herself.

Patients on Psychotropic Medication

The surgeon may recommend an operation for a patient who is known to be taking psychotropic medication. Such medication may have been prescribed for an episode of psychiatric illness which is current and active. On the other hand, the patient may be currently psychiatrically well but nonetheless taking a psychotropic drug regularly to prevent relapse of a remitting and recurring illness. Examples of such long-term treatment are lithium for a manic depressive illness, or flupenthixol for schizophrenia.

It is strongly recommended that no psychotropic medication, whether for current illness or for prophylaxis, should be stopped without first consulting the patient's general practitioner or psychiatrist. The main reason for this is that the stress of hospital admission may induce a psychiatric relapse in a patient made more vulnerable by withdrawal of powerful prophylactic drugs. Even anxiolytic drugs such as the benzodiazepines should not be stopped abruptly before admission, as withdrawal may lead to rebound anxiety or even withdrawal symptoms. Of course, oral psychotropic medication may have to be interrupted briefly before an anaesthetic, but rapid resumption of the medication will probably be desirable. There are of course certain classes of drug that need to be discontinued several weeks before anaesthesia, for example, monoamine-oxidase inhibitors (such as phenelzine or tranylcypromine) which should be stopped a fortnight before surgery. Decisions to stop such drugs should be taken well before admission, and in collaboration with the anaesthetist and the doctor prescribing the psychotropic medication.

Psychiatric Aspects of Pelvic Surgery

Before discussing links between psychiatric disorder and specific gynaecological operations, it is useful to know whether there is any evidence that women complaining of gynaecological problems are particularly prone to complain of psychiatric symptoms as well. If a significant association were found between the two types of complaint, this would again underline the need to distinguish between two possibilities: (1) that gynaecological pathology frequently induces psychiatric symptoms in the patient and (2) that a sizeable proportion of gynaecological patients have no significant pelvic pathology, but "their illness represents a psychic conflict sailing under a gynaecological flag" (Rogers 1950).

Prevalence of Psychiatric Disorder in Women with Gynaecological Symptoms

Psychiatric Disorder in Women Attending Gynaecology Outpatient Clinics

Psychiatric morbidity among women attending gynaecological clinics is often said to be high. Reference has already been made to the Australian study in which over half of a sample of gynaecological outpatients were found to be "probable psychiatric cases" as measured by the General Health Questionnaire (see p. 289) In gynaecological clinics in the United Kingdom, similar levels of morbidity have been found by psychiatrists who also used the General Health Questionnaire (Ballinger 1977; Byrne 1984). In Ballinger's study, the level of psychiatric morbidity was nearly double that in an age-matched sample of women from the general population (Ballinger 1975).

Of course, we cannot evaluate these findings properly unless we can compare levels of psychiatric disturbance amongst women attending gynaecological clinics with those found amongst women attending other outpatient clinics. There are a few reports suggesting that about one-third of patients attending general medical or dermatological outpatient clinics have significant psychological problems. Unfortunately, little can be inferred from these reports because they do not separate rates for males and females. It is well established that neurotic disorders are more frequent in women than in men, so it is still unknown whether the levels of psychiatric morbidity differ significantly between women attending gynaecological clinics and women attending other clinics.

Associations Between Gynaecological Complaints and Psychiatric Disorder Amongst Women in the General Population

It is of considerable interest to know whether there are significant associations between gynaecological complaints and psychiatric disorder amongst women in the general population (as opposed to women referred to gynaecologists). There have been very few epidemiological studies of this question. In a recent survey of women registered in two group practices in Oxford, a random sample of 521 women aged 35–59 were interviewed (Gath et al. 1987). Detailed psychiatric and gynaecological assessments were made. Psychiatric disorder was found to be significantly more frequent in four groups of women, namely those complaining of: premenstrual tension, dysmenorrhoea, heavy periods, and flushes and sweats at a perimenopausal age. Women with other types of gynaecological complaint did not show an increased prevalence of psychiatric disorder. The Oxford study also showed that the likelihood of referral to a gynaecological clinic was significantly greater in women who had both psychiatric symptoms and one or other of the four gynaecological complaints listed above.

Relationship Between Gynaecological Symptoms and Psychiatric Disorder

In the first part of this chapter, it was emphasised that the emotional disorders met in surgical patients may be either primary (that is, unrelated to the surgical condition) or secondary (that is, induced by the surgical condition). Of course, in an individual patient, both sets of factors may contribute to the aetiology of emotional disorder.

This principle is restated here because it is of particular importance in gynaecological surgery. Taking primary emotional disorder first, there can be no doubt that many women suffer from emotional disorders which are precipitated by environmental factors such as marital problems, financial worries, poor housing, problems with work and recent bereavement. In some women with such problems, psychiatric disorder may be independent of their gynaecological complaints. However, in many cases, the onset or worsening of an emotional disorder may lead to complaints about physical symptoms which were previously well tolerated.

If a patient presents with both gynaecological and emotional complaints and if there appear to be indications for gynaecological surgery, it is clearly important to decide how far emotional symptoms are inducing or aggravating gynaecological complaints. This is not an easy judgement to make, but certain guidelines may help: (1) the extent of any gynaecological pathology which might account for the gynaecological symptoms; (2) which came first, the gynaecological or the psychiatric symptoms; (3) whether the woman has experienced recent adversities or chronic social difficulties that might have induced the emotional disorder; and (4) whether the emotional problems seem to be largely related to the stresses of the gynaecological problem (see next paragraph).

There are several reasons why a gynaecological problem can be psychologically stressful to the patient. First, the gynaecological condition may itself lead to anxiety or depression, especially if it causes pain or discomfort, or social embarrassment (as in the case of urinary incontinence or menstrual flooding). Emotional symptoms are particularly common if such physical problems are chronic. Secondly, many women are made very anxious at the prospect of a gynaecological consultation or hospital admission. They may be particularly anxious about undergoing physical examination or discussing intimate symptoms with a stranger, or the possibility that the diagnosis will be cancer. Thirdly, on admission to hospital, anxieties may be focussed on many things, such as the prospect of postoperative pain or helplessness, lack of privacy in the ward, and the sight and sound of illness and distress in other patients. Fourth, anxieties about the consequences of surgery may be to do with possible disfigurement, loss of sexual function and loss of femininity.

As mentioned in the first part of this chapter, there can be little doubt that much anxiety or depression in patients can be avoided or reduced if the gynaecologist anticipates possible sources of distress and deals with them by explanation and reassurance.

This section has emphasised the complexity of the causal relationships between gynaecological and psychiatric symptoms, and has suggested some guidelines for evaluating these relationships in the individual patient. If the gynaecologist's enquiries leave him in doubt about the indications for surgery, it may be helpful to seek the opinion of a psychiatrist.

Psychiatric Sequelae of Gynaecological Operations

In this section, psychiatric sequelae of three gynaecological procedures will be discussed in some detail, namely hysterectomy, bilateral oophorectomy and elective sterilisation. These three procedures provide good examples of general principles, and they have been extensively studied by research psychiatrists. In the final section of this chapter, other pelvic operations will be discussed, especially those involving a major loss of function, for example, partial vaginectomy and vulvectomy.

Hysterectomy

It used to be said that hysterectomy was a common cause of psychiatric disorder, especially depression. In fact, early studies of hysterectomy did not justify this conclusion, because (1) they were retrospective; (2) they did not employ standardised measures to assess psychiatric disorder; and (3) they used mixed groups of patients undergoing hysterectomy for various indications, including malignancy. These earlier studies have been reviewed by Gath and Cooper (1982).

Recent studies from two centres (Oxford, UK, and St. Louis, United States) have used prospective designs, standardised assessment measures and homogeneous samples of women undergoing hysterectomy for menorrhagia of benign origin (dysfunctional uterine bleeding, fibroids or

endometriosis). These two studies have shown that the removal of the uterus in itself rarely leads to the onset of psychiatric disorder.

In the Oxford study 156 women undergoing hysterectomy for menorrhagia of benign origin were assessed 4 weeks preoperatively and again at 6 months and 18 months after hysterectomy (Gath et al. 1981a; Gath et al. 1981b). Standardised psychiatric measures of known reliability and validity were used, including the Present State Examination, or PSE (Wing et al. 1974). The PSE makes it possible to define patients as psychiatric "cases" or "noncases" for research purposes, and to compare the findings with the known data for other populations, such as psychiatric patients or the general population. In the Oxford study, 58% of the women were cases preoperatively; this proportion fell to 26% at 6 months and 29% at 18 months after the operation. In other words, the level of psychiatric morbidity was halved after hysterectomy. A salient finding was that hysterectomy was seldom followed by new psychiatric morbidity; of the 56 preoperative non-cases, only 9 had become cases at follow-up. There were many other indications that hysterectomy had a generally beneficial effect. For example, after hysterectomy psychosexual function improved in over half the women and deteriorated in only 17%. (This finding, like the findings on psychosexual outcome, was greatly at variance with the findings of earlier studies.)

The study in St. Louis was of similar design, but used different standardised measures (Martin et al. 1977; Martin et al. 1980). The preoperative level of psychiatric morbidity was similar to that found in the Oxford study, and again there was a reduction in psychiatric symptomatology after the operation.

Despite the substantial reduction in psychiatric disorder after hysterectomy, the Oxford study found a sizeable group of women who were psychiatric cases both before and after hysterectomy. It is obviously important to ask why some women remained psychiatrically unwell after the operation. It appeared from the Oxford study that a poor psychiatric outcome was not related to lack of demonstrable pathology in the uterus [a point of contrast with some of the earlier studies, such as those of Barker (1968) and Richards (1973)]. Furthermore, in the Oxford study, psychiatric outcome was not related to type of hysterectomy (abdominal or vaginal), age, childlessness or marital status.

In both the Oxford and St. Louis studies, and indeed in other studies, the most important determinant of psychiatric outcome after hysterectomy appeared to be preoperative psychiatric status. In the Oxford study, this was shown by a wide range of preoperative psychiatric measures, including the severity of psychiatric disorder shortly before hysterectomy, history of earlier psychiatric contact and high levels of neuroticism.

Against this background, it is interesting to turn to a study of the association between a woman's estimation of her menstrual blood loss and the actual blood loss as measured in the laboratory. In Oxford, Chimbira et al. (1980) measured objective blood loss over two menstrual periods in 92 women complaining of heavy periods for which no cause could be found. These investigators found that almost half the periods rated as heavy by the women involved blood loss below 80 ml, which is the level generally regarded as defining menorrhagia (Haynes et al. 1979). This study also showed that methods of assessing menstrual loss commonly used in gynaecological clinics (such as numbers of pads or tampons used, or length of periods) were poor predictors of actual loss.

If we combine these findings on measured menstrual loss with the findings of the Oxford hysterectomy study, we can speculate that women with prehysterectomy psychiatric disorder include two important subgroups: (1) Those with "true" menorrhagia on objective measurement of menstrual loss. In this group, prehysterectomy psychiatric disorder is likely to be secondary to the prolonged distress of heavy periods, and is likely to be relieved by removal of the uterus. (2) Those who do not have "true" menorrhagia on objective measurement. In this group, pre-existing psychiatric disorder may have led the patient to complain of levels of menstruation that were previously acceptable to her. Hysterectomy is much less likely to relieve the psychiatric symptoms in this group (who may benefit more from psychiatric treatment).

In the present state of knowledge, it is impossible to say whether many women fall into these groups; further research is needed to settle the question.

Bilateral Oophorectomy

There have been few reports of the psychiatric sequelae of bilateral oophorectomy, and it is difficult to draw any firm conclusions from them, for two reasons. First, bilateral oophorectomy is rarely performed without hysterectomy and it is therefore difficult to separate problems connected with loss of the ovaries from those related to loss of the uterus. Secondly, most studies on bilateral oophorectomy have been limited by retrospective design, small samples and assessments made at widely varying intervals after surgery.

The published research on bilateral oophorectomy has focussed mainly on the risks of subsequent psychiatric disorder and psychosexual problems. The four main studies of psychiatric sequelae have compared hysterectomy plus bilateral oophorectomy with hysterectomy alone. All four studies (two retrospective and two prospective) found no excess of psychiatric disorder in the hysterectomy plus bilateral oophorectomy group compared with the hysterectomy group (Barker 1968; Richards 1973; Martin et al. 1980; Gath et al. 1981b). However, Martin et al. did report an excess of headaches, fatigue and menopausal symptoms in the hysterectomy plus oophorectomy group.

All published studies on psychosexual function after bilateral oophorectomy have been retrospective and should therefore be interpreted with caution. The general conclusion from these studies seems to be that postoperative psychosexual function is no different after hysterectomy plus oophorectomy than after hysterectomy alone.

Further research is needed to confirm these tentative findings. However, it will only be possible to derive firm conclusions about psychiatric and psychosexual complications of bilateral oophorectomy from studies that are prospective, use standardised methods of assessment and employ large representative samples.

Sterilisation

In recent years, there have been changes in the practice of sterilisation in the United Kingdom. For example, the operation has increased in frequency and is much more commonly an elective interval procedure than it was formerly. Compared with 20 years ago, women undergoing sterilisation are younger and have fewer children. It is therefore of limited value to review pre-1970 studies on psychiatric disorder after sterilisation, though it is notable that quite a few earlier studies pointed to high rates of psychiatric morbidity after sterilisation. The early literature on psychiatric sequelae of sterilisation has been reviewed by Gath and Cooper (1982).

Most studies of psychiatric disorder after sterilisation have had the same limitations of method as the studies of hysterectomy and bilateral oophorectomy already described—namely retrospective design, mixed samples and lack of standardised assessment methods. Two recent studies attempted to avoid these methodological limitations, and both found that elective interval sterilisation as practised in the United Kingdom was very unlikely to cause psychiatric problems.

The first of these studies was carried out in Oxford (Cooper et al. 1981; Cooper et al. 1982). Nearly

200 women undergoing elective interval sterilisation were assessed before the operation, and 6 and 18 months afterwards. Before sterilisation, the level of psychiatric morbidity (as judged by the proportion of PSE cases) was not greater than in women in the general population, that is around 10%. This proportion had fallen to 5% at the 6-month follow-up, and did not exceed preoperative levels at the 18-month follow-up. As in the Oxford hysterectomy study described previously, amongst women who were psychiatrically well before sterilisation only a small proportion became psychiatric cases after the operation. In general, after elective sterilisation women had more frequent sexual intercourse than preoperatively and found it more enjoyable—a point of contrast with the findings of earlier retrospective studies. As predicted, postoperative regret at being sterilised was expressed mainly by women who had had preoperative psychiatric disorder.

The second study of elective sterilisation was done in Nottingham (Bledin et al. 1984). It differed from the Oxford study by the exclusion of women with previous psychiatric disorder and other health problems, and inclusion of women undergoing postpartum sterilisation as well as those undergoing interval sterilisation. The study also recruited two comparison groups of women who had not undergone sterilisation (from maternity wards and family planning clinics). As in the Oxford study of sterilisation, the Nottingham study found that sterilisation did not lead to psychiatric disorder, and that women with higher initial PSE scores were more likely to regret having being sterilised. Unlike the Oxford researchers, the Nottingham group found that sterilised women were more likely than the comparison group to report psychosexual problems at follow-up. These two studies show that elective interval sterilisation, as carried out at two teaching hospitals in the United Kingdom, does not lead to psychiatric disorder in previously healthy women at 6–18 months after the operation. The other important finding was that poor psychiatric outcome was predicted by preoperative psychiatric disorder, past psychiatric contact and neuroticism.

In general these findings resemble those of the Oxford hysterectomy study described above. The main difference is that women in the sterilisation studies showed far lower levels of preoperative psychiatric disorder than did the hysterectomy group.

The Oxford and Nottingham studies have implications for the selection of women for elective sterilisation. In assessing any woman who requests elective sterilisation, the gynaecologist should try to elicit any evidence of past or present psychiatric disorder. Any patient with such a history should be assessed with particular care, and the possibility of referral for a psychiatric opinion should be considered.

It is emphasised that the findings of these two recent studies relate only to elective sterilisation as practised in the United Kingdom; the psychiatric complications of sterilisation may be much different in other countries with different traditions.

Other Aspects of Gynaecological Surgery

Finally in this chapter, we discuss some psychological issues which are relevant to gynaecological surgery in general, but particularly to operations involving distortion of anatomical structures and loss of function. Here, as emphasised earlier in this chapter, an essential part of psychological management is to provide the patient with adequate information, explanation and reassurance (see p. 291).

Many women undergoing surgery to their reproductive organs or urinary system will be apprehensive about the possible effects on their femininity or their sexual functioning. These apprehensions may be increased because many women have limited knowledge of their pelvic anatomy, and therefore have inaccurate beliefs about the nature of various surgical procedures and the likely consequences. For example, it is not uncommon for a woman to believe that surgery for urinary incontinence will prevent her from having sexual intercourse. Whether their beliefs are accurate or inaccurate, many woman are afraid to express their fears about surgery and its outcome. For example, amongst women who remain sexually active in later life, it is not uncommon to feel ashamed of asking about the possible effects of surgery on their sexual activity. For the gynaecologist an important part of management is to encourage patients to express their fears, and then to help them with simple explanation, correction of any inaccurate beliefs and reassurance.

The nature of the explanation and reassurance required will depend on the extent to which surgery distorts the lower genital tract or impairs its functioning. With operations that do not involve such distortion of structure or function, it is unusual for women to experience loss of sexual functioning or of feelings of femininity as psychological reactions to the fact of having had pelvic surgery. Women in this group can therefore be reassured that their femininity and sexual functioning will not be impaired; indeed, they can be told that research has shown that sexual enjoyment is frequently enhanced after certain types of pelvic surgery.

The problem is different when a woman's fears of disfigurement and loss of sexual function or fertility are realistic. This problem arises with operations such as partial vaginectomy or vulvectomy which may radically change the appearance or function of the lower genital tract. It also occurs when gynaecological surgery results in loss of capacity for reproduction early in the patient's life—as in the case of a newly married young woman undergoing total pelvic clearance for carcinoma of the cervix. Patients with these problems are in particular need of sensitive and realistic explanations of the likely postoperative outcome. If the woman and her partner are still sexually active they may benefit from expert counselling about alternative means of obtaining sexual satisfaction, even if full intercourse is not possible. A couple who desire children but who cannot have them may need opportunities to express their grief to one another with the help of another person.

After operations such as partial vaginectomy, vulvectomy or total pelvic clearance, a woman is likely to go through a phase of mourning for her lost femininity and sexual and reproductive capacities. Psychiatrists have studied the grief reaction which often follows loss due to surgery such as amputation of a limb (Parkes and Napier 1970) or mastectomy (Renneker and Cutler 1952). Such grief reactions may occur immediately after the loss, or be delayed for several weeks or months, or even years. Grief reactions have certain features in common, whatever the loss. They include an initial sense of numbness or lack of feeling; denial that the loss has occurred; anger directed against medical staff, family, fate or God; guilt over real or imagined causation of the loss; and weeping, sleep disturbance, restlessness, poor concentration and poor memory. There may be a preoccupation with the anatomical part or the function that has been lost, and the woman may feel empty, hollow or incomplete. She may feel jealous of other women who still possess the parts and functions she has lost.

In the management of women experiencing structural or functional losses as a result of pelvic surgery, the assessment and treatment of emotional reactions should follow the principles outlined in earlier sections (see p. 288). It is generally helpful to encourage the patient to express the meaning of the loss to her, and then to discuss the problem with her, providing information and practical advice if required. The woman should be reassured that grief for a loss is natural, and may take several forms. Usually management needs to be no more sophisticated than this, and it is seldom necessary to prescribe psychotropic drugs for such patients. However, in some cases the patient's grief seems to be excessively severe or prolonged, and referral to a psychiatrist may then be indicated.

Conclusions

This chapter has emphasised a number of salient points, which can be summarised as follows. Levels of psychiatric morbidity are high amongst certain subgroups of gynaecological patients in the general population, in outpatient clinics and in surgical wards. It is important for the gynaecologist to detect and assess emotional problems in his patients for several reasons. One of the most important reasons is that an evaluation of emotional disorder may affect surgical management, including selection for surgery and the timing of the surgery. In making the evaluation, it is important to determine whether emotional complaints are secondary to gynaecological problems; or whether there is a primary emotional disorder, which may be quite unrelated to the gynaecological disorder, or may have led the patient to complain of gynaecological symptoms that were previously well tolerated. Even allowing for the pressures of working in gynaecological clinics and wards, it should be possible for the gynaecologist to make a good working assessment of emotional symptoms. The chapter has provided guidelines to such assessments.

One of the main determinants of psychiatric outcome and rehabilitation after surgery is the patient's psychiatric status before the operation, including mental state shortly before the operation, long-term history of psychiatric contact and the personality characteristic of neuroticism.

In women who are psychiatrically healthy before pelvic surgery, operations such as hysterectomy for menorrhagia, sterilisation and bilateral oophorectomy seldom lead to psychiatric disorder or other adverse sequelae, such as reduced sexual functioning. However, the situation is different with operations (such as partial vaginectomy or vulvectomy) that cause anatomical distortion or dysfunction of the lower genital tract; such operations may induce grief over lost femininity or sexual activity.

For all emotional disorders, whether preoperative or postoperative, it is extremely important to provide good explanation, advice and reassurance about gynaecological problems. Such simple counselling can be remarkably effective in reducing distress.

References

Ballinger CB (1975) Psychiatric morbidity and the menopause: screening of general population sample. Br Med J 3:344–346

Ballinger CB (1977) Psychiatric morbidity and the menopause: survey of a gynaecological out-patient clinic. Br J Psychiatr 131:83–89

Barker MG (1968) Psychiatric illness after hysterectomy. Br Med J 2:91–95

Bledin KD, Cooper JE, Mackenzie S, Brice B (1984) Psychological sequelae of female sterilisation: short term outcome in a prospective controlled study. Psychol Med 14 (2):379–390

Byrne P (1984) Psychiatric morbidity in a gynaecology clinic: an epidemiological survey. Br J Psychiatr 144:28–34

Chimbira TH, Anderson ABM, Turnbull AC (1980) Relation between measured menstrual blood loss and patients' subjective assessment of loss, duration of bleeding, number of sanitary towels used, uterine weight, and endometrial surface area. Br J Obstet Gynaecol 87:603–609

Cooper P, Gath D, Fieldsend R, Rose N (1981) Psychological and physical outcome after elective tubal sterilisation. J Psychosom Res 25:357–360

Cooper P, Gath D, Rose N, Fieldsend R (1982) Psychological sequelae to elective sterilisation in women: a prospective study. Br Med J 284:461–464

Eysenck HJ, Eysenck SBG (1963) The Eysenck Personality Inventory. University of London Press, London

Gath D, Cooper P, Day A (1981a) Hysterectomy and psychiatric disorder: levels of psychiatric morbidity before and after hysterectomy. Br J Psychiatr 140:335–342

Gath D, Cooper P, Bond A, Edmonds G (1981b) Hysterectomy and psychiatric disorder: demographic, psychiatric and physical factors in relation to psychiatric outcome. Br J Psychiatr 140:343–350

Gath D, Cooper P (1982) Psychiatric aspects of hysterectomy and female sterilisation. In: Granville-Grossman K (ed) Recent advances in clinical psychiatry, vol. 4. Churchill Livingstone, London, pp 75–100

Gath D, Osborn M, Bungay G, Iles S, Day A, Bond A, Passingham C (1987) Psychiatric disorder and gynaecological symptoms in middle aged women: a community survey. Br Med J 294:213–218

Gath D, Rose N (1985) Psychological problems and gynaecological surgery. In: Priest RG (ed) Psychological disorders in obstetrics and gynaecology. Butterworths, London

Gelder M, Gath D, Mayou R (1983) Oxford textbook of psychiatry. Oxford University Press, London

Goldberg DP (1972) The detection of psychiatric illness by questionnaire. Oxford University Press, London

Haynes PJ, Anderson A, Turnbull AC (1979) Patterns of menstrual blood loss in menorrhagia. Research Clinic Forums 1:73–78

Lipowski ZJ (1980) Organic mental disorders: introduction and review of syndromes. In: Kaplan HI, Freedman AM, Sadock BJ (eds) Comprehensive textbook of psychiatry, 3rd edn. Williams and Wilkins, Baltimore, pp 1359–1392

Lishman WA (1978) Organic psychiatry. The psychological consequences of cerebral disorder. Blackwells Scientific Publications, London

Maguire GP, Julier DL, Hawton KE, Bancroft JHJ (1974) Psychiatric referral and morbidity on two general medical wards. Br Med J 1:268–270

Martin RL, Roberts WV, Clayton PJ, Wetzel R (1977) Psychiatric illness and non-cancer hysterectomy. Dis Nerv Syst 38:974–980

Martin RL, Roberts WV, Clayton PJ (1980) Psychiatric status after hysterectomy-one-year prospective follow-up. JAMA 244:350–353

Parkes CM, Napier MM (1970) Psychiatric sequelae of amputation. Br J Hosp Med 4:610–614

Renneker R, Cutler M (1952) Psychological problems of adjustment to cancer of the breast. JAMA 148:833–838

Richards DH (1973) Depression after hysterectomy. Lancet 2:430–432

Rogers FS (1950) Emotional factors in gynaecology. Am J Obstet Gynecol 59:321–327

Smith DH (1979) Psychologic aspects of gynaecology and obstetrics. Obstet Gynaecol Ann 8:457–473

Wing JK, Cooper JE, Sartorius W (1974) The measurement and classification of psychiatric symptoms. Cambridge University Press, London

Worsley A, Walters WAW, Wood EC (1977). Screening of psychological disturbance amongst gynaecology patients. Aust NZ J Obstet Gynaecol 17:214–219

Subject Index